D1536207

CULTURAL, ETHNIC, AND RELIGIOUS MANUAL FOR HEALTH CARE PROVIDERS

Fourth Edition

Janice D. Andrews, RN, MSN, CTN –A
JAMARDA Resources, Inc.

Copyright © 1995 – 2013 by Janice D. Andrews, RN, MSN, CTN-A

All rights reserved. No part of this publication may be reproduced, copied, photocopied, or distributed in any form or by any means, stored in a database or retrieval system without the prior written permission from JAMARDA Resources, Inc.

Printed in the United States of America
First printing: December 1995
Second printing: April 1999
Third printing: March 2005
Fourth printing: May 2013

Contact Information

Mailing Address:
JAMARDA Resources, Inc.
931-B South Main Street #102
Kernersville, NC USA

Voice: 877.JAMARDA (877-526-2732)
Fax: 800.505.9450
Email: info@jamardaresources.com
Web: http://www.jamardaresources.com
Facebook: #JAMARDAResources
Twitter: @JAMARDAInc

ISBN-13: 978-1481197588
ISBN-10: 1481197584

This book is available through Amazon.com. We also offer an online subscription via our website and intranet licensing for corporate networks. Contact us for more information on subscription and licensing questions.

DISCLAIMER:

JAMARDA Resources, Inc. implies that the manual is to be used specifically as a reference manual and in no way should be used for prescriptive purposes of any kind, or as definitive medical, nursing, or other health care provisions for an individual or group.

"The world in which you were born is just one model of reality. Other cultures are not failed attempts at being YOU: they are unique manifestations of the human spirit."

—Wade Davis, Anthropologist

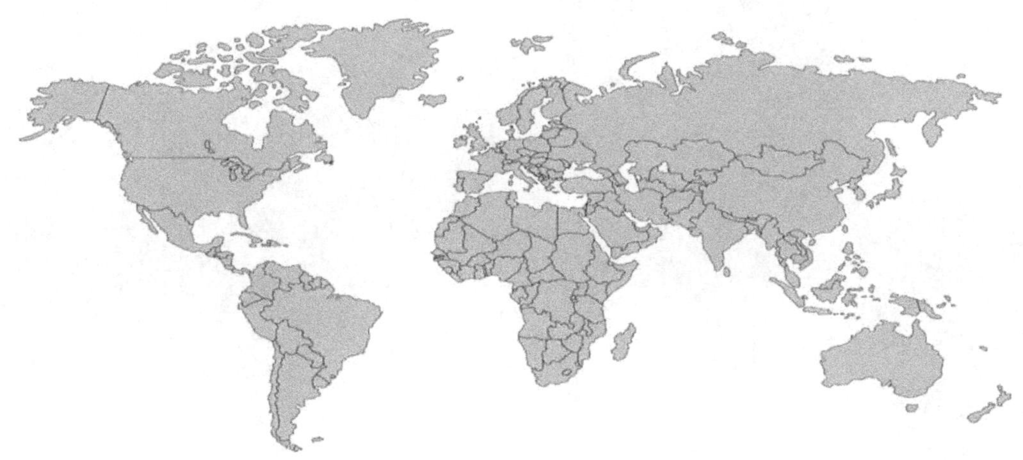

TABLE OF CONTENTS

ABOUT THE AUTHOR

Janice D. Andrews is a native of Birmingham, Alabama. She began her nursing career as a staff nurse in Washington, DC. There, while working in maternal-child nursing, she was challenged to provide nursing care to the culturally diverse people who make up the population of Washington, DC. While continuing her maternal-child focus throughout her nursing career, her interest in diversity led to the authorship of three previous editions of the *Cultural, Ethnic and Religious Reference Manual for Health Care Providers.* She is also the author of *Cultural, Ethnic and Religious Word Searches and Crossword Puzzles* and *Cultural, Ethnic and Religious Diversity Tests.*

Since 1978, Ms. Andrews has worked primarily in nursing education and leadership roles in acute care settings, where she gained first-hand knowledge of the challenges of diversity to health care providers. While continuing her nursing roles, she served for 11 years in the role of diversity facilitator, providing education to employees in a wide range of health care disciplines.

She holds a post-Master's certificate in transcultural nursing from the University of Northern Colorado–Greeley, Colorado and a specialty certification in transcultural nursing. She has memberships in a number of professional organizations. Ms. Andrews is the founder and President of JAMARDA Resources, Inc. An integral focus of her professional activities involves educating health care providers regarding diversity issues, transcultural nursing, and the provision of culturally congruent care through lectures, seminars, and workshops throughout the United States.

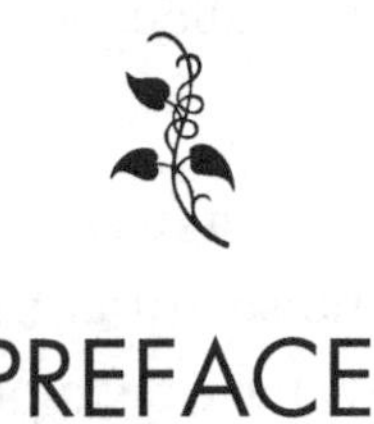

PREFACE

"Although we are in different boats, you in your boat and we in our canoe, we share the same river of life."

—Chief Oren Lyons, Native American Faithkeeper

The fourth edition of the *Cultural, Ethnic and Religious Reference Manual for Health Care Providers* has come to fruition as I continue my personal journey toward cultural competence. It is a never-ending journey because culture is dynamic. There is always something new and fascinating to discover about the unique living beings known as *humans*.

The world population stands at over 7 billion people–each of them unique. The population is estimated to reach 8 billion by 2025.[1] As health care professionals provide services globally, they are met with the challenges brought by diversity. On the other hand, the world has come to health care providers, as people continue to relocate to different parts of the world for various reasons and seek health care services. On a day-to-day basis, health care providers are faced with ever-increasing cultural quagmires. Although regulatory agencies are now bringing pressure to health care organizations to provide culturally competent environments, sadly, most providers have not received the needed formal education to prepare them for the challenges. It is encouraging that an increasing number of health care professional education programs are taking steps to integrate some aspects of cultural education in the curricula. Unfortunately, most of these courses do not provide the solid foundation needed for health care providers to develop cultural competence.

Each day, health care providers must balance the interplay of their personal culture, their professional culture, and the cultures of clients seeking services with unprecedented changes in health care. In the midst of increasing patient diversity, health care providers are caring for sicker patients, and sometimes working with staffing shortages, while attempting to meet the pressures to maintain high quantitative measures of productivity. How then, do health care providers cope with these enormous challenges without intensive education and training related to transcultural care?

In the 1950s, Dr. Madeleine Leininger, a nurse-anthropologist, began her untiring, lifetime efforts to establish and expand transcultural nursing as a distinct and formal area of study and practice. Her vision and efforts have been pivotal in advancing culture care not only in Nursing, but have also influenced other health disciplines, as well. Dr. Leininger passed away in 2012, but her legacy will live on through the many individuals she has impacted, who will carry on her quest to advance transcultural nursing. The term *culturally competent care* is often heard in health care facilities, but often without a clear knowledge of its meaning.

As regulatory agencies establish and enforce standards and requirements related to cultural competence, organizations will have to put forth increased efforts to achieve and maintain compliance. A critical ingredient of cultural exploration is sometimes omitted (i.e., the exploration of self), and on a broader basis, the exploration of the culture of health care institutions within the broader dominant society. We display our own ethnocentricism when we are only willing to study about others without studying ourselves at a personal, professional, institutional, and societal level, albeit sometimes uncomfortable and even painful. Without this level of exploration, we, as a group of health care professionals, will maintain our deficiencies in the provision of culturally congruent care. Cultural competence involves acquiring knowledge and developing skills, just as with any other area of study. It does not come with one class, one conference, one book, or one experience. Consequently, the same emphasis must be placed on its continuing development in our health care institutions, colleges, and universities.

In United States society, the statement is often heard, "Time is money." As would be expected, this value has been brought into the culture of health care facilities. However, maybe it is time that we add a twist to the above statement, "Time **not** spent, is money." I challenge health care administrators to quantitatively **and** qualitatively, explore the relationship of lack of cultural competence to measures such as length of stay, readmissions, patient satisfaction, patient safety, legal actions, misdiagnoses, etc., all of which are impacted by **cultural incompetence.** We cannot continue to espouse the notion of *quality care* without determining what *care* means to the patients and families that enter our facilities.

There are a number of comprehensive texts available now to assist health care providers with gaining cultural knowledge and skills. I strongly encourage individuals who use this manual to read further. As with previous editions of this manual, the intent is not to provide a comprehensive textbook related to transcultural care. As I continue my career and dialogue with other health care providers, there is an increased interest in learning to provide care to diverse clients. In the three previous editions of this manual, the format, conciseness, and focus on key points that are vital to patient care have proven to be helpful to busy health care providers in meeting the immediate cultural and religious needs of patients and their families. Therefore, I have kept that format in this fourth edition of the manual, revised and expanded existing chapters, and added new chapters.

As with the previous manuals, I urge health care providers to keep the uniqueness of each individual in the forefront of care. Although reference is made to groups of people who may have broad similarities, the health care provider must always remember that the information contained will not apply to **all** members of a certain group. There is great diversity within cultural and religious groups. The manual is meant to provide a quick, broad overview of key information that may help one to provide more culturally congruent care to the client/family seeking health care services. More in-depth knowledge should be gained about those cultural/ethnic groups that most often seek services at a given facility.

Our charge and challenge as health care professionals is to meet our ethical obligation to provide culturally congruent care to all individuals that enter our health care systems. It is the **right** of our patients to receive respectful and compassionate care, incorporating cultural aspects to the best of our ability. This is not an easy charge. But, most endeavors that lead to long-lasting pride and satisfaction are not easy. No health care professional can remember the cultural and religious needs of every cultural group. It is impossible! We can, however, begin the journey toward cultural competence through self-introspection, continuing education, and lots of creativity. We can lobby our legislators, health care administrators, and others to change some of the processes that do not support true individualization of care.

My journey will continue, for while others are the recipients of my efforts, I continue to stand in great awe and respect of the universality and diversity of my global family. I can only gain further enrichment and become a better person in my quest for learning and competence. I sincerely hope that the information in this manual will stimulate in the reader a desire to learn more about him/herself **first**, then the values, beliefs, and practices of various cultures, ethnic groups, and religions other than his or her own.

Janice D. Andrews, RN, MSN, CTN-A*
* (CTN-A = Certified Transcultural Nurse-Advanced)

[1] Worldometers. (2013). Current world population. Retrieved from http://www.worldometers.info/

DEDICATION AND ACKNOWLEDGEMENTS

In the beginning…

In Memory

of

Henry & Rosie Dobbins

Your Spirits Are Ever-present.

• • • • •

On my life's journey…

To

My Children and Their Spouses

I Have Been Generously Blessed With You.

In Loving Appreciation of Your Continuing Love, Support, and Kindness

• • • • •

Dreams for the future…

To

My Grandchildren

Bright Lights in My life; Immeasurable Joy in My Heart.

• • • • •

In humble recognition…

of

The healthcare providers who strive to provide excellent and compassionate patient care on a daily basis while meeting the challenges of diversity and an ever-changing healthcare environment.

·····

Special thanks to...

Deborah J. Gouge, RN, BSN, MA for your generous assistance with the research required for completion of this manual. I cannot express in words, my appreciation to you.

Claudia Cates for your editorial assistance in the preparation of the contents of this manuscript.

Andrea M. Weatherhead, Ph.D. for your late night, untiring efforts in the preparation of this manuscript for publication.

Dr. Madeleine Leininger (deceased) and my transcultural professors at the University of Northern Colorado – Greeley, CO, I am honored and humbled to have sat at your feet. Thanks also to the other transcultural pioneers who continue to inspire me.

Family, friends, and colleagues who have been unfaltering in their words of support and encouragement through this journey.

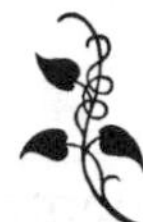

CULTURAL TERMINOLOGY

A

Acculturation

The process of adopting the social traits and patterns of another culture, generally the dominant culture. Involves adapting or borrowing aspects of another culture such as dress or speech.

Assimilation

The process of social and cultural adaptation and absorption of a minority group into the dominant culture. Forms of assimilation include *acculturation*, *identification*, *civic*, and *marital.*

Asylee

A person who seeks permission to reside in another country for protection from persecution and/or harm. Fear of returning to his or her homeland may be related to factors such as race, religion, political opinion, etc. The request for asylum is assigned after entering the receiving country.

B

Bat Gio

See *Pinching*.

Beliefs

Those things that are thought to be true.

Bicultural

Adjective describing a person who has adopted the values and lifestyles of two cultures.

Burning

Also known as *Poua*, a form of folk healing practiced among some Asian populations, particularly Hmong, Laotians, and Cambodians. It is a treatment of last resort and is used for the treatment of pain and failure to thrive. It appears as vertical rows of asymmetrical, superficial burns of approximately one-fourth inch on the front or back of the body, including the neck or a single burn may be seen in the center of the forehead. The joints will be burned when attempting to treat failure to thrive. The treatment is performed using a type of grass that has been dried, dipped in melted pork lard, ignited, then applied to the area of the body requiring treatment. The resulting marks on the body are often confused with intentional cigarette burns or child abuse. Poua is generally performed by a healer, but may be done by any experienced adult.[1,2]

C

Cao Gio

See *Coining/Coin Rubbing*.

Caring

Leininger refers to caring as "the essence of nursing." Caring refers to actions and activities that are directed toward assisting, supporting, or enabling another individual or group with evident or anticipated needs to ameliorate or improve a human condition or lifeway, or to face death.[3]

Cheut Sah

See *Coining/Coin Rubbing*.

Civic Assimilation

Involves members of an ethnic group who no longer make special claims on the political system based on the special needs of their particular ethnic group. This usually occurs when an ethnic group achieves an important measure of political power. See *Assimilation*.

CLAS

An acronym used in reference to the National Standards on Culturally and Linguistically Appropriate Services issued in December 2000. The fourteen standards were developed by the United States Department of Health and Human Services Office of Minority Health in an effort to assure that all people entering the United States health care system, regardless of culture, receive equitable and safe treatment in a manner that is culturally and linguistically appropriate. All healthcare facilities receiving federal funds are mandated to provide information regarding treatment, in the patient's preferred language. The standards have since been integrated with accreditation standards from the Joint Commission on Accreditation of Health Care Organizations (JCAHO). For more information about the CLAS standards, visit http://minorityhealth.hhs.gov.

Coining/Coin Rubbing

(Also referred to as *Cao Gio* – Vietnamese term. *Cheut Sah* or *Quat Sha* – Chinese term). A form of folk healing commonly practiced among some Asian populations, which involves rubbing the body with a coin or spoon. The coin/spoon is sometimes heated or oiled. The rubbing produces red welts on the skin, superficial ecchymosis, and non-painful areas with petechiae. These areas should not be mistaken for signs of abuse or signs of a specific disease process. The treatment is applied to the symptomatic area. The belief is that rubbing the coin against the skin draws illness out of the body of the individual and that the red welts will appear only on those individuals who are ill. Coining is done to treat illnesses such as colds, vomiting, headache, pain, heat exhaustion, and seizures. The practice is more common among Vietnamese, Chinese, Hmong, Cambodians, and Laotians.

Culture-Bound Illness

An illness that is only seen within a certain cultural population.

Cultural Competence

There are many definitions of cultural competence. Cross, Bazron, Dennis, & Isaacs (1989) apply the term to both individuals and organizations. Cultural competence is a continuing process and does not have an 'end point'. The importance of linguistics to cultural competence has been recognized. Andrews & Boyle (2012) define cultural and linguistic competence as, "the ability of health care providers and health care organizations to understand and effectively respond to the cultural and linguistic needs brought by clients to the health care encounter" (p.18). The health care provider must be cognizant of his or her own personal values and beliefs brought to each cultural interaction.

Cultural Imposition

The practice of imposing one's cultural beliefs upon others with the belief that they are best or superior.

Cultural Pain

The discomfort, suffering experienced by an individual or group resulting from the insensitivity of others who have different beliefs and/or cultural norms.[3]

Cultural Relativism

The attitude that the differences in ways of doing things hold equal validity.

Culture

The learned, shared, and transmitted values, beliefs, and practices of a particular group that guide thinking, actions, behaviors, interactions with others, emotional reactions to daily living, and one's world view.

Cupping

(Also referred to as *Ventouse*) – A form of folk healing commonly practiced among Asians, Latin Americans, and some Europeans. It involves heating a glass and placing it on the ill person's body. The vacuum created under the glass causes the skin to rise, leaving red marks on the skin of approximately two inches in diameter. The marks from cupping will typically be seen along the left and right sides of the chest, abdomen, and back. This treatment is generally performed only on adults. Cupping is done in an effort to equalize "hot" and "cold" body imbalances and to draw out evil spirits that are causing the illness.[1,5,6]

D

Discrimination

Referring to limiting opportunities, showing difference, limiting choices of a group or individual based on prejudice.

Dominant Culture

The culture of the dominant group within a society. It is not necessary that the dominant culture make up the majority of the population. In the United States, people of Anglo-European ancestry make up the dominant group. The critical difference related to dominant cultures is power, not numbers.

E

Emic

Referring to the insiders' views/perspectives of a culture.

Ethnic Group

A group of people who share cultural, racial, linguistic, and social heritage.

Ethnocentrism

The belief that one's own ethnic group, way of life, values, etc. are superior to others.

Etic

Referring to outsiders' views/perspectives of a culture.

Evil Eye

(Also referred to as *Mal Ojo* in Spanish.) A belief of some persons from Asia, Central America, the Middle East, Mexico, and Africa. The specific and associated practices may vary. However, the general concept is that one puts an evil spirit on a person by looking at the victim, causing the victim to become ill. The motive for placing the evil spirit on another person is generally envy. The concept is based on the ideal that there is a limited amount of good things in the world, such as intelligence, beauty, and wealth. If one person possesses one of these assets, other persons have less of the asset. Therefore, envy warrants giving the "evil eye" to the person who has the asset to cause illness. Some cultures believe that compliments cause the evil eye and have methods of neutralizing its effects.

F

Family of Orientation

Parents, siblings, and the individual.

Family of Procreation

Spouse, children, and the individual.

Folk Medicine

Practices within a cultural or ethnic group aimed at curing illness or preventing illness.

G

Geophagy

The eating of clay or dirt. Seen more commonly among African Americans, Africans, and Arab Americans.

H

Hot and Cold Health Concept

A health concept based on the ancient Greek concept of the four body humors: yellow bile, black bile, phlegm, and blood. A balance of these humors equates to health. The treatment of disease is accomplished through restoring the body's humoral balance through the addition or subtraction of substances that affect each of these humors. Disease conditions, foods, herbs, beverages, and medications are classified as hot or cold depending on their effect, not their physical temperature. Each cultural group defines what it believes to be hot and cold. The concept is found among Asians, Japanese, Blacks, Hispanics, Arabs, Muslim, and Caribbean cultures.[1]

I

Identification

Exists when members of an ethnic group share a perception of nationhood (e.g., "I am an American.") See *Assimilation*.

Immigrant

A person who voluntarily and legally immigrates to another country to become a resident. Undocumented immigrants are those who are living in a country without the permission of the government. Undocumented immigrants may be legal or illegal. Illegal immigrants have false or no immigration documents. Legal immigrants have temporary visas, but become undocumented when they stay past the expiration date of the visa.

K

Kosher Dietary Laws

These laws are based on humanness and practical reasons associated with health. The laws forbid eating pork, shellfish, non-kosher red meat, and poultry. Non-kosher meat is considered any meat obtained from an animal that was not killed with a single blow and/or was killed by strangulation. More than one blow to kill an animal is considered cruel because of the pain and suffering experienced by the animal between the first and final blows. Strangulation of an animal allows time for release of hormones that can be harmful to consumers of the red meat. Red meat must come from animals that chew their cud and have cloven hoofs. Any fish consumed must be of the type having fins and scales. Meat and dairy products cannot be eaten during the same meal; pots, utensils, plates cannot be used for both. Foods categorized as parve may be eaten with milk or meats dishes and include eggs, fruit, vegetables, and nuts.[7]

L

Lawful Permanent Resident

A non- United States citizen who has been granted the right to legally reside, work, study, and apply for United States citizenship according to established laws. The Bureau of Citizenship and Immigration Services issues to approved individuals, and an identification card commonly known as a 'green card.' The card must be in the individual's possession at all times. Permanent resident status can be obtained through several different paths such as family, certain jobs, etc. For detailed information about green cards, visit http://www.uscis.gov/portal/site/uscis.

Limited English Proficiency (LEP)

The term used to describe individuals whose native language is not English and who are limited in the ability to read, speak, and understand English.

M

Mal Ojo

See *Evil Eye*.

Marital Assimilation

Exists when members of two racial or ethnic groups live together as man and wife. See *Assimilation*.

Minority

A group or people who are singled out from others within a society in which they live, because of cultural characteristics, for unequal or different treatment. The members of the group regard themselves as objects of collective discrimination and exclusion from full participation in society life. This term may be offensive to some because of its perceived connection to discrimination and marginalization.

P

Pica

The craving and eating of non-food items such as laundry starch, clay, hair, burned matches, sand, grass, and plaster. The craving for ice is known as *pagophagia*. Persons with sickle cell anemia and those who are pregnant are known to eat clay and laundry starch with the belief that these substances will build the blood or keep an unborn baby's skin clean.

Bowel obstructions, lead poisoning, intestinal parasites, and other complications can occur. Pica occurring during pregnancy usually ends once the baby is born.

Pinching

A form of folk healing practiced among some Asian populations, particularly Hmong, Laotian, Vietnamese, and Cambodians. It consists of pinching any symptomatic area of the body, sometimes followed by pricking the area with a sharp needle. Conditions treated by pinching include localized pain, fever, coughs, poor appetite, dizziness, fainting, and blurred vision. It is practiced on children over ten years of age and on adults. Any adult may perform this treatment.[1,5]

Poua

See *Burning.*

Prejudice

Biased conclusions/perceptions about individuals or groups based on inaccurate information.

Q

Quat Sha

See *Coining/Coin Rubbing.*

R

Race

A group of people related by common descent of heredity who have similar physical characteristics such as skin color, facial form, eye shape, etc. The concept of 'race' continues to be challenged from purely biological or physical perspectives and is many times socially constructed.

Racism

The belief that race determines human capacities and that some races are superior to others.

Refugee

A person who seeks protection in a country other than his/her homeland because of fear of persecution or harm.

S

Smudging

A healing method used among Native Americans for the purpose of cleansing an individual of negative energies. Sage, tobacco or cedar, and sweet grass are burned in a bowl or pot. The smoke is fanned over the person, using an eagle feather. Smudging is often combined with other healing modalities such as fasting, praying, etc.[8, 9]

Stereotype

To label all persons of a cultural, ethnic, or racial group based on the assumption that all persons within that particular group share the same similarities, beliefs, and values.

Subculture

A large group of persons with shared characteristics that are part of a larger culture that does not share those characteristics. The group's characteristics distinguish them from the larger culture and are thought of as a subgroup of the primary culture.[1]

T

Time Orientation

How an individual or group of individuals behave in relation to the ordering of time – past, present, and future. Only among the American middle and upper class population, is time so highly valued. In many cultures, individuals' lives are not ordered by schedules, clocks, watches, etc.

1. **Present-oriented**: Persons generally do not value strict schedules. They perceive time as flexible. Present activities are generally more important than future or past activities. May be late for scheduled appointments, place little value on preventive health care practices, and resist rigid hospital schedules because the present moment in time is what is important.

2. **Past-oriented**: Individuals place great value on traditions and beliefs. They may be very hesitant to consent to new medical treatments.
3. **Future-oriented:** Persons generally "live by the clock and calendar." Many of these individuals mold their current behavior based on future goals and plans.

Transcultural Nursing

A field of study established by Dr. Madeline Leininger, nurse and anthropologist – "A substantive area of study and practice focused on comparative cultural care (caring) values, beliefs, and practices of individuals or groups of similar or different cultures with the goal of providing culture-specific and universal nursing care practices in promoting health or well-being or to help people to face unfavorable human conditions, illness, or death in culturally meaningful ways."[3]

Values

Personal standards of what is good or useful in relationship to oneself and to others.

Ventouse

See *Cupping*.

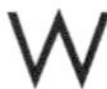

Worldview

One's perception or interpretation of phenomenon in the world around them, which forms the basis of actions.

Yin/Yang Health Concept

A Chinese concept of health. It is believed that the forces of nature are balanced to produce harmony. The Yin force represents the female aspect of nature. It is believed to be the negative pole and encompasses darkness, cold, and emptiness. The Yang force represents the male aspect of nature. It is believed to be the positive pole and encompasses fullness, light, and warmth. An imbalance of the Yin and Yang forces produce illness; an indication of disharmony. Therefore, illness is not thought of as an intrusion, but as a natural part of the life cycle. Illness is thought to be inevitable; perfect health is not the goal. Yin and Yang are assigned to certain diseases, health conditions, and body organs as indicated below.[1, 5, 10, 11, 12] The inside of the body and the front of the body is Yin. The surface of the body and the back of the body is Yang. Yin stores the vital strength of life. Yang protects the body from outside forces.[13]

Yin	Health Condition / Disease	Organs
	Cancer	Kidney
	Lactation	Liver
	Menstruation	Lungs
	Postpartum Period	Spleen
	Shivering	Spleen
	Wasting	
Yang	**Health Condition / Disease**	**Organs**
	Constipation	Bladder
	Hangover	Gallbladder
	Hypertension	Intestines
	Infection	Stomach
	Sore Throat	
	Toothache	
	Upset Stomach	
	Venereal Disease	
	Pregnancy	

1 Andrews, M. & Boyle, J. (2012). *Transcultural concepts in nursing* care. (6th ed.). Philadelphia, PA: Lippincott Williams & Wilkins.

2 Muecke, M. (1983). Caring for the Southeast Asian refugee patients in the USA. *American Journal of Public Health, 73*(4), 431-438.

3 Leininger, M. (1995). *Transcultural nursing: Concepts, theories, research and practices.* (2nd ed.). New York, NY: McGraw-Hill.

4 Cross, T., Bazron, B., Dennis, K., & Isaacs, M. (1989). *Towards a culturally competent system of care: Volume 1. Washington, DC: Georgetown University Child Development Center, CASSP Technical Assistance Center.*

5 Hansen, K. (1998). Folk remedies and child abuse: A review with emphasis on ciada de mollera and its relationship to shaken baby syndrome. *Child Abuse and Neglect, 22*(2), 117-127.

6 Galant, G. (2008). *Caring for patients from different cultures: Case studies from American hospitals.* (4th ed.). Philadelphia, PA: University of Pennsylvania Press.

7 Charnes, L. & Moore, P. (1992). Meeting patients' spiritual needs: The Jewish perspective. *Holistic Nurse Practitioner, 6*(3), 64-72.

8 Null, G. (1998). *Secrets of the White Buffalo: Native American healing remedies, rites and rituals.* Upper Saddle River, NJ: Prentice Hall.

9 Whiteman, W. (1992). *Sacred sage: How it heals.* Ashland, VA: Whiteman.

10 Giger, J.N.(2013). *Transcultural nursing: Assessment and intervention.* (6th ed.). St. Louis, MO: Mosby Elsevier.

11 Yanchi, L. (1988). *The essential book of traditional Chinese medicine, Volume I: Theory.* New York, NY: Columbia University Press.

12 Shealey, C. (1996). *Alternative medicine: An illustrated encyclopedia of natural healing.* New York, NY: Barnes & Noble Books.

13 Spector, R. (2004). *Cultural diversity in health and illness* (6th ed.). Norwalk, CT: Appleton & Lange.

BASIC STRATEGIES

General

- Persons from the same country may not necessarily share the same culture.
- Refrain from making assumptions relative to beliefs/practices based on an individual's cultural or religious affiliation. While there are commonalties among and across cultures, each individual is unique and interactions must be relative to his or her specific beliefs and practices. Individuals may accept the "official" doctrines, but practice in varying degrees.
- Be careful not to jump to conclusions concerning an individual's ethnicity based on appearance. Always ask. Emphasize this point with admission personnel who collect and enter data.

Communication

- Address **all** adults as Mr., Miss, Ms., or Mrs., unless otherwise instructed. Using a first name to address anyone other than family or a close friend is discourteous and inappropriate in most cultures. If there is frequent interaction with a specific cultural group, learning to address members of the culture using their formal titles helps to establish a positive rapport, especially among elders (e.g., Señor or Señora). Acknowledge family members in the room–particularly elders.

- Avoid using terms such as *boy*, *girl*, *gal*, etc. when addressing or referring to others–particularly non-African Americans to African Americans. Refrain from using terms of endearment such as *sweetie*, *honey*, or *baby* to address patients unless a positive rapport/relationship has been established and the use of the term is mutually agreeable.

- Many cultures highly value modesty and may be suspicious about personal questions. When conducting the admission assessment, the relationship between the medical problems and the need for asking personal questions should be explained clearly.

- Identify the primary decision-maker when there is a need to make a choice about treatment measures. In some cultures, the patient or parent of a child is not the primary decision-maker.

- Lack of eye contact may be a sign of respect instead of a lack of interest or untrustworthiness.

- Some languages lack pronouns that reflect sex. Pronouns such as "he" or "she" may not exist and will be confusing.

- **Gestures:**

Avoid using gestures when communicating. Note the difference in meanings of common gestures commonly used in the United States.[1,2]

- Beckoning with the index finger to come closer is a gesture used only in some cultures for the purpose of calling animals.

- The "okay" sign (thumb and index fingers together in a circle) is a sexual invitation in some cultures.

- The "thumbs-up" sign and the "V" sign for victory are insulting gestures in some cultures meaning the same as the raised middle finger in United States culture.

- Sitting with the soles of shoes visible toward persons of many Asian cultures may offend them because the feet are considered the lowest part of the body.

- Talking while the hands are in one's pockets or with arms folded is considered impolite in some cultures.
- Steady eye contact can be seen as rude or as a sexual invitation.

- Use objective descriptions instead of slang terms and phrases. For example, "cold feet" may be understood as vascular/circulatory problems. "Bagging", sometimes used to refer to manual ventilation, may be taken literally as placing the patient in a bag. The word "fanny" is a derogatory term in some cultures. "Rubber", commonly used in the US to refer to a condom, may be understood to be an eraser.[1] "Are you straight?" or 'I'm straight" may be an inquiry or affirmation about an individual's well-being or understanding of information instead of whether an individual is gay or non-gay.

- Avoid sentences or questions with negatives. The person may answer with an affirmative answer, meaning that you are correct that an event has not occurred (e.g., "You haven't had your bath yet, have you?" Instead ask, "Have you had a bath today?").

- Health care workers should take the time to assure that clients are familiar with the operation of electronic-based communication methods used in Western culture, including telephones, voice-mail, etc.

- If there are absolutely no available interpreter services, when speaking to persons who have limited English proficiency, speak slowly and clearly without raising the voice. Provide any instructions in the order that the steps will be performed.

- Some individuals may be able to read English better than they understand spoken English. Ask which language the patient prefers for communication in the health care setting.

- **Interpreters:**

  - **Anticipate that additional time will be needed to accomplish any interventions that require the use of an interpreter. It is critical that organizational administrators consider this need for additional time when planning staffing levels.**

  - **Interpreters should be included as critical members of the health care team. Consider the following guidelines when working with interpreters:**[3,4,5]

- Use only qualified interpreters trained in medical terminology or professional medical interpreter services. If using telephone or video interpreters, assure that patient confidentiality is maintained by using a private place for the conversation. Dual-receiver telephones are optimal for use during a telephone session requiring an interpreter. Staff members who are used as interpreters should have competency validated and documented.
- Use same-gender interpreters when translating matters that are of a private or sexual nature. In some cultures, it is inappropriate for persons of the opposite gender (including children) to discuss matters of this nature. Frequently, it is taboo for children to talk about subjects perceived as being of an intimate nature with adults. Avoid using family members as interpreters for any subject other than general, non-medical information, if at all possible to maintain patient confidentiality and to assure accuracy of communication. This includes having husbands translate for wives in areas such as Labor and Delivery, informed consent for surgeries related to reproductive organs, etc.
- Generally, older, mature interpreters are preferred. Do not assume that persons who can converse in a language, understand and can accurately communicate health-related information. Interpreters should be used to gain accurate health histories, to convey accurate medical information, and to participate in discharge teaching.
- Discuss the method of interpreting that the medical provider prefers prior to approaching the patient/family. **Consecutive interpretation** involves a pause after each sentence or phrase and is most often used in clinical settings. **Simultaneous interpretation** involves interpreting a few seconds behind as a person speaks. This type of interpreting tends to be confusing for patients. **Summary interpretation** involves summarizing long blocks of information. It carries the greatest risk of inaccuracies. If the information is simple and the interpreter is already familiar with the content, it may be an effective method.
- Ask the interpreter to introduce all persons who are present during the interaction.
- Request that the interpreter ask for clarification of any information that is not clearly understood.
- Speak to the patient or parent; not the interpreter. Maintain eye contact during conversation.
- Avoid the use of random gestures.

- Allow adequate time when speaking for interpretation to occur.
- Avoid the use of complex medical terms. If concerned about how the interpreter understands the medical terms, ask that the interpreter repeat the information back prior to communicating the information to the patient/family.
- Do not expect word-for-word interpreting. Some languages do not have words for medical terminology. What is said to the patient through the interpreter may take significantly longer to convey an accurate message.
- Ask the interpreter to share the meaning of any nonverbal behaviors that may be culturally-based.
- Offer interpreters to deaf or hard-of-hearing persons. Sign languages of various countries are not mutually understandable.[6]

Health and Illness

- When assigning patients in semi-private rooms, avoid placing patients in the same room who are from countries having negative or volatile relationships (i.e. war, political/religious conflicts, etc.).

- If members of the clergy routinely visit clients who are hospitalized, clients should have this practice explained prior to the visit since persons of some cultures associate visits by the clergy with imminent death.

- The common practice of sending flowers to hospitalized clients is not a practice in some cultures and is frequently associated only with rites for the dead.

- Pain is culturally expressed varying from stoic to very expressive. Do not assume that the 'quiet' patient is not experiencing pain. Some may attach spiritual and religious meanings to pain and how it should be endured. Medications that cloud consciousness such as narcotics may be rejected in some instances. Explore medication alternatives and non-pharmacologic comfort approaches.

- Self-treatment for illness episodes is common among most cultures. Herbal treatments can be toxic, particularly among children. Always include assessment questions related to what has been used for treatment of an illness prior to presenting to mainstream health facilities.[3]

- Persons may have family members send medications, herbs, and other substances for folk treatments to them from their native country. The names of those medications and herbal preparations may not be congruent with the names in the current country of residence. Consult medical provider or pharmacist for presence of any possible adverse effects or interactions with prescribed medications.

- Members of some ethnic groups believe that illness is caused by supernatural sources or by environmental factors such as cold air, impurities in the air, etc. and seek folk healers to cure illness. It is important that health care workers not dismiss these beliefs as 'old wives tales,' 'silly,' or 'strange' as they play important roles in individuals' lives.

- Individuals often carry or wear religious symbols. Symbols that absolutely have to be removed for diagnostic purposes, should be removed gently, respectfully, and kept in contact with the patient's body if at all possible. The person and/or family should be given an explanation of why the symbol needs to be removed prior to any attempts to remove it. Following are some spiritual/cultural symbols:

  - A rosary or jewelry with images of the Virgin Mary or Saints may be worn or images may be placed in the hospital room or the home. This is commonly seen among Catholics.

  - Sacred threads or pouches may be worn around arms, neck, and other areas of the body.

  - Native Americans may carry or wear medicine bags.

  - Small red ribbons or strings may be worn, often on the wrist, for protection from evil.

  - A special charm or pouch/bag on a chain or cord may be worn around the neck, wrist, or waist. Various items are added and are thought to be protective.

- Cutting or shaving hair from the body and/or head is forbidden in many cultures. This should be considered when there is a need to shave or cut a patient's hair in preparation for procedures.

- In some cultures, particularly Asian, elimination is considered unclean and, therefore, should not be done in bed. In the native country, bowel elimination is sometimes accomplished by squatting over a hole in the ground. If the family has a toilet, it is often located separately from the tub or sink. The individual may place the feet on the toilet seat and squat to have a bowel movement. Patients who are forced to use a bedpan in the hospital may insist on getting out of bed, if at all possible, and may squat over the bedpan to have a bowel movement.[1]

- Families should be asked how they wish to participate in preparation of the body after death. In some cultures, the family "washes" the body of a relative after death and may consider it an infringement if health care personnel proceed with the usual preparations for the morgue. Funeral directors should be notified prior to transport of the body to the funeral home if the preparation of the body is different from mainstream practices.

Family/Children

- Many cultural groups emphasize the family over the individual and inter-dependence over independence. Self-care is not an important concept in most other cultures.
- When complimenting babies and children of cultures that believe in the evil eye concept, watch for non-verbal cues from the mother. If she seems uncomfortable with your compliments, she may believe in the evil eye. For Mexican Americans who believe in the evil eye, touching the infant or child while offering the compliment neutralizes the effects of the evil eye.
- When assessing the growth status of children, it is important to remember that standard growth charts in the United States have been developed based primarily on growth patterns among White Americans. Children of various ethnic groups may exhibit growth patterns that may not be considered "normal" according to United States standards. Therefore, the overall status of the child must be assessed before a conclusion is drawn.

Birth Control

- Always approach discussions about birth control cautiously. Some religions do not support artificial forms of birth control. In some cultures, the number of children sired or borne is a major source of self-esteem.

- When discussing birth control, it is necessary to know the cultural beliefs related to handling the genitals, discussing birth control measures, etc. Birth control measures such as diaphragms, spermicidal foams, etc. will be unacceptable in many cultures because of extreme modesty and the belief that the genitals are dirty areas of the body. Abstinence or the rhythm method may be more acceptable.

Food and Nutrition

- The belief that certain foods are considered edible or inedible is primarily influenced by culture. Do not assume that the client shares your beliefs about which foods are edible or inedible.

- Consider typical ethnic diets when discharging patients with special dietary restrictions. Length of time in a given country affects acculturation. Staple foods of an individual's country of origin will generally be the last eliminated from the diet. Older individuals are more likely to maintain traditional diets.[7,8]

- Do not assume that persons from other countries eat the usual three meals a day as many United States Americans eat or at similar times of the day. When teaching about medications that must be taken with food, it is important to be specific in saying to take the medication the designated number of times/per day with food, rather than instructing the patient to take the medication with meals (assuming that all persons eat three meals a day).

- During nutritional assessments, be specific when inquiring about types of foods consumed. For instance, a patient may respond that 'red meat' is not consumed because s/he only consumes the meat when it is 'brown' after being cooked.

Discharge/Patient Teaching[9]

- Plan for the teaching session to last at least twice as long as usual.

- Speak slowly and use simple words.

- Avoid the use of technical terms (e.g., heart instead of cardiac).
- Provide instructions for any procedures/treatments in the same sequence that the patient should carry out the steps.
- Ask the patient to give a return demonstration or explanation of the procedure.
- Include family members in the teaching process.
- Calendar date sequences differ in other countries. Assure clarity by writing out the full name of the month and weekday.
- Be specific about recommended times of day to take medications instead of only stating how many times/day. Include visuals as adjuncts to teaching about medication administration. Use caution when using the written word *'once'* in instructions for medications, treatments, etc. "Once" in Spanish means eleven (11).
- When possible, flexibility should be built into appointment times, including the availability of walk-in clinics, evening, and weekend hours. For persons who do not have telephones in the home, arrange for the patient/family member to call the office or clinic at a specified time. Provide a toll-free number, if applicable. For migrant workers, it is helpful to obtain the phone number of the crew leader or person who is providing jobs to the migrant workers.[3]
- For migrant workers or homeless persons, provide portable medical records that indicate, minimally, immunizations given, allergies, prescribed medications, critical health problems, etc.[3]
- Some patients/families do not own clocks or watches. Inquire about availability of time devices if discharge components are time-dependent.

---

1 Galanti, G. (2008). *Caring for patients from different cultures.* (3rd ed.). Philadelphia, PA: University of Pennsylvania Press.

2 Pease, A. & Pease, B. (2006). *The definitive book of body language.* New York, NY: Bantam Books.

3 American Academy of Pediatrics & Migrant Clinicians Network (2000). *Guidelines for the care of migrant farm workers' children.* Elk Grove Village, IL & Austin, TX: American Academy of Pediatrics and the Migrant Clinicians Network.

[4] Massachusetts General Hospital. (2002). *Medical interpreter services.* Retrieved from http://www2.massgeneral.org/interpreters/index.asp

[5] Andrews, M. & Boyle, J. (2012). *Transcultural concepts in nursing care.* (6th ed.). Philadelphia, PA: Lippincott Williams & Wilkins.

[6] Crystal, D. (2010). The *Cambridge encyclopedia of language.* (3rd ed.). New York, NY: Cambridge University Press.

[7] Burrowes, J. (2004). Incorporating ethnic and cultural food preferences in the renal diet. *Advances in Replacement Therapy, 11*(1), 97-104.

[8] Kittler, P.G. & Sucher, K.P. (2008). *Food and culture* (5th ed.). Belmont, CA: Thomson Higher Education.

[9] Tripp-Reiner, T. & Afifi, L. (1989). Cross-cultural perspectives on patient teaching. *Nursing Clinics of North America, 24*(3), 613-619.

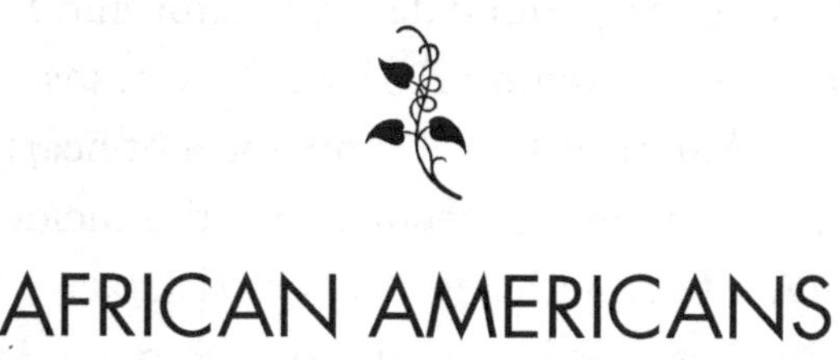

AFRICAN AMERICANS

Background

The majority of African American ancestors were victims of the largest forced migration in world history, the African slave trade. The slave trade lasted for four centuries, spurred originally by the spread of sugar production after Christopher Columbus introduced sugar cane into the New World. One in six Africans died en route to the Americas. In spite of the high mortality rate, ten to twelve million Africans survived the trip to the Americas. They were members of the numerous heterogeneous tribes living along the West Coast of Africa.[1,2,3] Africans were delivered to the Caribbean, Portugal, Brazil, Spanish America, and North America to work as slaves.[2,4]

Approximately 90 percent of African Americans in the United States have some Anglo ancestry; at least 25 percent have Native American ancestry.[5] The genetic strains found among African Americans number more than one hundred.[6]

There is tremendous diversity among African Americans, comprising about 13 percent of the United States population. They live in all areas of the United States and come with preparation at all educational levels. African Americans are represented in all socioeconomic levels. However, as of 2010, almost one-third lived at poverty level. The median age is 29.5 years. Over 50 percent of African Americans live in Southern states. The ten states with the largest populations of African Americans are New York, Florida, Texas, California,

North Carolina, Illinois, Maryland, Virginia and Ohio. African Americans make up 51 percent of the population in the District of Columbia.[7,8]

In spite of advances in health care and technology, African Americans are still faced with numerous health disparities and have a life expectancy approximately six years less than Whites. As a group, they are confronted with high morbidity and mortality rates from a number of diseases. The causes of these disparities are multi-factorial. The leading causes of death among African Americans are heart disease, cancer, stoke, injuries, diabetes, kidney disease, lower respiratory disease, homicide, septicemia and HIV/AIDS. The disparities in prevalence of some health issues among African Americans are note-worthy. Approximately 40 percent of African Americans have some form of heart disease. Strokes are more severe, often resulting in disability and mortality, and the incidence of strokes is twice as high when compared with White Americans. A major risk factor for stroke is hypertension. One in every three African Americans is hypertensive. African Americans are almost twice as likely to have diabetes. Among those greater than 20 years of age, almost 15 percent are diabetic.

As age increases, so does the incidence of diabetes, especially among women. Twenty-five percent of African American women above 55 years of age are diabetic. Among women and men, complications of diabetes are more severe and sometimes life-threatening. Of further concern is the high rate of obesity, especially among African American women with four of every five women classified as overweight or obese. Diabetes and hypertension are contributing factors to a high incidence of kidney disease.

Cancer statistics reflect similar disparities. The highest death rate from cancer of any ethnic group in the United States occurs among African Americans. Once diagnosed, they also have the shortest survival rates. HIV/AIDS continues to be a major cause of death among African Americans and, according to the most recent statistics, accounts for more than 40 percent of newly diagnosed cases. Moreover, African American women are disproportionately affected, accounting for more than half of the newly diagnosed cases of HIV/AIDS. Most are infected through heterosexual sexual contact. It is the leading cause of death among African American women, ages 25-34.

Lastly, in spite of extensive research, pre-term birth and infant mortality remain highest among African Americans. Furthermore, Sudden Infant Death Syndrome (SIDS) occurs among African American babies at a rate that is twice that of non-Hispanic Whites. Other health risks include sickle cell disease, homicide, and occupational injuries.[8,9,10,11,12,13,14]

Language/Communication

- The dominant language among African Americans is English. However, there are a number of Black dialects and pidgins spoken, sometimes reflecting the combination of various native African languages and languages of other cultures. Gullah, a Creole language derived from West African languages, is the first language of some African Americans along the coast of Georgia and South Carolina.[6, 15] There may be frequent use of words that are classified as "slang," especially among teenagers and young adults. Confirm meanings and context of words without using a condescending approach.

- Clarify the meanings of terms that may be used to describe an illness. For example, "low blood" might refer to anemia or to low blood pressure; "sugar" might refer to diabetes.

- Speech may be accompanied by animated non-verbal gestures (e.g., hand movements, touching, etc.). The voice may become louder with excitement/other emotions and gestures more animated, which is sometimes mistaken for aggressiveness or anger.

- African Americans may sometimes refer to each other using terms such as "Boy," "Girl," etc. Nicknames are also frequently used. Health care providers should not assume that they can use the same terms without negative repercussions.

- Consistent eye contact and other signs of listening valued by many members of the dominant culture may not be seen among some African Americans. This may be related to factors such as historical influences or to upbringing where consistent eye contact may be seen as a sign of disrespect especially from younger to older individuals. Use open-ended questions; ask the individual to express or demonstrate his or her understanding of information discussed.

Time Orientation

- Many African Americans are present-oriented, being faced with an uncertain future in the face of poverty and life-threatening environments. However, there may be strong future-oriented behaviors such as saving for a college education for children, purchasing insurance policies to cover funeral and burial costs, etc. Elders may place a great deal of value on past experiences, which are frequently shared with younger individuals. In general, there is a great deal of variation in time orientation.

- For African Americans who are more present-oriented and see time as 'flexible', allow flexibility in treatment approaches, if appropriate. For those medical activities where adherence to scheduled times is important such as medications, appointments, etc., stress that adherence is critical.[15]

Worldview/Religious Beliefs

- Health and happiness are connected to living a life that is pleasing to God.
- Many African Americans have strong ties with the church and will wish to have friends, the minister and/or other church officials visit and offer prayers for recovery. Communion may be offered to hospitalized individuals or those confined to the home because of illness. There is a strong belief in the healing powers of God.
- Most African Americans are Protestants. A growing number of African Americans follow Islam and other religions.[16]
- In addition to specific religious observations, Kwanzaa and Juneteenth celebrations will be important to many African Americans. Kwanzaa, celebrated between December 26th and January 1st, is a celebration of the New Year, while reminding African Americans of their African cultural roots. It reinforces seven principles—*unity, self-determination/persistence, collective work/responsibility, collective economical efforts, purpose, creativity,* and *faith.* Consistent practice of these seven principles is thought to strengthen African Americans as a group. Juneteenth is celebrated on June 19th in commemoration of the ending of slavery in the United States. Although the Emancipation Proclamation was official January 1, 1863, it was two and a half years later that Union soldiers arrived in Galveston, Texas to announce that slaves were free. This occurred on June 19, 1865.[17,18]
- Because of years of oppression, discrimination, etc., African Americans may have a general suspicion and non-trust of White healthcare providers. This may negatively impact preventive health screenings, acceptance of treatment options, compliance with treatment regimens, and end-of-life decision-making.[19]

Health Beliefs/Practices

- There is tremendous variation in health beliefs. Examples of common health beliefs among African Americans are:[6,15,20]
  - Incorporation of some hot and cold principles.
  - Everything has an opposite, such as for every birth, there must be a death.
  - Trouble and pain are God's will. Health is a gift from God; illness is punishment from God for some past wrongdoing, worry, overindulgence, or exposure to environmental elements such as cold air.
  - Illness may result from supernatural and magical causes, including hexes. May practice folk medicine and/or visit 'root doctors' or a person knowledgeable of curing the effects of hoodoo.
  - Women are more susceptible to illness at certain times such as during menstruation or after having a baby. Babies and children are weaker than adults.
- Health and illness may be influenced by astrological forces. Attention to 'the signs' is common. Each of the twelve astrological signs is thought to influence the health and functions of specific parts of the body.[15]
- Prayer is a common method for treating illness. Prayer cloths may be placed on the bed or gown of an ill person.[15] It is important not to remove the prayer cloth.
- May be suspicious of the health care system. African Americans are sometimes resistant to hospitalization believing that, once an individual enters a hospital, he or she will not come out alive.[21,22]
- May use various home remedies for illnesses and not seek medical care until a crisis occurs. Some African Americans believe that certain persons have the power to heal illnesses or family disharmony and will consult these persons prior to seeking a mainstream practitioner.[23]
- **Blood/Blood Products:** Generally acceptable unless religiously prohibited.

Expression of Pain

- Varies from stoic to very expressive.

Male-Female/Kinship/Social Relationships

- Females head 45 percent of African American households. Maternal parents may play a strong role in decision-making.
- Immediate and extended family are important. "Family" titles may be attached to friends of the family such as *Aunt*, *Uncle*, *play mother*, *play sister or brother*, *adopted mother*, *daughter*, or *son*. These persons are considered members of the family and will be as important for support as blood kinship. Members of the church may be referred to as *Brother* or *Sister*.[24,25]
- The elderly are generally highly respected. Younger persons often refer to elders as *Miss* or *Mr.* (person's first name) as a sign of respect. For example, Miss Sarah or Mr. James.
- African Americans may resist placing loved ones in nursing homes, etc., instead opting to involve family members and friends to assist in caring for the relative in the home. It is likely that even children in the home will assist in care of the individual to the extent of their abilities.
- Health care providers will be evaluated by their actions as well as their words. In non-emergency situations, provide care in an unhurried manner and with full, honest explanations.
- Older African Americans generally prefer to be addressed as *Mr.* or *Mrs.*, followed by their last name. Subsequent interactions may be compromised by assuming that use of a first name is acceptable.[22,26]

Birth/Children

- Common beliefs/practices surrounding childbirth include:[6,24,27]
  - Reaching above the head during pregnancy will cause the umbilical cord to wrap around the unborn baby's neck.

- Pictures taken during pregnancy will cause a stillbirth.
- The mother should stay inside for six weeks after the baby is born to prevent unnecessary exposure to 'air'.
- Birthmarks present on the infant at birth may be attributed to the baby being 'marked' because the mother ingested or craved certain foods during the pregnancy.

- Bellybands made from clean white cotton may be placed on the baby until the umbilical cord falls off. This is believed to contribute to a non-protruding umbilical area. Castor oil and coins (particularly or half-dollar coins) may also be applied to the cord until it falls off. Some persons believe that the dried umbilical cord should be burned when it falls off.

- Mongolian spots are found in at least 90 percent of African American newborns. They are most often found in the lumbosacral and gluteal areas, but are not limited to these areas. These should not be confused with bruises. They begin to fade during the first two years of life but may persist into adolescence.[28]

- There is a higher incidence among African Americans of placing their infants in the prone position for sleep. SIDS is higher among African American babies. The prevalence of prone positioning is thought to be, in part, a contributing factor to this higher incidence of SIDS. Reinforce the importance of placing infants in supine position for sleeping and the potential benefit to the baby in decreasing risk of Sudden Infant Death Syndrome.[11]

- Infants are often started on solid foods at an early age, sometimes within a few weeks after birth. Generally, if this occurs, it is baby cereal that is mixed with the formula and given by bottle. This is more likely to occur with the belief that formula is insufficient to relieve the baby's hunger and that the baby will sleep through the night with the addition of cereal to the formula. Provide counseling to parent(s) about the negative effects of beginning early solid foods.[6]

- Post-neonatal follow-up care is important. The post-neonatal mortality rate for African American children is twice as high as for White infants.[9]

- The hair of male infants and toddlers may be braided or plaited through two years of age or later.[29]

- Children may be spanked as a method of discipline, following the writings in the Holy Bible of "spare the rod and spoil the child."

Death

- Expressions of grief vary widely.
- **Organ Donation/Transplants**: African Americans are underrepresented as organ donors.[30]
- **Autopsy**: Some African Americans may be resistant to autopsies, believing that the relative's body will be mutilated.

Patient Teaching/Dietary Considerations

- African Americans are frequently lactose-intolerant.
- Diets are frequently high in fat and sodium, and low in fiber. Determine foods that are usually eaten and how they are prepared, and then negotiate substitute methods of preparing foods in a healthier manner without sacrificing taste. Consider the cost of recommended foods, whether the individual will be able to afford the foods, and/or if there are resources to assist in the purchase of foods.[6, 31]
- Laxatives may be used as a method of keeping the system clean and open. Assess frequency of use.[31]
- African Americans may expect almost immediate improvement in their medical condition or lose faith in the medical system. It is important to thoroughly explain the disease process and the expected course of improvement.

Other Considerations

- African Americans have traditionally been underrepresented in clinical trials of drugs. More recently, studies suggest that African Americans respond to and metabolize certain drugs differently from Whites. Examples of such drugs include alcohol, anti-hypertensives, some psychotropics, antidepressants, beta-blockers, and drugs used for dilating pupils. Side effects may be more pronounced, or the expected positive drug effects may not occur. Closely monitor individuals for expected drug effects and for side effects.[6]

- African American skin color varies widely. Skin not exposed to the sun will appear lighter than exposed skin. Lip and gum color may vary from pink to almost purple. Flat, darker pigmented birthmarks occur in approximately 20 percent of African Americans and can be present on any part of the body. Skin discolorations often seen among African Americans include dark streaks on the nails, dark spots on the palms and soles of the feet, and gray or dark areas on the buccal mucosa and gums. Albinism (the skin is unable to produce melanin) and vitiligo (results in loss of melanocytes) may be seen among African Americans. Determine if the areas in question are new findings or normal for the individual. Assure that skin assessments are carried out under good lighting. In dark-skinned individuals, inspect the oral mucosa and conjunctivae for central cyanosis; inspect the sclera of the eyes for jaundice.[6,15,32]

- Trauma to the skin can result in the formation of *keloids*, raised areas of scar tissue that overgrow the boundaries of the original injury and do not spontaneously shrink in size. Keloids can occur after skin piercing, surgical incisions, lacerations, etc. Among some male African Americans, close shaving sometimes leads to *pseudofolliculitis barbae* (razor bumps), a condition caused by the facial hair growing back into the skin when cut short, causing a skin reaction and possible infection. Inquire about usual items used for shaving.[15,32]

- Hair texture varies widely among African Americans, and consequently, requires diverse care approaches. Ask the patient or family members about usual hair care. In addition to the usual combs that are available in health care facilities, have larger, wide-toothed combs available for hair grooming.

- When considering implementation of community health programs for African Americans, involve churches in planning since pastors and the church can often play an important role in the success of the programs.

---

1 Franklin, J. & Moss, A. (1994). *From slavery to freedom: A history of African Americans* (7th ed.). New York, NY: McGraw-Hill.

2 Bennett, L. (1998). *Before the Mayflower: A history of black America*. New York, NY: Penguin Books.

3 Quarles, B. (1987). *The Negro in the making of America*. New York, NY: Simon & Schuster.

4 Klein, H. (1986). *African slavery in Latin America and the Caribbean*. New York, NY: Oxford University Press.

5 Davis, F. (1991). *Who is Black? One nation's definition*. University Park, PA: Pennsylvania State University Press.

[6] Campinha-Bacote, J. (2013). People of African American heritage. In L. Purnell, *Transcultural health care: A culturally competent approach* (4th ed.), (pp. 91-114). Philadelphia, PA: F. A. Davis Company.

[7] The Office of Minority Health. (2012). *African American profile.* Retrieved from http://minorityhealth.hhs.gov/templates/browse.aspx?lvl=2&lvlID=51

[8] DeNavas, C., Proctor, B. & Smith, J. (2011, September). *Income, poverty, and health insurance: Coverage in the United States.* Washington, DC: U. S. Census Bureau.

[9] Centers for Disease Control and Prevention. (2012). *Minority health.* Retrieved from http://www.cdc.gov/minorityhealth/populations/REMP/black.html#10

[10] American Cancer Society. (2011). *Cancer facts & figures for African Americans.* Atlanta, GA: Author. Retrieved from http://www.cancer.org/acs/groups/content/@epidemiologysurveilance/documents/document/acspc-027765.pdf

[11] Hauck, F., Moore, C., Herman, S., Donovan, M., Kelelkar, M., Christoffel, K. & Rowley, D. (2002). The contribution of prone sleeping position to the racial disparity in sudden infant death syndrome: The Chicago infant mortality study. *Pediatrics, 110*(4), 772-780.

[12] National Stroke Association. (2012). *African Americans and stroke.* Retrieved from http://www.stroke.org/site/PageServer?pagename=aamer

[13] American Diabetes Association. (2012). *African Americans and complications.* Retrieved from http://www.diabetes.org/living-with-diabetes/complications/african-americans-and-complications.html

[14] Smedley, B., Stith, A. & Nelson, A. (2003). *Unequal treatment: Confronting racial and ethnic disparities in health care.* Washington, DC: The National Academies Press.

[15] Cherry, B. & Giger, J.N. (2013). African-Americans. In Giger, J.N. *Transcultural nursing: Assessment and intervention* (6th ed.). (pp.162-206). St. Louis, MO: Mosby Elsevier.

[16] Pinn, A. (1998). *Varieties of African American religious experience.* Minneapolis, MN: Fortress Press.

[17] Riley, D. (1995). *The Complete Kwanzaa: Celebrating our cultural harvest.* New York, NY: HarperCollins.

[18] *Juneteenth World Wide Celebration.* (n.d.). Retrieved from http://www.juneteenth.com

[19] West, S. & Levi, L. (2004). Culturally appropriate end-of-life care for the Black American. *Home Healthcare Nurse, 22(*3), 164-168.

[20] Fishman, B., Bobo, L., Kosub, K. & Womeodu, J. (1993). Cultural issues in serving minority populations: Emphasis on Mexican Americans and African Americans. *The American Journal of the Medical Sciences, 306*(3), 160-166.

[21] Washington, H.A. (2006). *Medical apartheid: The dark history of medical experimentation on Black Americans from colonial times to the present.* New York, NY: Doubleday.

[22] Brown, J. (1990). Social work practice with the terminally ill in the Black community. In J. Parry, *Social work practice with the terminally ill: A transcultural perspective* (pp. 67-82). Springfield, IL: Charles C. Thomas, Publisher.

[23] Spector, R. (2004). *Cultural diversity in health and illness* (6th ed.). Stamford, CT: Appleton and Lange.

[24] Slicer, E. (1977*). Ethnic medicine in the Southwest.* Tucson, AZ: University of Arizona Press.

[25] Diller, J. (2004). *Cultural diversity: A primer for the human services.* Belmont, CA: Brooks/Cole-Thomson Learning.

[26] Fongwa, M. (2002). Overview of themes identified from African American discourse on quality of care. *Journal of Nursing Care Quality, 16*(2), 17-38.

[27] Morgan, M. (1996). Prenatal care of African American women in selected USA urban and rural cultural contexts. *Journal of Transcultural Nursing, 7*(2), 9.

[28] Dinulos, J. & Graham, E. (1998). Influence of culture and pigment on skin conditions in children. *Pediatrics in Review, 19*(8), 268-275.

[29] Joyner, M. (1988). Hair care in the black patient. *Journal of Pediatric Health Care, 2*(6), 281-287.

[30] Ford, D. & Steele-Moses, S. (2011). Predictors for African Americans' willingness to donate organs: A literature review. *Nephrology Nursing Journal, 38*(5), 405-410.

[31] Lassiter, S. (1994). Black is a color, not a culture: Implications for health care. *The Association of Black Nursing Faculty, 5*(1), 4-9.

[32] Lang, P. (2000). Dermatoses in African Americans. *Dermatology Nursing, 12*(2), 87-90, 93-100.

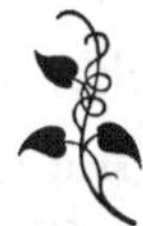

AFRO-CARIBBEAN RELIGIONS

Haitian Vodou, Santeria, Candomblé

Background

Afro-Caribbean religions evolved as a result of the forced transport of millions of Africans to the Americas during the Atlantic slave trade period. Most came from West Africa and West-Central Africa.[1,2] Over one hundred African ethnic groups were a part of this mass displacement of people. Millions of slaves were taken to work in the Caribbean sugar plantations of Cuba, Jamaica, and Hispaniola. Many more were taken to Brazil and other places to work the sugar plantations, coffee groves, silver mines, and other businesses. Among the most prominent African groups were the *Fon*, *Yoruba*, *Kongo*, *Ibo*, *Ewe*, and *Hausa*.

As the slaves were distributed to their various destinations, European slave owners purposely mixed the various African ethnic groups in an effort to decrease the possibility of like tribesmen uniting against their owners. However, the slaves originated from powerful African kingdoms and were determined to preserve a bit of their humanity. The religious and ancestral spirits that were an integral part of their lives in Africa were all that they had to connect them with their homeland.[3,4,5] Although faced with unimaginable hardships and abuse, the Africans proved to be quite clever and creative. They used these skills to form bonds with each other through their African religious spiritualism.[3,4]

The European slaveholders prohibited the slaves' religious practices, forced them to be baptized, and to "become Christians." Although Europeans believed that their mission had been accomplished, Africans actually used the cover of components of Catholicism as a method of practicing their own religion. The various Catholic saints came to represent African spirits with similar symbolic and mythological characteristics. Contact with Natives that already inhabited the Americas led to the incorporation of some components of the Natives' religious practices.[4, 5, 6, 7] The fusion of these religious beliefs and practices led to common roots, but different religious pathways such as Vodou in Haiti, Candomblé in Brazil, Santeria in Cuba, Orisha/Shango in Trinidad, and other Afro-Caribbean religious groups.[6, 8, 9]

These religions have survived years of persecution and inaccurate media depictions. Even today, the religions carry labels such as witchcraft, sorcery, devil worship and are identified with wanton animal sacrifice and zombies. The rich history and complexity of the religious beliefs are left unexplored for understanding. Therefore, many of the religious practices are still carried out in secret.

In spite of the elements of secrecy, Afro-Caribbean religions continue to attract many new members. There are millions of adherents, including many that practice an Afro-Caribbean religion concurrently with Catholicism. Membership in Afro-Caribbean religions is not limited to persons of African descent, but is embraced by many ethnic groups. In the United States, Afro-Caribbean religions are most prevalent in New York, Miami, and Los Angeles.[8, 10]

Vodou

There are a number of variations on the spelling of the word Vodou. The spellings include *Vodou*, *Vodoun*, *Vodun*, *Vaudoux*, and *voodoo*. Most scholars today agree that the spelling *vodou* most appropriately reflects its evolution from Africa to Haiti, more accurately reflects the correct pronunciation, and gives distance to the many negative and incorrect distortions that have been associated with the word voodoo.[4,5,7,10] The word comes from the Fon language and means *spirit*, *god*, or *image*.[4, 10, 11]

Vodou has been practiced for at least four thousand years in parts of Africa.[8] Since many of the slaves brought to Haiti originated from the Fon and Yoruba tribes, Vodou remains an integral part of the religious life of the majority of Haitians.[12] Reportedly, more than fifty million people are followers of Vodou.

The word *voodoo* most often refers to practices and traditions in New Orleans and other southern United States. Many of the practices differ from Vodou practices in Haiti and Africa.

Voodoo in New Orleans has become associated with magical charms, magical potions, and voodoo dolls, although many of the true religious components remain out of the public view.[4, 13, 14] The word *hoodoo* is often used interchangeably with the word *voodoo*. *Hoodoo* most often refers to a tradition among some African Americans involving folk magic, magical practices, and herbal medicine.[4, 13, 15]

Santería (the Way of the Saints) and Palo Monte ('sticks of the forest')

Santeria is also known as *Lucumi* and *Regla de Ocha*. The name Regla de Ocha is used to distinguish Santeria from Palo Monte, a Cuban Afro-Caribbean religion whose primary African influence is from the people of the Congo. Santeria's primary African influence is that of the Yoruba slaves.[4, 16, 17] Millions of people practice Santeria and come from all walks of life.[18, 19]

Candomblé

Candomblé is also primarily based on Yoruban beliefs. Candomblé retained more African influences than any of the other African-based religions. Its practitioners most strongly resisted the pressures of Catholicism. Today, Candomblé practitioners seek to maintain their ties to Africa by making pilgrimages to Africa to increase their knowledge and understanding of its religious beliefs and practices. There are several types of Candomblé called *nacões* (nations). They include Candomblé de Ketu, Candomblé de Angola, Candomblé de Congo, Candomblé de Jeje, Candomblé de ljexá, and Candomblé de Caboclo, referring to the origins of the deities, chants, etc. of each group.[2, 4] Candomblé is seen more often in Brazil, but is practiced in other countries as well.

Other

Persons associated with magical spells designed to do harm to others or take away harmful spells have long been associated with Afro-Caribbean religions. This sector has also received the most public and media attention. These persons do not reflect the true essence of the Afro-Caribbean practices. Their work is seen as having temporary outcomes vs. the long-term outcomes of priests and priestesses. They are considered to be on a lower spiritual level than priests and priestesses.[20]

Religious Representatives[2, 4, 12, 20, 21, 22, 23]

Haitian Vodou

- **Priest** (Houngan/oungan) or **priestess** (manbo): Often called "Papa Loa" or "Mama Loa," respectively. Both males and females perform the same functions and have equal power. The primary role of the priest/priestess is to serve as intermediary between the spirits (lwas) and the people who belong to their temple. He or she officiates at rituals, serves as leader of the temple, advisor, healer, and therapist within his or her Vodou community. Priests and priestesses undergo many years of spiritual and practical training prior to initiation into the priesthood.

- **Laplas**: Male assistant to the priest/priestess.

- **Oungenikon**: Female assistant to the priest/priestess.

- **Prèt Savann** (bush priest): An unordained Catholic priest. Usually this priest is Haitian, but is not in official standing in the Catholic Church. Officiates at ceremonies requiring Catholic rites such as baptism, prayers in French/Latin, hymns, or benedictions. The prêt savann serves in a symbolic capacity as a link to the Catholic Church, but is not required for ceremonies.

Santeria

- **Babalawo**: High priest of the religion. May be consulted by santeros and santeras for extremely difficult issues. Only men serve in this role.

- **Santero/Santera**: Priest and priestess, respectively. They may also be called 'omo' plus the name of their orisha, such as "Omo-Changó."

- There are twelve ranks among followers of Santería and several categories of santeros or santeras.

Palo Monte (Regla de Conga)

- **Palero**: Functions as a group leader and has powers to communicate with the spiritual world and with God. The title of palero is sometimes affectionately preceded by *tata* (papa) and *yaya* (mama). The palero leads ceremonies and performs healing rituals among other duties.

Candomblé

- **Mãe-de-santo/pao-de-santo**: Mother/Father of saints.

Worldview/Religious Beliefs [2, 4, 5, 7, 12, 14, 16, 22, 23, 24, 25, 26, 27]

- Most Afro-Caribbean religions share the following:
  - **Belief in a Supreme God**: A popular misunderstanding of Afro-Caribbean religion is that its followers do not believe in a Supreme God. Vodou, Santeria, and Candomblé all recognize one Supreme God, comparable to the God of Christianity, Allah of Islam, etc. In Haitian Vodou, He is called *Bondye*, *Le Bon Dieu* (the Good God), or *Gran Mèt* (the Grand Master); in Santeria–*Olódùmarè* or *Olórun*; in Candomblé–*Olórun*; in Palo Monte–*Zambi*. God is seen as the Creator of all things. He is manifested in anything in nature that cannot be controlled (e.g., the cycles/forces of nature, the cycle of life and death, the tides and flow of oceans, etc.). He is manifested in anything that is greater than humans. He is believed to be too great and too busy to be involved with the everyday issues and problems of humans. A follower should know God, but not expect to connect with Him on a personal level. God's will is non-negotiable; therefore, there is no need to plead with Him or to make offerings to Him. It is not meant for humans to understand His will. One must accept and adapt to it. Followers of these religious groups consider themselves good Christians and, if asked, will often identify themselves as Catholic.
  - Because of the greatness and remoteness of God, humans are not meant to connect with Him directly. He has delegated the work for helping humans with everyday issues to powerful spirits or angels who possess supernatural powers. The spirits were

created by God to communicate His will, express His significance in nature, and to guide or protect mankind. They serve as intermediaries between the Supreme God and humans. In Haitian Vodou, the spirits are call *lwa*; in Santeria *Orishas*; in Candomblé–*Orixás*; in Palo Monte–*minkisi* and *mpungas*. Spirits of dead family members are not honored outside of the family.

- Belief that the spirits are the immortal souls of the great ancestors–people who were once alive. The term 'gods' is not an appropriate reference to the spirits. They must be honored and served, not worshiped. The more powerful spirits may have once been powerful people, such as kings and queens or great warriors. Or, they may be people, now dead, who have come to be served by many people, placing them in a higher level among the hierarchy of spirits. God has placed some spirits closer to Him and given them more power in the complex hierarchy of the spiritual world. Each spirit has a specific function in the lives of the followers and has certain preferences for types of offerings, colors, days of the week, etc.

- Each individual's life is overseen by a spirit or a 'guardian angel' that guides and protects the individual, regardless of the individual's religious preferences.

- Reverence to the dead and their spirits.

- Service to the more powerful intermediary spirits through offerings or celebrations. One must live their lives and give service to the spirits in such a way that the spirits are pleased with the follower. Failure to do so can result in anger and sometimes punishment from the spirit.

- The belief that the spirits must be fed to maintain their strength and energy. The offerings may include food, drink (especially raw rum) or the blood of a sacrificed animal, which is seen as a powerful offering to a spirit. Various spirits have preferences for the type of animal offered. In many instances, especially in rural areas, the animal is cooked after the sacrifice. The meat of the sacrificial animal is seen as sacred and provides physical and spiritual nourishment for the followers.

- The belief that one can be 'possessed or mounted' by a spirit for the purpose of communicating to the followers.

- The use of drums (considered sacred) to assist in calling forth the spirits during ceremonies.

- Use of divination methods by priests/priestesses, to assist with predicting or resolving life events.
- Catholic saints may be used to represent African spirits.

Sample Representations

Religion	Spirit/Loa/Orisha	Catholic Saint
Haitian Vodou	**Ezili**: Represents motherhood, beauty, love; rules over the home.	The Virgin Mary
	Papa Legba: Keeper of the crossroads. Guards the gate between the human and spirit world.	St. Peter: A cross may also be used to represent the crossroads.
	Ogou: Protects those at war, ruler over fire, metal, war, male fertility.	St. Jacques
Santeria	**Elegguá**: Opener of the ways.	St. Anthony
	Babalù-ayé: Viewed as a kind father figure, but also feared. He can both send or cure illness, particularly infectious ones.	St. Lazarus
Candomblé	**Yemanjá**: Female orixa of the sea, saint of the fisherman.	The Virgin Mary
	Oxalá: Represents love and peace. Is always dressed in white.	Jesus Christ
	Iansã: Associated with storms, lightning, and wind.	St. Barbara

- No formal religious creed. Practices may vary from locale to locale. Knowledge of religious practices is passed down orally and through strong mentorship. Those persons who practice Catholicism and Afro-Caribbean religion concurrently, will also adhere to the religious creeds of Catholicism.[4, 10]

- Life is not a struggle between good and evil, rather it is a mixture of good and evil, with more or less of either distributed to individuals during their lifetime. There is no heaven or hell. Suffering to some extent cannot be avoided.[12]

Special/Religious Observations

- Many of the traditional Catholic religious observations are recognized.
- Numerous celebrations in honor of the spirits.
- **Vodou**: July 16th - Pilgrimage to Saut d'Eau to pay homage to the spirit Elizi. Persons cleanse themselves in a pool beneath a waterfall that is thought to have the power to heal physical and spiritual illnesses. Followers in New York simulate this pilgrimage by taking part in a parade to a church located in Harlem.[4, 6]
- **Vodou**: July 25th - Pilgrimage to Plaine du Nord in Northern Haiti to take baths in a mud pool thought to have healing powers. Also called the Feast of St. James.[4, 6]

Health Beliefs/Practices

- The religions also serve as medical systems. Priests and priestesses have extensive knowledge of plants for medicinal purposes. Persons will many times consult the priest/priestess before consulting mainstream medical personnel. Always ask what treatments have been used for treatment of an illness and what is believed to have caused the illness.[2]
- During psychosocial assessment, the patient or family may be reluctant to associate themselves with one of the religions because of fear of ridicule.
- Psychiatric, seizure disorders, and other illnesses may be attributed to the individual's weakened spirit, punishment, an angry spirit, an enemy, or because of the evil eye-particularly among persons in rural areas or the uneducated. Among the educated, the germ theory is readily accepted. However, the question of why one person becomes ill while another individual stays well may require the assistance of a priest or priestess.[4, 19]

- Cubans may refer to the effects of the evil eye as having been "celebrated." The resulting illnesses include headache, depression, fever, diarrhea, or depression. Generally, the illness lasts no longer than one week.[19]

- Protective bracelets, sacred necklaces or plants may be worn or taken in a small bag. Do not remove from the body unless absolutely necessary. If necessary to remove, do not discard or misplace items. Give to a trusted family member.[19]

- Religious altars may be visible in the home.

- Herbal/cleansing/luck baths are popular treatment measures for illnesses and neutralizing negative influences.[19, 24]

- Mercury is used frequently in rituals and in amulets because it is thought to have magical properties. Children are particularly vulnerable to the effects of mercury exposure.[28, 29]

Birth/Children

- In Vodou, twins are seen as sacred and endowed with great powers. They must always be treated equally to avoid angering one. The twin may use its power in a negative manner during anger. A child born immediately following twins is thought to have even **greater powers.**[4]

- Children and pregnant women are often believed to be especially susceptible to the effects of the evil eye.[19]

Death

- Death is not seen as the end of life, but as a change from a physical to a spiritual state as an immortal spirit that will remain active in the everyday lives of the family.[4, 20]

- Families may request Catholic rites associated with terminal illness and death.

- Special rites may be performed to assure that the dead person's soul departs appropriately to the spiritual realm. These rites may be quite complex and may vary based on locale. Family members must assure that rites are carried out completely. Ask the family about their desires to participate in preparation of the body. Provide privacy as needed. Do not remove any sacred items (e.g., necklaces, threads, etc.) from the body without the permission of family members.[4, 24]

Other

Obeah (Obi)

- *Obeah* refers to a set of practices originally used among Africans who were enslaved in British-controlled Jamaica. The term is thought to have been derived from West African ethnic groups.
- Obeah practices called upon supernatural and magical forces to assist people in gaining or keeping control over certain aspects of their lives or when assistance was needed in facing life events. It could also be used to assist with regaining or maintaining health as well as a way to gain good fortune. On the other hand, it could allow individuals to gain revenge or justice.
- Obeah was feared by the colonists because it was thought to facilitate slave resistance and revolts. The practices were greatly misunderstood by the British and were labeled evil. That label has persisted throughout the years, but the perception is lessening. Individuals today, still seek Obeah services for similar reasons.
- Obeah lacks the usual characteristics of an organized religion, but it can incorporate some religious traditions and teachings. It lacks a central set of beliefs; there are no congregations, no designated buildings for ceremonies, no public rituals, and no specific deity.
- A practitioner is called an 'Obeah-man' or 'Obeah-woman'. The practices and art of Obeah are mainly passed down through oral means and through working with experienced practitioners. Although the practices are cloaked with secrecy, its practitioners' services are commonly sought by individuals throughout the Caribbean and by people of many socio-economic levels, ethnic groups, and religions. The practices used are based on the needs and desires of the individual seeking help. These may include summoning forces from

the supernatural world for the benefit of individuals, the use of prayer, charms, protective items, herbals, sacrifices, spiritual services, and 'readings' to foretell the future, etc. Clients may be required to undergo steps for purification prior to major interventions from the practitioner.

- Generally, the services of Obeah practitioners for illness are sought when other avenues have failed to bring positive results. As a result of the diaspora of Caribbean peoples to locations around the world, the practice of Obeah is no longer limited to the Caribbean.[23,30]

---

[1] Klein, H. (1986). *African slavery in Latin America and the Caribbean.* New York, NY: Oxford University Press.

[2] Voeks, R. (1997). *Sacred leaves of Candomblé: African magic, medicine, and religion in Brazil.* Austin, TX: University of Texas Press.

[3] Burdick, J. (1992). The long night of slavery. *Report of the Americas, 25*(4), 38-39.

[4] Turlington, S. (2002). *The complete idiot's guide to voodoo.* Indianapolis, IN: Alpha Books.

[5] Galembo, P. (1998). *Vodou: Visions and voices of Haiti.* Berkeley, CA: Ten Speed Press.

[6] Hurbon, L. (1995). *Voodoo: Search for the spirit.* New York, NY: Harry N. Abrams, Inc. Publishers.

[7] Wucker, M. (1999). *Why the cocks fight: Dominicans, Haitians, and the struggle for Hispaniola.* New York, NY: Hill and Wang.

[8] Henning, C. & Oberländer, H. (1996). *Voodoo: Secret power in Africa.* New York, NY: Benedikt Taschen Verlag.

[9] Houk, J. (1995). *Spirits, blood, and drums: The orisha religion in Trinidad.* Philadelphia, PA: Temple University Press.

[10] Desmangles, L. (1992a). *The faces of the Gods: Vodou and Roman Catholicism in Haiti.* Chapel Hill, NC: The University of North Carolina Press.

[11] Dayan, J. (1997). Vodoun, or the voice of the gods. In M. Olmos & L. Paravisini-Gebert (Eds). *Sacred possessions: Vodou, Santeria, Obeah, and the Caribbean* (p. 13-36). New Brunswick, NJ: Rutgers University Press.

[12] McCarthy-Brown, K. (1991). *Mama Lola: A Vodou priestess in Brooklyn.* Los Angeles, CA: University of California Press.

[13] Davis, R. (1999). *American Vodou: Journey into a hidden world.* Denton, TX: University of North Texas Press.

[14] Pinn, A. (1998). *Varieties of African American religious experience.* Minneapolis, MN: Fortress Press.

[15] Haskins, J. (1990). *Voodoo & hoodoo.* New York, NY: Scarborough House.

[16] Vega, M. (2000). *The altar of my soul: The living traditions of Santeria.* New York, NY: The Ballantine Publishing Group.

[17] Barnet, M. (1997). La regal de ocha: The religious system of Santeria. In M. Olmos & L. Paravisini-Gebert (Eds). *Sacred possessions: Vodou, Santeria, Obeah, and the Caribbean* (p. 79-100). New Brunswick, NJ: Rutgers University Press.

[18] Núnez, L. (1992). *Santeria: A practical guide to Afro-Caribbean magic.* Woodstock, CT: Spring Publications, Inc.

[19] Pasquali, E. (1986). Santeria: A religion that is a health care system for Long Island Cuban-Americans. *Journal of the New York State Nurses Association, 17*(1), 12-15.

[20] Glassman, S. (2000). *Vodou visions: An encounter with divine mystery.* New York, NY: Villard.

[21] Métraux, A. (1959 – translated in 1972 by Hugo Charteris). *Voodoo in Haiti.* New York, NY: Schocken Books.

[22] Deren, M. (1953). *Divine horsemen: The living gods of Haiti.* Great Britain: Jarrold and Sons, Ltd.

[23]. Murrell, N.S. (2010). *Afro-Caribbean religions: An introduction to their historical, cultural, and sacred traditions.* Philadelphia, PA: Temple University Press.

[24] González-Wipper, M. (1994*). Santeria: The religion.* St. Paul, MN: Llewellyn Publications.

[25] Fleurant, G. (1996*). Dancing spirits: Rhythms and rituals of Haitian Vodun, the Rada rite.* Westport, CT: Greenwood.

[26] Canizares, R. (1999). *Cuban Santeria: Walking with the night.* Rochester, VT: Destiny Books.

[27] St. Clair, D. (1971). *The drum and candle.* Garden City, NY: Doubleday & Company, Inc.

[28] Riley, D., Newby, C., Leal-Almeraz, T. & Thomas, V. (2001). Assessing elemental mercury vapor exposure from cultural and religious practices. *Environmental Health Perspectives, 109*(8), 779-87.

[29] Forman, J., Moline, J., Cernichiari, E., Sayegh, S., Torres, J., Landrigan, M., Hudson, J., Adel, H. & Ladrigan, P. (2000). A cluster of pediatric metallic mercury exposure cases treated with meso02,3-dimercaptoduccinic acid (DSMA). *Environmental Health Perspectives, 108*(6), 575-77

[30] Bilby, K.M. & Handler, J.S. (2004). Obeah: Healing and protection in West Indian slave life. *The Journal of Caribbean History, 38*(2), 153-183.

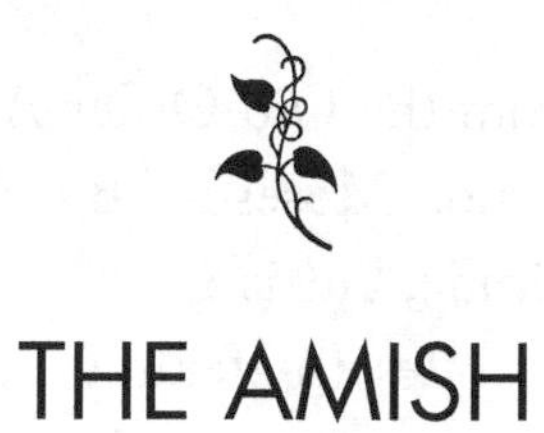

THE AMISH

Background

The Amish derive their name from Jacob Ammann, a prominent Anabaptist elder. They are a branch of the Mennonite Church and are descendants of the Swiss Anabaptists who settled in Pennsylvania during the 1700s. Groups settled in Indiana and Ohio in the 1800s.[1,2]

Their conservative lifestyle shuns modern technologies, higher education, adornments such as makeup/jewelry, and modern dress. The Amish way of plain dress is symbolic of non-conformity, humility, and modesty, based on their interpretation of Biblical scriptures. Farming and agriculture are the primary occupations.[2,3,4]

The current population of Amish in North America is approximately 261,000, with at least half of the total population being less than eighteen years of age. As of 2011, the largest Amish populations are found in Pennsylvania, Ohio, Indiana, Wisconsin, and New York, respectively. New communities are established almost annually and can be found in many other areas of the United States, Canada, and Latin America. Only Beachy Amish reside outside of North America. Although there are many basic similarities among Amish groups, there are at least two dozen branches and some practices may differ. Some major Amish groups include:[5,6,7,8]

- The **Swartzentruber** and **Andy Weaver Amish**: These groups practice strict shunning and are ultra-conservative in their use of technology. Andy Weaver Amish are allowed to use battery lights; Swartzentruber Amish are not.

- **Old Order Amish** compromise the largest group. They have little or no use of modern technology (including driving cars and other motorized vehicles). They are allowed to ride in motorized vehicles, including automobiles, trains, and airplanes. Public electricity services are not used.

- The **Beachy Amish** separated from the Old Order Amish over a period of years, beginning in 1927, and were led by Bishop Moses M. Beachy. The group resembles Old Order Amish in dress and general attitude, but is more relaxed in discipline.[1] Beachy Amish permit the ownership of automobiles (preferably black), meeting houses are used for religious services, English is used in ceremonial functions, and public electric services are used.

- The **New Order Amish** group, formed in the 1960s, has more liberal views related to technology, including the use of telephones and electricity. They do not permit ownership or driving of cars or use of meeting houses for worship services. High moral standards are still emphasized.

Religious Representatives

- **Bishop** (Voelliger-Diener or "minister with full powers"): Performs baptisms, marriages, ordinations, rites of communion and is considered the spiritual authority. Families may want to consult the bishop when major decisions must be made related to medical care.[2]

- **Preacher/Minister** (Diener zum Buch or "minister of the book"): Assists in communion/other services and delivers sermons.[2]

- **Deacon** (Armen-Diener or "minister of the poor"): Collects and distributes funds to the needy, assists the Bishop by investigating disputes between members and serves as a mediator/counselor, confirms parental approval for marriage from the bride's family, and assists with some religious ceremonies.[4]

Religious Beliefs

- Sunday is observed as the Sabbath. Church services are generally held every other Sunday. The Holy Bible is used.
- Time is set aside daily for prayer and reading of the scriptures. Allow privacy.
- Core religious practices include:[6, 9]
  - Adult baptism
  - **Gelassenheit** meaning 'submission' or yielding to a higher authority. It involves a strong sense of community and is expressed through simplicity, obedience, and humility.
  - **Ordung** consists of rules regarding expected behavior that is usually passed orally instead of in a written form through generations.
  - Imposing **meidung** (shunning/social avoidance of adult community members who violate community rules/values).
- The Amish believe that its members are joined together in an effort to become righteous Christians. Modern technology and 'worldliness' will lead them away from true Christianity. Groups live in 'settlements,' 'church districts,' or 'communities' that are somewhat isolated from the dominant culture. Worship takes place in private homes among more conservative groups. Beachy and New Order groups may hold services in meeting houses.[8]
- Typically, Amish do not marry non-Amish. This has led to a smaller gene pool. Several recessive hereditary genetic conditions are seen within the group–some more common within certain Amish communities. **Early screening and treatment is critical for early recognition and treatment/supportive interventions**. Disorders more commonly seen among the Amish population include:[6, 8, 10, 11, 12, 13, 14, 15]
  - Hemophilia B (particularly in Ohio)
  - Cystic fibrosis (particularly in Ohio)

- Dwarfism syndromes such as Ellis-van Creveld Syndrome (Lancaster County, PA) and *cartilage hair hypoplasia* (most Amish communities in the United States and Canada).
- PKU
- Pyruvate kinase anemia
- Type 1 glutaric aciduria, a metabolic disorder
- Nemaline myopathy
- Amish lethal microcephaly syndrome with 2-ketoglutaric aciduria (Lancaster County, PA–called "small headed" children among the Amish).
- Infantile Refsum disease has been recently reported among four Amish siblings. It is expected that this disorder will be seen in subsequent generations.

- Farming and traffic accidents are additional health risks, particularly among children.

Special/Religious Observations

- Communion services are held twice a year, generally once in the Spring and Fall. Preparation includes prayer, fasting, and meditation. Washing one another's feet is part of the service and ritualizes the virtue of humility.[2, 4]
- Holidays are observed in various ways among Amish groups, which include Christmas, Thanksgiving, Easter, Good Friday, Ascension Day, and Pentecost.[8]

Language

- **Deitsch**: A German dialect also known as *Pennsylvania Dutch* or *Pennsylvania German* is generally used in communicating with other Amish. English is used in communicating with non-Amish. In church services, the scriptures, prayers, and songs are generally conducted in German.[16]

- Preschool children may need parents to translate for them. Fluent English is learned after entering school. German is also taught in school.[9,16]

- Typically, Amish individuals do not participate in verbal confrontations. Therefore, silence is often used to convey anger, disappointment, or as a signal that another individual needs to change his or her behavior. Silence may be exhibited by not speaking or by simply ignoring an individual.[2]

Health Beliefs

- The body is the temple of God, and each individual has responsibility for personally promoting health and well-being.[10]

- Illness affects everyone and must be endured with faith and patience. The inability to perform one's daily work constitutes illness. Good mental and physical health is considered a gift from God. Hard work, 'clean' living, and a well-balanced diet contribute to good health. Mainstream preventive healthcare may not be deemed important. Individuals often utilize the mainstream health care system only during an emergency for health crises.[6]

- Home remedies, chiropractors, and folk healers within the community are frequently used before seeking mainstream medical treatment. *Brauche* is often sought as a method of treatment. Brauche (also referred to as *powwowing)* involves physical manipulation similar to therapeutic touch in which the healer places his or her hands near the patient's head or abdomen to draw illness from the body.[10,17] When taking health histories, explore types of herbal preparations taken and other folk remedies/treatments.

- Generally, technology used within the hospital for treatment purposes is accepted as long as it benefits the client.

- There are no religious prohibitions against the use of tobacco. However, opinions concerning its use vary among the Amish. Some Amish men smoke cigars, pipes, or brown-wrapped cigarettes. Commercial white-wrapped cigarettes are frowned upon because they are seen as 'worldly.'[9]

Expression of Pain

- Stoic, even among children.
- Narcotics are prohibited. Seek other pharmacologic and non-pharmacologic methods of pain management.[6]

Kinship/Social Factors

- Expect multiple visitors from the community. It is likely that a hospitalized individual, particularly a child, will not be left alone. Family and members of the community will want to participate in care.[12]
- Generally, all members of the group contribute money to pay for the treatment of members.
- The family pattern among the Amish is known as *freindschaft*, referring to a three-generational family structure.[10] Families often live in adjoining houses on a farmstead. The concept of 'family' extends beyond the immediate to include members of the community. There is strong respect for elders. The Amish are committed to caring for members throughout the life cycle, including the sick, elderly, orphaned, and mentally challenged. Placement in outside facilities will be refused.[6]
- Most Amish groups do not participate in insurance plans or government subsidies such as Social Security, Medicaid, and Medicare.[16] Taking oaths of loyalty, military service, holding public office, membership in political organizations, and/or government jobs are prohibited. Amish members are allowed to vote, and they do pay taxes.[8]
- Modesty is highly valued. Provide same-sex caregivers if at all possible. Protect privacy. May be reluctant to discuss personal issues, especially those of a sexual nature until trust has been established.
- Amish women wear head coverings (called *kapps*, *prayer veilings*, *head caps*, *coverings*, or *prayer coverings*). Styles will vary. The coverings are worn at all times that women are in the presence of men or when praying. Some women always wear a covering–even to bed–since they can never be certain when there may be the need to pray. Collaborate

with family about how this need can be met if there is an **absolute** need to remove the covering.[2]

- Females do not cut their hair. If there is an **unavoidable** need to cut the hair, thorough explanations should be given to the individual/family prior to the cutting. Give the hair that has been cut to the family.

- Affection between husband and wife or other adults, is rarely displayed in public. This is seen as a private matter.

- Married men and single men over forty years of age wear full beards; single men under age forty are clean-shaven. Mustaches are forbidden.[17]

- Will require **very careful** explanations relative to the need for treatments, tests, etc. because of reluctance to spend money unnecessarily.

- Photographs are generally not permitted. Mirrors are not permitted in the homes. Both practices are related to *Gelassenheit.*[6] Tape recorders, CD players, television, and films/videos are also prohibited.[4] Some Amish individuals are familiar with cell phone and Internet use, especially those who own or work in businesses. Inquire about availability in the home.[18]

Birth/Children

- All children are viewed as a gift from God.

- Use of birth control is uncommon. Women are likely to be multiparas. Large families are the norm among the Amish. The average number of live births per Amish couple is seven.[8]

- The Amish have the highest incidence of twins of any known population.[8]

- Alpha-fetaprotein testing will be rejected since elective termination is unacceptable. Fetal monitoring is acceptable since it helps to ensure a positive birth outcome.

- Although some Amish women seek prenatal care late in pregnancy, or not at all to minimize costs and inconveniences, most are receptive to prenatal care to assure good pregnancy outcomes. If late prenatal care is sought, it is likely because complications or abnormalities are suspected. Individuals may choose not to attend classes that involve videos as a form of conveying information. Provide information by alternative means.[10,19] Home deliveries are often preferred, particularly after the first baby.[20] Will likely want to be discharged from the hospital as soon as possible after birth.

- There is a strong belief that children learn what they see role-modeled by adults. Children are taught to be respectful and obedient to adults. Corporal punishment may be used.

- It is important to question parents about the status of children's immunizations.[21]

- Education past the eighth grade is prohibited because of religious beliefs and work ethics. The United States government has exempted Amish youth from attending school past the eighth grade.[5] The Amish have their own schools.[9]

- Children are at risk for accidents related to farming since they may be expected to assist with farm chores and operate farm equipment at a young age.[17] During assessment of children, ask what the child's responsibilities are at home. This may provide an opportunity to teach about risk factors for childhood accidents.[14]

- Appropriate toys for hospitalized children include dolls without facial features, blocks, balls, etc. Videotapes, video games, and television should not be used for diversion unless parental permission is given. Group activities are permissible as long as religious prohibitions are observed (e.g., board games involving dice, etc. are not acceptable). **If in doubt, ask!**[12]

- Parents may want to bring plain gowns from home for hospitalized children in lieu of the child wearing the usual colorful pediatric gowns with prints. Keep girls heads covered based on parents' wishes.[12]

- Since photographs are forbidden, provide explanations other than "take your picture" to describe x-rays.[12]

- Teenagers and unmarried young adults in some Amish groups may experiment with cigarettes, alcohol, and other chemical substances. This behavior is seen by some Amish as experiencing worldliness before joining the Amish Church (most renounce such practices after joining the church) and is referred to as *Rumspringa*. Assess persons of this age group for evidence of substance abuse.[7,16]

Patient Teaching/Dietary Consideration

- Diets tend to be high in fats, carbohydrates, and sugar–sometimes leading to obesity, particularly among women. However, because of regular exercise gained through daily work activities, obesity is not seen to the degree that it is seen among the general population.
- Educational methods should focus on reading, demonstration, and return demonstration by the patient/family since TV, videotapes, and computers are prohibited. Be sure that written materials are at a level congruent with eighth-grade reading levels. Use simple, non-technical terminology.
- Determine access to a telephone in case of emergencies since telephones may not be found in most Amish homes.[16] Inquire about the family's acceptance of cell phone use as it may serve as a form of communication with the family, if needed; particularly for emergencies.[2]
- Consider that travel to and from hospital and follow-up appointments may be difficult and expensive for families of more conservative groups. They will generally have to either pay someone to bring them or ride the bus. Group appointments if possible.
- Electricity may or may not be available in the home. Consider alternative sources of power for home equipment.

Death

- Death is seen as entrance to a better life – an eternal life with God. The Amish prefer to die at home. Death only occurs in hospitals when it is unavoidable.[9] Relatives and friends may not display true emotions in the presence of health care workers.[17, 22]
- **Autopsy**: Seldom done, but permitted in case of medical necessity or legal requirement.[6]
- **Organ Donation/Transplants**: No religious prohibition, but generally do not participate in donation or transplants.

- Burial clothes are made by the Amish women. The deceased person is dressed after the body has been embalmed.

- Burial often occurs on the third day following death.

Other Considerations

- Clocks are set either slower or faster than 'worldly' (mainstream) time, generally by one-half hour. When making appointments, determine if the client uses "fast" or "slow" time, and set appointments accordingly.[8]

- **Blood/Blood Products**: Permitted

- **Vaccines:** Permitted. Health care providers should include questions during initial assessments concerning the status of immunization.

---

[1] Mead, F. & Hill, S. (1995). *Handbook of denominations in the United States.* Nashville, TN: Abingdon Press.

[2] Rensberger, S. (2003) *The complete idiot's guide to understanding the Amish.* New York, NY: Alpha Books.

[3] Scott, S. (1997). *People's place book No. 7: Why do they dress that way?* Intercourse, PA: Good Books.

[4] Kraybill, D. (1993). *The riddle of Amish culture.* Baltimore, MD: The Johns Hopkins University Press.

[5] Noit, S. (1992). *A history of the Amish.* Intercourse, PA: Good Books.

[6] Andrews, M. & Boyle, J. (2012). *Transcultural concepts in nursing care* (6th ed.). Philadelphia, PA: Lippincott.

[7] Elizabethtown College: The Young Center for Anabaptist and Pietist Studies at Elizabethtown College. (2012). *Amish studies.* Retrieved from http://www2.etown.edu/amishstudies/Index.asphttp://www2.etown.edu/amishstudies/Index.asp

[8] Hostetler, J. (1993). *Amish society* (4th ed.). Baltimore, MD: The Johns Hopkins University Press.

[9] Kraybill, D. (1993). *Old order Amish: Their enduring way of life.* Baltimore, MD: The Johns Hopkins University Press.

[10] Wenger, A. and Wenger, M. (2013). The Amish. In L. Purnell, *Transcultural health care: A culturally competent approach* (4th ed.). (p.115-136). Philadelphia, PA: F. A. Davis.

[11] Ontario Consultants on Religious Tolerance. (2006). *The Amish.* Retrieved from http://www.religioustolerance.org/amish5.htm

[12] Banks, M. & Benchot, R. (2001). Unique aspects of nursing care for Amish children. *American Journal of Maternal-Child Nursing, 26*(4), 192-196.

[13] Johnston, J., Kelley, R., Morton, D., Agarwala, R., Koch, T., Schaffer, A., ...Biesecker, L. (2000). A novel nemaline myopathy in the Amish caused by mutation in troponin T1. *American Journal of Human Genetics, 67*(4), 814-821.

[14] Bader, P., Dougherty, S., Cangany, N., Raymond, G., & Jackson, C. (2000). Infantile Refsum disease in four Amish sibs. *American Journal of Medical Genetics, 90*(2), 110-114.

[15] Rhodes, D. & Hupcey, J. (2002). Farm injuries among Old Order Amish children. *Clinical Excellence for Nurse Practitioners, 6*(3), 49-54.

[16] Beachy, A., Herschberger, E., Davidhizar, R., & Giger, J. (1997). Cultural implications for nursing care of the Amish. *Journal of Cultural Diversity, 4*(4), 118-126.

[17] Brewer, J. & Bonalumi, N. (1995). Cultural diversity in the emergency department. *Journal of Emergency Nursing, 21*(6), 494-497.

[18] Amish America. (2010). *Do the Amish use computers and the internet?* Retrieved from http://amishamerica.com/do-the-amish-use-computers-and-the-internet/

[19] Campanella, K., Korbin, J. & Acheson, L. (1993) Pregnancy and childbirth among the Amish. *Social Science Medicine, 36*(3), 333-342.

[20] Palmer, C. (1992). The health beliefs and practices of an Old Order Amish family. *Journal of the American Academy of Nurse Practitioners, 4*(3), 117-122.

[21] Briss, P., Fehrs, L., Hutcheson, R., & Schaffner, W. (1992). Rubella among the Amish: Resurgent disease in a highly susceptible community. *The Pediatric Infectious Disease Journal, 11*(11), 955-959.

[22] Adams, C. & Leverland, M. (1986). The effects of religious beliefs on the health care practices of the Amish. *Nurse Practitioner, 11*(3), 58, 63, 67.

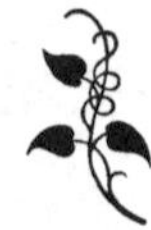

APPALACHIAN AMERICANS

Background

Scholars have given a number of geographical definitions of Appalachia. The definitions have changed a number of times over the years.[1] According to the federally supported Appalachian Regional Commission (ARC), Appalachia encompasses 205,000 square miles and 420 counties in thirteen states. All of West Virginia and portions of Alabama, Georgia, Kentucky, Maryland, Mississippi, New York, North Carolina, Ohio, Pennsylvania, South Carolina, Tennessee, and Virginia occupy Appalachia. In addition, Appalachia is divided into five sub-regions based on common demographics and economic measures.

- **Northern**: Includes the southern portion of New York through most of Pennsylvania, parts of Ohio, Maryland, and West Virginia.
- **North Central**: Includes most of West Virginia and portions of Ohio.
- **Central**: Includes portions of Kentucky, Tennessee, West Virginia, and Virginia
- **South Central**: Includes portions of Tennessee, North Carolina and, Virginia.
- **Southern**: Includes portions of Mississippi, Alabama, Georgia, and South Carolina.[2]

Some areas of Appalachia have a well-developed infrastructure and modern amenities, while other locations remain quite isolated without what is often considered basic conveniences such as water and sewer services. In these areas, easily traveled roads may be nonexistent and access to medical care miles away.

The members of the Cherokee Nation were the majority residents of Appalachia until the early 1700s. At that time, settlers began to migrate to the area because there were fewer people residing there and cheap land was available. Most of the people who migrated were of Scotch-Irish, German, English, and French origins. During the past thirty years, the ethnic diversity of Appalachia is expanding secondary to the increase in immigration to the United States as a whole.[1,3,4]

Years of economic instability have resulted from exploitation of Appalachia by outsiders because of its rich natural resources such as lumber, coal, and valuable land at cheap prices. This contributed to an initial distrust of 'outsiders' and bureaucracies.[5] In addition, the exploitations were catalysts for the out-migration of millions of Appalachians during mid-century to cities such as Cincinnati, Columbus, Pittsburgh, Cleveland, and Detroit where jobs were more plentiful. Fortunately, this out-migration has declined and most of Appalachia is experiencing a healthier growth rate.[6]

Approximately twenty-five million people reside in Appalachia. However, the region contains few large metropolitan cities. Approximately 36 percent of Appalachian residents live in non-metropolitan areas. The mountainous Appalachian terrain has contributed to isolation of some of the inhabitants and limited access to health care. Socioeconomic status varies greatly in Appalachia. By reputation, Appalachia has been portrayed as extremely poor. Based on ARC data published in 2011, the average poverty rate in Appalachia from 2005–2010 was 15.6 percent, which was comparable to the overall average poverty rate in the United States. The overall poverty level in Appalachia is in decline, but the distribution of poverty shows marked differences in the overall region. Poverty levels are highest in Central Appalachia and lowest in Northern Appalachia. In 2012, based on per capita income and high rates of poverty, 96 counties in Appalachia are designated as 'distressed,' down from 223 in 1965. Kentucky has the highest number (41), followed by Mississippi (17) and Tennessee (17) with equal numbers. Other states with counties designated as distressed include West Virginia (8), Ohio (7), Alabama (4), with North Carolina and Georgia having one designated county each.[2,7]

Many negative, narrow stereotypes about Appalachia and its inhabitants are popular and still depicted in the media, as well as professional literature. Appalachians today are quite diverse. However, common values include loyalty to family, independence, self-reliance, modesty, pride, love of the homeland, strong connection to religion/faith, dislike of assertiveness/aggressiveness, minding one's own business, equality, and avoidance of disagreements. The cultural identity of urban Appalachians may be impacted by factors such as their generation of heritage, social class, and degree of assimilation.[8, 9, 10] Middle and upper classes of Appalachia may tend to share values and behaviors of members in similar social classes in the rest of the United States; however, their connection to the homeland remains strong.[10]

Major risk factors for Appalachians, especially residents of rural areas, include cancer, obesity, high prevalence of tobacco use, heart disease, hypertension, stroke, accidental injury including mining accidents, respiratory illnesses, diabetes, disabilities, and infant/child mortality.[4, 11, 12] Factors such as higher rates of poverty, limited access to medical care, and lower education rates place many residents of Appalachia at a higher risk for morbidity and mortality as a result of these diseases. Vision and dental problems may also be prevalent as a result of lack of preventive and ongoing care.[13, 14] Some studies suggest that women and children in isolated rural areas may be at a higher risk of all types of abuse with less access to ongoing support.[15] Mental health disorders and suicide are other risks of concern. In recent years, there is an increasing incidence of substance abuse involving alcohol and opiates, particularly prescription drugs for pain. Consequently, deaths related to drug overdoses are at an increased level.[16]

Language

- Appalachians speak English; however, there are a number of dialects spoken. Do not judge an individual's intelligence based on use of dialects unfamiliar to the health care provider.
- Be cognizant that non-English-speaking individuals who are not Appalachians also reside in Appalachia, and interpreters may be needed to support effective communication.
- Health care providers should ask the meaning of words that are misunderstood rather than making assumptions about the meaning. Continue to use the language of the person unless there is some strong reason to correct the person's language or to substitute scientific language.[17]

- Clarify meanings of descriptions of health problems during the assessment phase and for discharge education. Common terms include:[10, 18, 19]
  - **High or low blood**: Refers to blood volume vs. high or low blood pressure
  - **Running off**: Diarrhea
  - **Grippe**: Flu
  - **Dropsy**: Heart disease
  - **Leader**: Ligament/tendon
  - **Kernel**: Swollen lymph node in armpit
  - **Fallen off/falling off**: Weight loss
  - **Corruption**: Pus
  - **Smothering/drawing spell**: Labored breathing/an episode of labored breathing
  - **Bold hives**: Croup
- When taking health histories, be aware that some individuals from underserved areas may not be familiar with mainstream medical terms and, therefore, may not be able to verbalize names of family members' diagnoses.[20]

Time Orientation

- Appalachians tend to be present oriented. However, based on the exposure to everyday mainstream activities, this may vary. Consider that those living in isolated areas may not follow clock time.[18]
- When planning for health appointments, allow flexibility in scheduling since family commitments may supersede the importance of keeping an appointment at the designated time. Consider that travel may be difficult and the need to meet every day financial needs may not allow time to take off from work. Group appointments for persons who have travel difficulties.[18, 21]

Worldview/Religious Beliefs

- Many religious denominations are represented in Appalachia. Baptist (many different subgroups), Pentecostal, Methodist, and Catholic are the major religious groups.
- One form of old-line fundamentalism has been over-sensationalized by the media, though the practices involve a very small population of people. Worship services involve handling poisonous serpents, fire, and/or drinking poisonous solutions such as strychnine, battery acid, or lye. The practices are based on a passage from Mark 16:17-18, as well as some other passages in the King James Bible. The few individuals who are injured during these services generally treat themselves through prayer and other means and do not come to hospitals even when faced with extreme pain and a high probability of death.[1,22,23]
- Most Appalachians have very strong religious beliefs and faith in the power of prayer in overcoming illness. It is important to allow the patient to have a Bible close by and to allow the 'church family' to visit liberally. Allow privacy for prayer. Church officials commonly perform anointing of the sick with oil. Prayer cloths may be left with the patient. Assure that prayer cloths are not discarded.[24]
- Health is a result of chance, sickness is God's will and largely out of the hands of the individual; healing is a sign of forgiveness. Illness may result from influences such as exposure to cold temperatures, lifestyle, etc.[8,9,18]
- Life and its events are predestined with the individual having little control over events in life. This may impact adherence to maintenance medications for conditions such as diabetes, hypertension, etc.[9]
- May have a strong sense of spiritual connection to nature. A patient room with a view of trees, flowers, etc. may be comforting.[25]

Health Beliefs/Practices

- Superstitions may influence beliefs about health and healing. Folk medicine is often practiced, including herbal preparations, turpentine, kerosene (coal oil), vinegar, honey, onions, baking soda, etc. Individuals will often try folk remedies and consult with family members or folk healers before visiting a formal medical setting for treatment.

Medications may be shared with other family members who are ill prior to consulting a medical provider. During the assessment phase, determine prescription drugs taken, herbal preparations and other folk treatments for illnesses or preventive health.[4, 9, 14, 26]

- Health and illness may be influenced by astrological forces. Attention to 'the signs' is common. Each of the twelve astrological signs is thought to influence the health and functions of specific parts of the body.[19]

- Hospitals may be feared and viewed as places where one comes to die, thereby contributing to persons coming to the hospital only when a health crisis occurs.[27]

- A state of illness may only be perceived as illness if the person subjectively *feels* ill and is unable to meet personal and family basic needs. Mental illness sometimes carries a stigma and may be described as the person having a case of "nerves," "odd-turned," "acting peculiar," or "just getting old." In some areas of Appalachia, *mentally ill* or *crazy* are seen as unacceptable and therefore, other more acceptable terms are substituted. Individuals may be reluctant to seek professional help or discuss issues surrounding mental health.[8, 17, 28, 29]

Expression of Pain

- May appear stoic, relying on the health care provider to interpret nonverbal cues. May have difficulty precisely describing emotions or types of pain.[10]

Male-Female/Kinship/Social Relationships

- In rural Appalachia, men tend to make major decisions in the family. However, females have strong influence on the male's decision and generally serve as the health care resource for the family.[8, 18]

- Elders are valued, honored, and respected. They are likely to be cared for by family members when no longer able to be independent.[17]

- Strong sense of familism. Health care decisions may be delayed until family members can be consulted. 'Family' may extend to church members who may also sometimes be asked to participate in health care decisions.

- At least one family member is likely to accompany the client to the health care facility. If an individual is hospitalized, a number of family members will likely come to the facility and wish to stay with the hospitalized person. Accommodate family members staying with the patient as much as possible. Their presence will provide comfort for the patient. During illness, involve family members in the patient's care as much as possible.

- Health care providers may need several social patient interactions before the patient will be willing to discuss personal issues and problems that need interventions. Individuals are often judged on how they act and relate to the patient/family, instead of on their title.[21,30] Inquire about less sensitive issues before proceeding to more sensitive/complex issues. Consistency in caregivers will contribute to establishment of trust. Be a good listener so that the health care provider can "start where the client is."

- The health care provider should exhibit an unhurried approach. Personalism is valued among many Appalachians. Allow the patient and family adequate time to describe issues and problems within the context that they see them.[31]

- Direct eye contact may be interpreted as impolite. Some Appalachians engage in direct eye contact primarily during states of aggressiveness.[8] May avoid eye contact with nurses, physicians, and other health care providers out of respect.[17]

Birth/Children

- Birth seen as a normal process and a satisfying human need.[32] Children are highly valued.

- Breastfeeding is supported, but prevalence of breastfeeding in Appalachia as a whole is lower than national levels.[33] Assess for barriers to successful initiation and maintenance of breastfeeding. Educate the mother regarding resources that can be accessed to support successful breastfeeding.

- Purnell (2008) identifies the following pregnancy-related beliefs that may be encountered when providing care to Appalachian women:
  - One can determine the sex of the child by the shape of the mother's abdomen and whether the baby is carried 'high' or 'low.'
  - Having a picture taken can cause stillbirth.
  - A pregnant woman reaching above her head can cause the umbilical cord to strangle the fetus.
  - Wearing an opal during pregnancy can lead to fatal harm.
  - Being frightened by a snake, eating certain fruits, or craving certain foods and not eating the food will cause birthmarks.
  - Congenital anomalies can be caused by the mother experiencing tragedy.
- Additional beliefs may include:[19]
  - Dental work or other medical procedures during pregnancy may lead to deformities or illness in the baby.
  - Unkind remarks made during pregnancy about a disabled person will lead to disability in the baby.
  - Giving birth when the astrological sign is in the loins is unfavorable.
  - A knife placed under the bed mattress during labor will decrease pain and bleeding.
  - It is bad luck to cut a newborn's nails during the first few weeks of life. Mothers may attempt to bite the nails instead to shorten them. Teach safety measures.
  - Cutting an infant's hair is bad luck. If hair must be cut for procedures, return hair to the parent(s).
- Mothers may place bellybands on babies in an effort to prevent umbilical hernias. Asafetida bags may be placed on babies and children to prevent contagious diseases. (Asafetida is a **strong-smelling** plant from which the resin of the plant, the root, and other parts

of the plant is mixed sometimes with herbs, to be placed in a small pouch for placement around the neck.) Asafetida is also sometimes dissolved in water or liquor. A drop or two is sometimes given to babies to relieve colic.[4]

- Infants may be fed solid foods earlier than recommended by nutritionists.[34]
- Generally, mothers are the primary caregivers for children. This is changing among urban Appalachians.
- Discipline of children may seem harsh to non-Appalachians. Corporal punishment is sometimes used, adhering to the Bible reference of "spare the rod and spoil the child."[31]

Death

- Reactions to the death of a loved one and expressions of grief may seem extreme or exaggerated to non-Appalachians.[35,36]
- Allow time for relatives and friends to visit with the deceased prior to moving the body to the morgue or calling for the funeral home.[37]
- May be very hesitant to consent to autopsies and organ donations.[37]
- Earth burial is the most common form of interment. Cremation is infrequent.[36]
- May wish to take photographs of the body after it has been dressed as a form of remembrance.[36]

Patient Teaching/Dietary Considerations

- Written teaching methods will not be effective among persons who cannot read and effectively process information in the written documents. Use alternative methods of teaching, such as demonstrations, oral communication, videos, etc. Consistently assess understanding.

- Patient education must be consistent with the client's frame of reference (perception of the etiology of the disease/condition, treatment that would typically be used at home, etc.) or suggestions/instructions may be rejected.[10]

- Take advantage of all opportunities to share information about free or low-cost preventive/ medical care, prescriptions, etc. as indicated by the individual's socioeconomic status.

- Diet is often high in fat, sugar, and sodium.

- For rehabilitation purposes, explore the client's skills other than those of his/her former occupation. Other skills may be built upon if primary skills have been lost because of disability.[38]

- When teaching about medications, stress that prescribed medications such as those for hypertension, diabetes, etc. are to be taken not only when the patient feels bad, but even after he or she begins to feel better. Also, stress that because the prescribed dosage brings about improvement in symptoms, double doses of the medicine will not make one feel twice as good. Ask about the availability of a clock in the home.[17]

- Assure that indoor plumbing and electricity are available in the home. Ask what type of fuel is used to heat the home. This may impact the type of medical equipment and/or treatment used in the home.

---

1 McCauley, D. (1995). *Appalachian mountain religion: A history*. Chicago, IL: University of Illinois Press

2 The Appalachian Regional Commission. *The Appalachian region*. Retrieved from http://www.arc.gov

3 Shackelford, L. & Weinberg, B. (1997). *Appalachia*. New York, NY: Hill and Wang.

4 Purnell, L. (2013). *Transcultural health care: A culturally competent approach* (4th ed.). Philadelphia, PA: F.A. Davis Company.

5 Rosswurm, M., Dent, D., Armstrong-Persily, C., Woodburn, P., & Davis, B. (1996). Illness experiences and health recovery behaviors of patients in Southern Appalachia. *Western Journal of Nursing Research, 18*(4), 441-459.

6 Isserman, A. (1996). *Socio-economic review of Appalachia: An update of "the realities of deprivation" reported to the president in 1964"*. Retrieved from http://www.arc.gov/assets/research_reports/SocioeconomicReviewofAppalachiaThenandNow.pdf

7 DeNavas-Walt, C., Proctor, B.D., & Smith, J. C. (2011, September). *U.S. Census Bureau current population report: Income, poverty, and health insurance coverage in the United States: 2010*. Washington, DC: U.S. Government Printing Office.

8 Diddle, G. & Denham, S. A. (2010). Spirituality and its relationships with the health and illness of Appalachian people. *Journal of Transcultural Nursing, 21*(2), 175-182. doi:10.1177/1043659609357640

[9] Helton, L. (1996). Folk medicine and health beliefs: An Appalachian perspective. *Journal of Cultural Diversity, 3*(4), 123-128.

[10] Tripp-Reimer, T. & Friedl, M. (1977). Appalachians: A neglected minority. *Nursing Clinics of North America, 12*(1), 41-54.

[11] Borak, J., Salipante-Zaidel, C., Slade, M.D., & Fields, C.A. (2012). Mortality disparities in Appalachia: Reassessment of major risk factors. *Journal of Occupational & Environmental Medicine, 54*(2), 146-156. doi:10.1097/JOM.0b013e318246f395

[12] Halverson, J., Barnett, E., & Casper, M. (2002). Geographic disparities in heart disease and stroke mortality among Black and White populations in the Appalachian region. *Ethnicity and Disease, 12*(4), 82-91.

[13] Rochman, S. (2010). The culture and cancer of rural poverty. *American Association for Cancer Research: CR Magazine, 5*(2), 30-39.

[14] Huttlinger, K., Schaller-Ayers, J. & Lawson, T. (2004). Health care in Appalachia: A population-based approach. *Public Health Nursing, 21*(2), 103-110.

[15] Denham, S. (2003). *Describing abuse of pregnant women and their healthcare workers in rural Appalachia, 28*(4), 264-269.

[16] National Opinion Research Center. (2008). *An analysis of mental health and substance abuse disparities & access to treatment Services in the Appalachian region.* Bethesda, MD: Author.

[17] Lewis, S., Messner, R., & McCowell, W. (1985). An unchanging culture. *Journal of Gerontological Nursing, 11*(8), 20-26.

[18] Giger, J.N. (2008). *Transcultural nursing: Assessment and intervention* (6th ed.). St. Louis, MO: Mosby Elsevier.

[19] Abramson, R. & Haskell, J. (Eds.). (2006). *Encyclopedia of Appalachia.* Knoxville, TN: The University of Tennessee Press.

[20] Schoenberg, N.E., Howell, B.M., & Fields, N. (2012). Community strategies to address cancer disparities in Appalachian Kentucky, *Family Community Health, 35*(1), 31-43.

[21] Bauer, W. (2003). Rehabilitation counseling in Appalachian America. *Journal of Rehabilitation, 69*(3), 9-15.

[22] Kimbrough, D. (1995). *Taking up serpents: Snake Handlers in Eastern Kentucky.* Chapel Hill, NC: The University of North Carolina Press.

[23] Burton, T. (1993). *Serpent-handling believers.* Knoxville, TN: The University of Tennessee Press.

[24] Simpson, M. & King, M. (1999). "God brought all these churches together": Issues in developing religion-health partnerships in an Appalachian community. *Public Health Nursing, 16*(1), 41-49.

[25] Burkhardt, M. (1993). Characteristics of spirituality in the lives of women in a rural Appalachian community. *Journal of Transcultural Nursing, 4*(2), 12-18.

[26] Cavendar, A. (1992). Theoretic orientations and folk medicine research in the Appalachian South. *Southern Medical Journal, 85*(2), 170-178.

[27] Barnette, D., Bauer, A., Baker, B., Ehrhardt, K., & Stoller, S. (1994). A case for naturalistic assessment and intervention in an urban Appalachian community. In K. M. Borman & P. J. Obermiller (Eds.). *From mountain to metropolis: Appalachian migrants in American cities.* (pp. 94-104). Westport, CT: Greenwood Publishing Group.

[28] Slusher, I.L., Withrow-Fletcher, C., & Hauser-Whitaker, M. (2010). Appalachian women: Health beliefs, self-care, and basic conditioning factors. *Journal of Cultural Diversity, 17*(3), 84-89.

[29] Griffith, B.N., Lovett, G.D., Pyle, D.N., & Miller, W.C. (2011). Self-rated health in rural Appalachia: Health perceptions are incongruent with health statue and health behaviors. *BMC Public Health, 11*(29). Retrieved from http://www.biomedcentral.com/1471-2458/11/229

[30] Helton, L., Barnes, E., & Borman, K. (1994). Urban Appalachians and professional intervention: A model for educators and social service providers. In K. M. Borman & P. J. Obermiller (Eds.). *From mountain to metropolis: Appalachian migrants in American cities.* (pp. 1-5, 120). Westport, CT: Greenwood Publishing Group.

[31] Helton, L. (1995). Intervention with Appalachians: Strategies for a culturally specific practice. *Journal of Cultural Diversity, 2*(1), 20-26.

[32] Horton, C. (1984). Women have headaches, men have backaches: Patterns of illness in an Appalachian community. *Social Science Medicine, 19*(6), 647-654.

[33] Wiener, R.C. & Wiener, M.A. (2011). Breastfeeding prevalence and distribution in the USA and Appalachia by rural and urban setting. *Journal of Rural and Remote Health Research, Education, Practice and Policy, 11*(1713). Retrieved from http://www.rrh.org.au/publishedarticles/article_print_1713.pdf

[34] Flasher, W. (2010). *Cultural diversity: Eating in America–Appalachian.* Retrieved from http://ohioline.osu.edu/hyg-fact/5000/pdf/5252.pdf

[35] Weller, J. (1965). *Yesterday's people: Life in contemporary Appalachia.* Lexington, KY: The University Press of Kentucky.

[36] Crissman, J. (1994). *Death and dying in Central Appalachia: Changing attitudes and practices.* Chicago, IL: University of Illinois Press.

[37] Obermiller, P. & Rappold, R. (1994). The sense of place and cultural identity among urban Appalachians: A study of post death migration. In K. M. Borman & P. J. Obermiller (Eds.). *From mountain to metropolis: Appalachian migrants in American cities.* (pp. 25-31). Westport, CT: Greenwood Publishing Group.

[38] Blakeney, A. (1987). Appalachian values: Implications for occupational therapists. *Occupational Therapy in Health Care, 4*(1), 57-71.

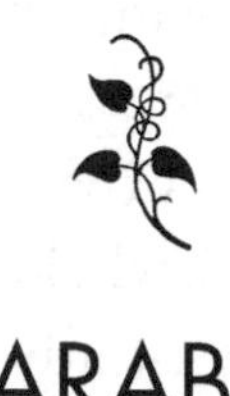

ARABS

Background

Arab refers to an individual who speaks Arabic and shares the values and beliefs of Arab culture.[1] Although there are commonalties among the Arab people, there are unique cultural beliefs, values, and practices among the people of each Arab country. The Arabic speaking world includes the following:[2,3,4]

- Algeria
- Bahrain
- Comoros
- Dijibouti
- Egypt
- Iraq
- Jordan
- Kuwait
- Libya
- Mauritania
- Morocco
- Oman
- Portions of Lebanon
- Portions of Palestine
- Qatar
- Saudi Arabia
- Somalia
- Sudan
- Syria
- Tunisia
- United Arab Emirates
- Yemen

Arabs reside in numerous areas of the world. Approximately 1.7 million Arabs reside in the United States and almost one million in Canada. Population estimates vary widely. In Canada, the largest numbers reside in Ontario. In the United States, two-thirds of the Arab population resides in ten states with one-third of the total residing in California, Michigan, and New York.

United States metropolitan areas with large concentrations of Arabs include Chicago, Detroit, Los Angeles, New Jersey, New York, and Washington, DC. States with the highest population of Arabs are California, Michigan, New York, Florida, and Texas, respectively. Arabs of Lebanese heritage make up the largest percentage of Arabs living in the United States. Arabs living in the United States and Canada tend to be well educated, with almost half over the age of twenty-five holding a bachelor's degree or higher. Arabs are employed primarily in professional, high-tech, administrative careers, or self-employed.[4,5]

Most Arabs living in urban areas have a deep appreciation of Western medicine. However, in rural areas, persons are still at risk for diseases such as malaria, tuberculosis, cholera, and dysentery. As Arabs adopt more Western practices, the incidence of cardiovascular disease, hypertension, diabetes, and cancer increases. Since the September 11, 2001 terrorist attacks, many Arabs have experienced high levels of stress related to their heritage and assumptions about their religious affiliation. The higher stress levels may, in turn, contribute to increased health risks.

Diseases of genetic background include thalassemia, various anemias, sickle cell disease, and Mediterranean fever. Vitamin D deficiency, particularly among women, is a health risk and, left untreated, may contribute to serious health problems. In the Arab world, infant mortality rates remain high. Newly immigrated Arabs of lower socioeconomic and educational status are at risk for all health problems that are secondary to poverty.[6,7,8,9,10]

Language

- Arabic is the official language of the Arab world. It is written and read from right to left. There are several branches of Arabic–formal classical (the language of the Qur'án), modern classical (language of most books, newspapers, etc.), and regional Arabic dialects (for everyday communicating). The Egyptian Arabic dialect is spoken by many Arabs because the majority of Arab films and television dramas are produced in Cairo.[3,5,11] Many Arabs also speak English and other languages.

- Conversation is often accompanied by touching (between members of the same sex), animated gestures, and rising of the voice to emphasize certain points. These actions may be erroneously interpreted as anger and/or aggressiveness.[7]

- Comfort distance during conversation is approximately two feet.[12, 13]

- Sitting with the soles of the feet visible, or leaning against the wall with hands in one's pockets may be considered impolite.[13]

Worldview/Religious Beliefs

- Worldwide, the majority of Arabs are Muslims. In the United States, the majority are Christians.

- One's destiny is pre-determined by God. Life is controlled by fate with humans having little control. However, the individual should strive to live a life of obedience.[2]

- Individual actions reflect on the entire family. Family concerns override individual concerns.

- Relationships are valued over tasks.[13] Social status and family background is important.[2]

Health Beliefs/Practices

- Illness can result from bad luck or disobedience. God inflicts and heals illness; outcomes are in His hands–"*inshallah.*" If this belief is present concerning illnesses, self-care and preventive interventions may be difficult to implement. Set short-term instead of long-term goals.[6]

- The belief that energy must be conserved for recovery may interfere with early/frequent ambulation regimes advocated in most Western medical facilities.[7]

- Belief in the evil eye is not uncommon. Amulets and/or charms may be worn as protection from harm. These may be placed on infants shortly after birth.

- Incorporation of hot and cold principles. Illness can result from imbalances within the body.

- Descriptions of illnesses may be vague and generalized since disease is seen as affecting the entire body. Explore further with patient in an effort to determine if mental health issues are contributing to symptoms, particularly among women. There may be hesitancy to discuss mental health problems since they may be seen as private and only to be discussed among family.[14]

  The left hand is considered unclean, being used for unclean tasks such as toileting, etc. The right hand is used for handshakes, eating, etc. Consider these factors when choosing IV sites, etc.

- Folk healers, herbal, and folk remedies may be utilized for treatment of illnesses and/or as preventive medicine, particularly in rural areas. Treatments may include cupping, cauterizing, spiritual interventions, etc. Boiled mint, sage, thyme, and chamomile may be used to relieve menstrual pain.[15,16]

- The family may be opposed to telling a family member the full extent of a grave prognosis. It is believed that hope helps a patient to cope with an illness, it will be upsetting to the patient, and only God can determine if hope is futile. Any grave information should not be communicated solely to the patient, but should include the family spokesperson–often, the eldest male. A plan of care/communication about the disease process should be developed.[6,12,17]

- Privacy is highly valued among Arabs. Provide continuity of caregivers as much as possible to establish a trusting relationship with client and family. Individuals may be reluctant to share personal information with strangers. Provide thorough explanation concerning the need to ask such questions. Keeping one's word is a component of the value of honor. Providers should assure that commitments and agreements are fulfilled. Individuals and/or family members may insist on speaking directly with a physician or other persons seen as authority figures.[6,7]

- May believe that intramuscular and intravenous medications are more effective than oral medications.[1]

- May place heavy importance on ingestion and elimination, equating the condition of the alimentary tract with the overall health of body systems.[18] Food deprivation is considered a precursor to illness. Carefully explain the need to be NPO (nothing by mouth).

Expression of Pain[19]

- Expressive and may expect immediate intervention to relieve pain.
- Assess pain level at frequent intervals. Offer pain medication prior to pain becoming intense.
- Include family members in notifying providers of early signs of discomfort.

Male-Female/Kinship/Social Relationships

- Women may decline shaking hands with men outside the family circle.[6]
- Marriages may be arranged, particularly among Arabs living in more traditional settings. In this instance, marriage may occur during the early to late teen years. This practice has changed significantly among Arabs who have become more acculturated to Western life styles.[6]
- Family is of utmost importance, including extended family. Households may be multigenerational. Allow liberal visitation. Family members will likely desire to stay with a hospitalized relative at all times. Involve in care as much as possible. Females may not answer questions directed to them; the husband or family spokesperson will answer. The family will often relay any patient needs rather than the patient doing so.[3] This should not be mistaken for powerlessness.
- Titles are important, often point back to an individual's family ties, and are often recognized in everyday interactions. Older non-relatives are sometimes called 'aunt' or 'uncle' as a sign of respect. When addressing an individual, the oldest son's name is sometimes used preceded by the word *Umm* and *Abu*, meaning "mother of" or "father of," respectively (e.g., *Abu Mohammad*, meaning *Father of Mohammad*). A man's given name may be

followed by the word *bin* and his father's name, meaning "son of." Individuals with Arabic names may be addressed in several different ways. Inquire about individual's preference for name to be addressed by while in the health care facility.[4,6]

- Gender roles vary among Arab groups and regions. Often, males are authority figures and make or communicate important family decisions. In the absence of a father or husband, this role may fall to the oldest son or brother. Women are very much a part of the decision-making, but not publicly. Elders will be consulted for decisions, as they are highly respected members of the family.[6]

- Beards worn by Arabic men carry cultural and religious meanings. Avoid touching or shaving without asking permission and unless absolutely medically necessary.[16]

- Status and authority is gained with aging, particularly women. Women who have sons gain even more status. Adult sons will make every effort to accommodate the wishes of their mother.[20]

- Direct eye contact between a male and female may be interpreted as an invitation of a sexual nature instead of as directness.

- Family honor is tied to female purity. **Extreme** modesty and sexual segregation are required among Muslims. Men may have less respect for the female nurse or physician because duties of these professions require that the woman look at and touch the bodies of naked strangers, which violates the laws of the Qur'án. Female patients will not be in the presence of a strange male without being fully dressed or covered. Provide covering for hair, if needed. If the woman is accustomed to her face being covered and is to have surgery, a towel, surgical mask, or sheet may be used until time for anesthesia induction.[13] Same-sex nurses and physicians should care for Arab Muslim patients, if possible. Housekeepers, lab technicians, etc. should also be of the same sex as the patient, if possible.

- Men and families may be perceived as demanding, particularly when an individual requires hospitalization. The family will indulge patients. Self-care may not be a goal.

- Out-of-wedlock pregnancies are viewed as a disgrace to the males of the family, who are charged with protecting the female's honor. The female may be punished severely or even killed.

- In traditional Arab culture, unmarried female teens and young women generally do not discuss issues such as menstruation with males. Because of the high value placed on virginity, tampons and douches may be unacceptable and sanitary pads preferred.[15]
- Family members, regardless of the care demands, will care for the sick and elderly.
- Women generally, do not change their last name when they marry.

Birth/Children

- Traditional female genital surgery is practiced among some Arab groups. Determine if this surgery has been performed as early as possible in the pregnancy to plan for any additional measures that may need to be taken for delivery of the baby.[15] (See *Traditional Female Genital Surgery*.)
- In traditional Arab culture, pregnancy is seen as a natural condition and children are highly valued – especially males. Prenatal care may be delayed. Advice about pregnancy care is often sought from female relatives and friends. This practice may vary based on degree of acculturation and other factors. However, pregnancies are valued and, therefore, mothers are expected to eat a nutritionally-sound diet. Spicy foods, sour foods, and other strong-flavored foods may be avoided.[15]
- Expressive of discomfort during labor. May refuse epidurals because of fear of paralysis.[15]
- Lack of planning ahead for delivery (i.e., layettes, baby showers, nurseries, etc.) should not be seen as a sign of the family not wanting the new baby. Such planning may be viewed as negatively affecting the future by interfering with God's will.[1, 15]
- A common belief is that birthmarks are present on the baby as a result of unsatisfied food cravings during pregnancy.[4]
- Husbands may choose not to participate in labor and delivery. In many instances, females are support persons during labor and delivery, as well as during the postpartum period. A lying-in period of up to forty days may be observed.[15]
- Breastfeeding may be delayed until the second or third day with the belief that the mother needs to rest and that colostrum is not good for the baby.[4]

- May avoid showering for several days following birth preferring sponge baths instead. Will prefer warm teas, soups, etc. during post-partum period.
- May use bellybands on newborn babies because of the belief that cold can enter through the baby's abdomen.[7]
- Post-discharge, mothers with new babies may apply *ko'hl* (a charcoal-like substance used for cosmetic purposes in the Middle East) to the umbilical cord to facilitate drying of the cord. Mothers should be cautioned about using ko'hl on children because of its high lead content.[20]
- Male children may receive preferential treatment, especially the firstborn male because in traditional Arab culture, males provide security for parents during old age.[15]
- Children will likely view the mother as the source of comfort since fathers are generally seen as the authoritarian and disciplinarian in the family. Maternal bonds with eldest son will be especially strong.[21]
- Spanking and shaming may be used as methods of discipline. Adults expect obedience and respect from children and generally do not try to reason with small children.[2, 22]

Death

- Based on individual's religious preference.

Patient Teaching/Dietary Considerations

- Based on individual's religious preference.
- Dates are generally a popular food, but are high in potassium. Must be limited for those patients requiring restricted potassium.
- Foods considered either 'hot' or 'cold.' Hot foods are avoided during warm seasons. Cold foods are avoided during cold seasons. Common hot foods are beef, potatoes, and most protein-rich foods. Common cold foods are chicken/fish, fruit, and beer.

[1] Meleis, A. (1981, June). The Arab American in the health care system. *American Journal of Nursing*, 1180-1183.

[2] Nydell, M. (1996). *Understanding Arabs: A guide for Westerners*. Yarmouth, MA: Intercultural Press, Inc.

[3] AbuGharbieh, P. (1998). Arab-Americans. In L. Purnell & B. Paulanka, *Transcultural health care: A culturally competent approach*. (pp. 137-162). Philadelphia, PA: F. A. Davis Company.

[4] The Canadian Arab Friendship Association. (2012) Retrieved from http://www.cafaedmonton.ca/

[5] The ArabAmerican Institute. (2012). *Demographics*. Retrieved from http://www.aaiusa.org/pages/demographics/

[6] Haddad, L. & Hoeman, S. (2000). Home healthcare and the Arab American client. *Home Healthcare Nurse, 18*(3), 189-197.

[7] Kulwicki, A. & Ballout, S. (2013). People of Arab heritage. In L. Purnell, *Transcultural health care: A culturally competent approach* (4th ed.) (pp. 159-177). Philadelphia, PA: F. A. Davis Company.

[8] Kulwicki, A., Khalifa, R. & Moore, G. (2008). The effects of September 11 on Arab American nurses in metropolitan Detroit. *Journal of Transcultural Nursing, 19*(2), 134-139.

[9] Hobbs, R. D., Habib, Z., Alromaihi, D., Idi, L., Parikh, N., Blocki, F. & Rao, D.S. (2009). Severe Vitamin D deficiency in Arab-American women living in Dearborn, Michigan. *Endocrine Practice, 15*(1), 35-40.

[10] Saadi, H.F., Kazzam, E., Ghurbana, B. & Nicholls, M.G. (2006). Hypothesis: Correction of low vitamin D status among Arab women will prevent heart failure and improve cardiac function in established heart failure. *European Journal of Heart Failure, 8*, 694-696.

[11] Butt, G. (1997). *The Arabs: Myth and reality*. New York, NY: I. B. Tauris, Publishers.

[12] Lipson, J. & Meleis, A. (1983). Issues in health care of Middle Eastern Patients. *The Western Journal of Medicine, 139*(6), 854-861.

[13] Sheets, D. & El-Azhary, R. (1998). The Arab Muslim client: Implications for anesthesia. *Journal of the American Association of Nurse Anesthetist, 65*(3), 304-312.

[14] Hamdan, A. (2009). Mental health needs of Arab women. *Health Care for Women International, 30*, 595-613. doi:10.1080/07399330902928808

[15] Kridli, S. (2002). Health beliefs and practices among Arab women. *American Journal of Maternal Child Nursing, 27*(3), 178-182.

[16] Al-Shahri, M. (2002). Culturally sensitive caring for Saudi patients. *Journal of Transcultural Nursing, 13*(2), 133-138.

[17] Ali, N. (1996). Providing culturally sensitive care to Egyptians with cancer. *Cancer Practice, 4*(4), 212-215.

[18] Ramer, L. (1992). *Culturally sensitive caregiving and childbearing families*. New York, NY: March of Dimes Birth Defects Foundation.

[19] Andrews, M. & Boyle, J. (2003). *Transcultural concepts in nursing care* (4th ed.). Philadelphia, PA: Lippincott Williams & Wilkins.

[20] Luna, L. (1989) Transcultural nursing care of Arab Muslims. *Journal of Transcultural Nursing, 1*(1), 22-25.

[21] Luna, L. (1994). Care and cultural context of Lebanese Muslim immigrants: Using Leininger's theory. *Journal of Transcultural Nursing, 5*(2), 12-20.

[22] Khoury-Dassabri, M. (2010). Attitudes of Arab and Jewish mothers towards punitive and non-punitive discipline methods. *Child and Family Social Work, 15*, 135-144. doi: 10.1111/j.1365-2206.2009.00667.x.

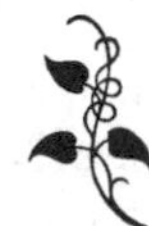

ASIAN INDIAN HINDUS

Background

India is located in south Asia and is the seventh largest country in the world in land area. It is approximately one-third the area of the United States, and had an estimated population in 2011 of over 1.2 billion people. The median age of the people of India is 26.2 years, and the birth rate is 20.6/1000. However, the infant mortality rate is more than double the birth rate at almost 46.07/1000 live births. More than half of the population is literate. The life expectancy is approximately 67 years of age. Over 80 percent of the population is Hindu. Other major religious groups in India are Muslim (13.4 percent), Christian (2.3 percent), and Sikh (1.9 percent).[1,2]

Asian Indian Hindus have migrated to the western countries from all areas of India. In the United States, the largest numbers are concentrated in California and New York. They are the second largest Asian group in the United States. Because of immigration requirements in the United States, most individuals that have come to the United States from India since 1965 are well educated, with 70 percent ages twenty-five and older holding a bachelor's degree or higher. Asian Indians, as a whole, have one of the highest incomes in the United States.[3,4,5,6]

Cardiovascular disease, diabetes, cancer, and sickle cell disease are risk factors among Asian Indians. Persons living in rural areas of India and immigrating from these areas are more at risk for malaria, rheumatic heart disease, respiratory infections, parasitic infections, dental caries, and gum disease.[7, 8, 9, 10, 11, 12]

Language

English is one of India's official languages. Hindi is spoken by approximately 41 percent of India's population. There are fourteen other languages recognized as official ones in India. Other principal languages in order of most spoken are: *Bengali*, *Telegu*, *Marathi*, *Tamil*, *Urdu*, *Gujarati*, *Kannada*, *Malayalam*, *Oriya*, *Punjabi*, *Assamese*, and *Maithili*. Almost six percent of the people speak other languages. Hindustani is not an official language, but is widely spoken in northern India.[2]

In addition, there are more than 1,600 dialects spoken. The majority of Asian Indian Hindus who came to western countries because of special educational and professional qualifications, speak English well or very well. However, relatives granted visas because of marriage or other family relationships, such as parents, may not have the same English language proficiency.[2, 4, 7]

Worldview/Religious Beliefs

- See *Hinduism*

Health Beliefs[8, 9, 10, 13]

- Health-seeking behaviors may be influenced by multiple healthcare systems (mainstream Western medicine and traditional Indian medicine) factors such as education, level of acculturation, etc.[14]
- Health encompasses three governing principles in the body—*vata*, *pitta* and *kapha*. Vata is responsible for movement, pitta controls metabolism and, heat kapha supplies the body structure and solidity. When these three principles are balanced, the body functions normally and health is optimal. Balanced vata creates energy and creativity; balanced pitta creates optimal digestion, balanced kapha provides strength, stamina, immunity, and even

temperament. Imbalances of these principles cause illness and disease. Illness may also be attributed to the effects of karma. (See *Hinduism*)

- The *hot* and *cold* theory applies to foods, medications, illnesses, environments, etc. Perceptions of what foods are hot or cold vary among regions of India. Compliance with taking medications may be influenced by whether the patient believes the medication supports this balance.[14]

- Health is related to the connectedness of the body, mind, and spirit. Mind-body practices such as yoga, meditation, etc. may be practiced as ways of maintaining balance of the three systems.

- Mental illness is not readily accepted and is sometimes considered a defect in the individual's strength, or character and reflects negatively on the family's honor. Symptoms may be expressed with non-specific physical descriptions. Health care providers will need to explore symptoms further to gain more specific information.[14]

- Inquire about use of herbal supplements and treatments using folk medicine. These approaches may be used for illness prevention, health maintenance and treatment of illnesses. The degree of use may be influenced by the individual's access to mainstream health care and other factors. Collaborate and negotiate with the individual and family members to repattern any health care practices that may be harmful to the individual's health and well-being.

- Modesty and personal hygiene are **highly** valued. A bath is required at least daily, but generally not following a meal.

- Among some more traditional South Asians, menstruation and childbirth place the female in an 'unclean' state. In some instances, the female is not allowed to cook and may be segregated from other family members until ritual purification baths are taken.[7, 15]

- Healthcare providers should inquire about compliance with preventive cancer screenings such as mammography, Pap smears, etc. Modesty, particularly among women, may serve as a barrier to having such screenings.[12, 14]

- The right hand is believed to be clean and is used for handling items such as religious books and eating utensils. The left hand is used for handling the genitals and other items considered dirty. Consider these factors when choosing IV sites, etc.

Expression of Pain

- Asian Indians are generally stoic related to the value of self-control. Observe non-verbal behavior. Offer comfort measures and medications, even if not requested.

Male-Female/Kinship/Social Relationships[7, 13, 14, 16, 17, 18]

- Although the caste system (dharma), based on four colors (varnas), has been legally abolished in India, there are strong evidences that this practice still exists in traditional family life and behaviors. Dharma required persons to remain in the caste that was assigned at birth. Caste categories were as follows:
  - **Brahmins**: Priests who occupied a position of prestige and influence. White was the distinguishing color.
  - **Kshatriyas**: Ranked second to the priests. Red was the distinguishing color. Military and political leadership was an obligation.
  - **Vaisyas**: Made up the largest caste. Members in this group were involved in commerce such as raising cattle, shop keeping, farming, and lending money. Yellow was the distinguishing color.
  - **Sudras**: Members of this group were servants of the higher groups. Most were poor farmers or artisans. The distinguishing color was black.
  - **Harijans** (Untouchables): Members of this group were not allowed to live within the community boundaries. They performed duties considered unclean such as handling the dead, handling garbage, executing criminals, and tanning leather.
- Family highly valued and will be an integral part of decision-making. Policies concerning confidentiality may not be readily accepted and understood among family members. Family members will desire to stay with the hospitalized client continuously and will be included in personal care of the client. Courtesy is particularly valued among Asian Indians.

- In an effort to protect a family member, full disclosure of the severity of illness may not be supported among family members. Health care providers will need to explore such issues with the patient and family early during a hospital stay.

- The husband is the primary decision-maker and spokesperson for his family, although he may confer with his mother, father, and wife. Wives will frequently not answer questions if the husband is present in the room. Direct questions to the husband, who will confer with his wife, then answer the question.

- Mothers-in-law are considered authoritative in issues related to female health. Include in teaching sessions and other health-related conversations unless there are objections by the wife or husband.

- Elders are highly respected. Married sons may continue to live with parents. Parents maintain authority.

- Generally, there is limited direct eye contact from women to men. Direct eye contact is acceptable from men to men. Initiation of direct eye contact (male to female) other than from the female's husband is unacceptable.

- In traditional families, wives may exhibit deference to their husbands, and men may be considered superior to women. A woman is to be protected always. As a girl grows, she is protected by her father and brothers until she is married. Her husband assumes the role of protector and, ultimately, her sons if her husband precedes her in death. Women are not passive, but see their role as an intricate part of marriage, nurturing children, and caring for the home. The traditional hierarchical structure is being tested in some instances as families adopt more Western behaviors.

- Public expressions of affection such as touching are considered disrespectful.

- Among traditional Asian Hindus, it is taboo for a man, other than the woman's husband, to extend his hand toward the woman for greeting purposes. During introductions of male to female clients, the greeting should be addressed to the husband or eldest female companion first.

- May meditate. Provide a quiet environment without interruptions during meditation.

Birth/Children[9, 18]

- Pregnancy is considered a normal physiologic condition. Use of mainstream health care practitioners for prenatal care varies based on socioeconomic status, access to care, etc. Elder women are considered sources of information or assistance during pregnancy. A popular belief among women with more traditional beliefs is that the woman has little or no control over the outcome of the pregnancy.

- Pregnancy is considered a 'hot' condition. Foods with hot properties such as animal products, chili, spices, eggs, and gas-producing foods will be avoided. Eggs and mangos are sometimes thought to contribute to abortion. It is believed that *hot* foods eaten early in pregnancy cause miscarriages and fetal anomalies. *Hot* foods may be eaten during the last weeks of pregnancy to facilitate the expulsion of the baby.[9] *Cold* foods are believed to strengthen and calm the pregnant woman. Among foods that are considered cold are milk products, foods sour in taste, and most vegetables.

- The post-partum period is considered a cold condition warranting the consumption of foods with hot properties, staying warm, etc. Showers may be avoided; warm sponge baths may be substituted for hygienic purposes.

- There may be a risk of inadequate nutrition during pregnancy as a result of fasting during pregnancy, and the traditional practice of women eating after the children, elders, and men have eaten their meal. There may be less than adequate food left for the pregnant woman. Some women will purposely eat smaller amounts of food for the purpose of having a smaller baby.

- In traditional families, women assist during labor and delivery. Husbands may not desire to participate in these phases. Provide ongoing reports of the wife's labor status, even if the father does not ask.

- Mongolian spots are common among babies, especially among those of darker skin tones. Mongolian spots are more common in the lumbosacral and gluteal areas, but can be found on other areas of the skin. They should not be confused with bruising.

- Breastfeeding is widely supported, although some mothers may not wish to breastfeed until "real milk" comes in because of beliefs surrounding the impurity of colostrum.

- Various methods may be used to ward off the evil eye or other harm to the baby. Do not remove articles placed on the baby for this purpose.
- If family members are available, they may do all infant care with the exception of feeding the baby in observance of the mother's "lying-in" period. The lying-in period varies from seven to forty days.
- Children are deeply loved and treated with indulgence. However, they are expected to be obedient and respectful toward adults. Corporal punishment is rarely used.
- Children may appear to have closer relationships with the mother. Children will rise out of respect when the father enters the room.
- Male children may receive preferential treatment, especially the firstborn male.[7, 19]
- Modesty training for girls will begin at approximately two years of age.

Death

- See *Hinduism.*

Patient Teaching/Dietary Considerations

- Generally vegetarian. Some may eat fish, eggs, or chicken. Beef is forbidden. Foods may be spicy, and frying is a common cooking method. Explore dietary choices with patient.[20]
- The religious practice of fasting is significant and is crucial to consider in diet teaching for pregnancy and specific diseases such as diabetes.
- There is a common incidence of lactose intolerance among Asian Indians.

Other

- Monitor responses closely when psychotropic drugs are prescribed. Lower doses may result in desired effects. Asian Indians may also exhibit a higher sensitivity to alcohol.

---

1 Williams, B. (1993). *The Kingfisher reference atlas: An A-Z guide to countries of the world.* New York, NY: Kingfisher Books.

2 The Central Intelligence Agency. (2012). *India.* Retrieved from http://www.cia.gov

3 Lessinger, J. (1995). *From the Ganges to the Hudson: Indian immigrants in New York City.* Boston, MA: Allyn & Bacon.

4 Barringer, H., Gardner, R. & Levin, M. (1993). *Asians and Pacific Islanders in the United States.* New York, NY: Russell Sage Foundation.

5 *Migration Information Source.* (2013). Retrieved from www.migrationinformation.org

6 Indian Americans top in income and education. (2012, June 20). *NY Daily News.* Retrieved from http://india.nydailynews.com/newsarticle/e8faab16334706cfa07731c5da6e3098/indian-americans-top-in-income-and-education

7 Jambunathan, J. (2013). People of Hindu Heritage. In L. Purnell. *Transcultural health care: A culturally competent approach* (4th ed.) (pp. 288-309). Philadelphia, PA: F. A. Davis.

8 Larson-Presswalla, J. (1994). Insights into Eastern health care: Some transcultural nursing perspectives. *Journal of Transcultural Nursing, 5(*1), 21-24.

9 Choudhry, U. (1997). Traditional practices of women from India: Pregnancy, childbirth, and newborn care. *JOGNN, 26*(5), 533-539.

10 Choudhry, U. (1998). Health promotion among immigrant women from India living in Canada. Image: *Journal of Nursing Scholarship, 30*(3), 269-274.

11 Mathews, R. & Zachariah, R. (2008). Coronary heart disease in South Asian immigrants. *Journal of Transcultural Nursing,19*(3). 292-299. Doi: 10.1177/1043659608317448.

12 Palaniappan, L., Mukherjea, A,. Holland, A., & Ivey, S.L. (2010). Leading causes of mortality if Asian Indians in California. *Ethnicity & Disease, 20*(1), 53-57.

13 Giger, J. & Davidhizar, R. (2013). *Transcultural nursing: Assessment and intervention.* (6th ed.). St. Louis, MO: Mosby.

14 Gupta, V. B. (2010). Impact of culture on healthcare seeking behavior of Asian Indians. *Journal of Cultural Diversity, 17*(1), 13-19.

15 Mahon, T. & Fernandes, M. (2010). *Menstrual hygiene in South Asia: A neglected issue for WASH (water, sanitation, and hygiene) programmes.* Retrieved from http://www.wateraid.org/documents/plugin_documents/menstrual_hygiene_in_south_asia_1.pdf

16 Khilnani, S. (1997). *The idea of India.* New York, NY: Farrar, Straus, Giroux.

17 Ramamurthi, B. (1995). Mentality and behaviour in India. *ACTA Neurochirurgica, 132*(4), 199-201.

18 Mahat, G. (1998). Eastern Indians' childbearing practices and nursing implications. *Journal of Community Health Nursing, 15*(3), 155-161.

19 Ahmad, N. (2010). Female feticide in India. *Issues in Law & Medicine, 26*(1), 13-29.

20 Sekhon, S. (1996). Insights into South Asian culture: Food and nutrition values. *Topics in Clinical Nutrition, 11*(4), 47-56.

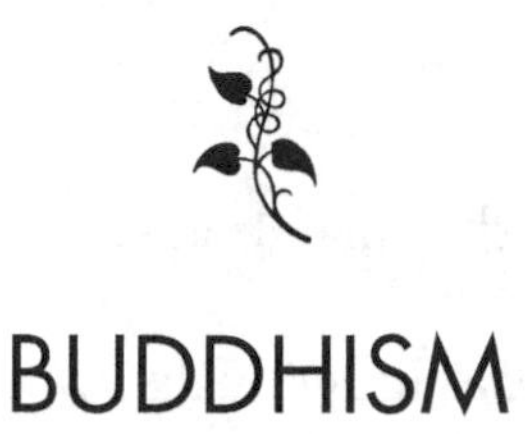

BUDDHISM

Background

Buddhism was founded by Siddhartha Gautama in northeastern India about 500 BC.[1, 2] The religion is based on the life and teaching of this spiritual leader. Siddhartha Gautama was given the title of *Buddha* (the Awakened or Enlightened One) after reporting that he had gained knowledge of the true nature of reality. He preached that all of life involves suffering. The cessation of suffering (nirvana) is the goal of all human efforts. When an individual reaches nirvana, all human qualities become perfect and the cycle of rebirth is broken. The Buddha is not seen as a God, but an example of a way of life. The word Buddha is a *title*, and therefore should always be preceded by a word such as 'the' or 'a'.[3, 4, 5, 6]

There are two main divisions of Buddhism—*Theravada* (the Way of the Elders) *Buddhism* and *Mahayana* (the Great Vehicle) *Buddhism*. The two groups have differing approaches to spiritual life, but share broad beliefs of the religion.[7] Theravada Buddhism is the more conservative and most widely practiced form of the religion today.[2] Mahayana Buddhists assert that Buddha Siddhartha Gautama is one of many Buddhas of the past, present, and future. Mahayana Buddhism is further divided into *Vajrayana/Tantric Buddhism* (Tibetan Buddhism), *Pure Land Buddhism* and *Zen Buddhism*.[4, 5, 8, 9]

The most fundamental and basic characteristics of Buddhism is the promise of enlightenment.[10] There are several Buddhist sects. The most well-known ones include Zen, Pure Land, and Nichiren. There are approximately five hundred million followers of Buddhism worldwide.[11]

Religious Representatives

- Priest
- **Temple President**: A layperson that may lead services in the absence of a priest.[12]
- **Buddhist monks and nuns**: These individuals live in monasteries or nunneries and are allowed to own only eight items. Their time is spent studying sacred texts, working in the community, caring for the sick, etc.[5]

Religious Beliefs

- **Religious texts**: The only complete collection of Buddhist scripture is the **Pali Canon.**[2, 13] Other authoritative texts are used among various Buddhist groups.
- Buddhists believe in the laws of Karma and cause and effect.[4]
- Buddhism is seen as the "eternal truth about reality" (Dharma). It is believed that Dharma, over long periods of time, is forgotten and rediscovered by beings that have fully awakened to reality as it is and are, therefore, called *Buddhas* (awakened ones).[14]
- The teachings of the Buddha included the *Four Noble Truths* and *Noble Eightfold Way*. The philosophies dictate one's response to health and illness. The Four Noble Truths are the foundation of Buddhism. They are as follows:[2, 5, 9, 14]
  - **The truth of suffering**: The Buddha taught that everything is *duhkha*, meaning that there is some degree of pain whether physical, mental, or within one's heart associated with all existence. As long as an individual grasps for lasting satisfaction and gratification, duhkha will exist. This concept is also known as the universal law of impermanence.

- **The truth of the origin of suffering (tahna)**: Suffering is the result of cravings and greed for the purpose of self-fulfillment. It also results from those things in life that are less than perfect.
- The truth that suffering can be destroyed through final liberation or Nirvana.
- The way that leads to the cessation of pain is the Noble Truth of the Eightfold Way.

- The Noble Eightfold Way dictates practical rules. An individual should precede these steps with the 'right association,' realizing that one may be influenced both positively and negatively by social surroundings. The Buddha teaches that an individual should associate with persons who are wise, patient, responsible, noble, and understanding. After the 'right association' is accomplished, the Noble Eightfold Way specifies: right views, intention, speech, action, livelihood, effort, mindfulness, and concentration.
- Buddhism prohibits killing, stealing, sexual misconduct, lying, the ingestion of alcohol, eating during prohibited hours, participating in amusements, use of perfumes and ointments, and accepting money for one's services. A Buddhist is expected to sacrifice oneself, if needed, for the happiness of others.

Special/Religious Observations[5, 12, 15]

- Buddhist celebrations vary from country to country and from one Buddhist school of thought to another. Most Buddhists follow the lunar calendar for religious celebrations.
- Buddhists have many celebrations. Most are celebrated during the time of a full moon because it is believed that the Buddha was born and died at a full moon. Some of the major celebrations are:
  - **Uposatha**: Holy days observing the new moon, full moon days of each lunar month, the eighth day following the new moon, and full moon days. Fasting may be associated with these holy days.
  - **Anniversaries of Buddha's Life (Vesek)**: His birth, his Enlightenment, and his entrance into final Nirvana. Usually celebrated in April. In some countries, the

anniversaries may be celebrated on separate dates (or different dates): April 8, December 8, and February 15, respectively.

- **Vassa**: Observation of the beginning and end of Vassa-a period of meditation, study, and renewed dedication. The period of time encompasses July to October–the rainy season.
- **All Souls Festival**: The purpose of this festival is to remember the dead, free the spirits of those who could not be buried because of an accident, and allow them to experience heavenly peace.
- New Year Festival

Health Beliefs/Practices

- Illness is believed to be a trial to aid development of the soul.
- Medical interventions may be refused on holy days.
- **Medical Procedures/Interventions**: The emphasis within Buddhism is on the individual living *now* and the attainment of Nirvana. Extremes in anything are to be avoided. Generally, any treatment that will contribute to the attainment of Nirvana is acceptable.[3, 16]
- Provide a quiet, uninterrupted environment when an individual is meditating, chanting, and/or prayer. The goal of meditation is to gain a state of peacefulness during which the mind is void of conflicting thoughts. Buddhists may use a certain object, including prayer beads, or assume a certain position to assist them in focusing appropriately during meditation. Do not move personal objects without first asking. Assist to desired meditation position as needed.[5]

Dietary Considerations

- Buddhists are often vegetarians but may follow food preferences related to ethnic background.[16] Buddhists will generally avoid any alcoholic beverages so that the mind is not clouded. Foods containing alcohol may be refused.

- Make patient aware of any medication with an alcohol base to allow for a choice in taking the medication or requesting an alternate. Stimulants may also be avoided.

Death

- Aggressive treatments to prolong an individual's life whose condition is terminal may not be acceptable since such treatments are seen as increasing suffering and interfering with a peaceful death.[17]

- Buddhists believe that humans are dying from moment to moment, based on the belief in the impermanence of everything. Individuals are believed to be reborn into another life based on their deeds and actions in this life. One's existence is a cycle of birth, death, and rebirth. In this belief system, life does not end at the time of death and should not be viewed as an end point, but a natural part of life.

- The state of mind during the time that a person is dying is extremely important in determining his or her rebirth. Offer pain medication, though the patient may refuse medications that cloud the mind. Consider that extreme pain may also disturb the patient's mental state and some analgesia may be needed.

- Facilitate a peaceful environment. Allow relatives at the bedside of the individual for recitation of scriptures and other acts of devotion, including assisting in the care of the dying person. To be with the dying person during the last moments of life is believed to later bring happiness to the people who are present at the time of death. Because mental peace may be disturbed by the dying patient seeing/hearing open expressions of grief by family members, those family members who cannot remain calm may leave the room until composure can be regained. Calmness of family and relatives is seen as a symbol of "letting go" of the dying person.[18,19,20,21]

- Last rites given by a Buddhist priest may be desired at the time of death. The family may request that the body be left undisturbed and in quietness for several hours since only the person's body has died. Some level of 'consciousness' is believed to still exist as the deceased person's soul passes through the several stages of afterlife (*bardos*) to final reincarnation. Explore preferences with family prior to handling and removing the body.[22] The deceased may be cremated or buried.

- **Elective Pregnancy Termination**: Possibly acceptable based upon the situation.[18]
- **Autopsy**: Acceptable
- **Organ Donation**: Individual choice

Other Considerations

- **Pain**: Individuals may be reserved in requesting analgesics that are likely to decrease clarity of the mind. Chanting and medication may be used as a method of pain control. Offer pain medications and collaborate with the physician or pain management team regarding the use of pain medications that are least likely to affect clarity.[19]
- In most Buddhist homes, a statue of a Buddha will be found. Some homes also have shrines in a separate room for worship purposes.[18]

---

[1] Overmyer, D. (1986). *Religions of China*. New York, NY: HarperCollins Publishers.

[2] Littleton, C. (1996). *The sacred East: Hinduism, Buddhism, Confucianism, Daoism, Shinto*. London, England: Duncan Baird Publishers.

[3] Green, J. (1989). Death with dignity: Buddhism. *Nursing Times, 85*(9), 40-41.

[4] Pollock, R. (2001). *The everything world's religions book*. Avon, MA: Adams Media Corporation.

[5] Meredith, S. & Hickman, C. (2001). *The Usborne Internet-linked encyclopedia of world religions*. London, England: Usborne Publishing, Ltd.

[6] Buddhism. (2013). Retrieved from http://buddhism.about.com/

[7] Toropov, B. & Buckles, L. (2011). *The complete idiot's guide to the world's religions* (4th ed.). New York: Alpha Books.

[8] Burke, T. (1996). *The major religions: An introduction with texts*. Cambridge, England: Blackwell Publishers.

[9] Smith, H. & Novak, P. (2003). *Buddhism: A concise introduction*. New York, NY: HarperCollins Publishers.

[10] Das, S. (1997). *Awakening the Buddha within*. New York, NY: Broadway Books.

[11] CIA World Factbook. (2012). *World: People and society*. Retrieved from https://www.cia.gov/library/publications/the-world-factbook/geos/xx.html

[12] Matlins, M. & Magida, A. (2003). *How to be a perfect stranger: A guide to etiquette in other people's religious ceremonies*. Woodstock, VT: Skylight Paths Publishing

[13] Goring, R. & Whaling, F. (Eds.). (1994). *Larousse dictionary of beliefs and religions*. New York, NY: Larousse Kingfisher Chambers, Inc.

[14] Fenton, J., Norvin, H., Reynolds, F., Miller, A., Nielsen, N., Burford, G. & Forman, R. (1993). *Religions of Asia* (3rd ed.). New York, NY: St. Martin's Press.

[15] Warrier, S. & Walshe, J. (2001). *Dates and meanings of religious and other multi-ethnic festivals: 2002–2005*. New York, NY: Foulsham Educational.

[16] Andrews, M. & Boyle, J. (2012). *Transcultural concepts in nursing care* (6th ed.). Philadelphia, PA: Lippincott Williams & Wilkins.

[17] Kongsuwan, W., Keller, K., Touhy, T. & Schoenhofer, S. (2010). Thai Buddhist intensive care unit nurses' perspective of a peaceful death: An empirical study. *International Journal of Palliative Nursing, 16*(5), 241-247.

[18] Keene, M. (1993). *Seekers after truth: Hinduism, Buddhism, Sikhism.* Great Britain: Cambridge University Press.

[19] Wilkins, A., Mailoo, V. J. & Kularatne, U. (2010). Care of the older person: A Buddhist perspective. *Nursing and Residential Care, (12)*, 295-297.

[20] Shubha, R. (2007). End-of-life care in the Indian context: The need for cultural sensitivity. *Indian Journal of Palliative Care, 13*(2), 59-64.

[21] Wada, K. & Park, J. (2009). Integrating Buddhist psychology into grief counseling. *Death Studies, 33*(7), 657-683.

[22] Morrisey, B. (2010, September 14). *Buddhist funeral rites.* Retrieved from http://www.facingbereavement.co.uk/buddhist-funeral-rites.html

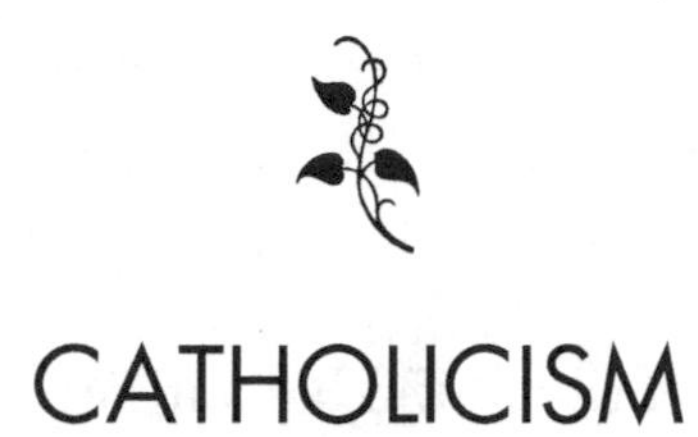

CATHOLICISM

Background

The Roman Catholic Church is one of three major branches of Christianity. The original Christian Church began approximately two thousand years ago in Palestine. Early Christians believed that even though Christ had left the earth (after His crucifixion), He was continuing His mission through a new physical body of which He remained the head. The Holy Spirit was the soul of the Church.[1]

The message of Christianity was carried to places such as Greece and Rome. With the Roman Conquest of the Greek East, a firm Graeco-Roman civilization was formed. The Roman Empire was eventually divided and essentially had two capitals; one located in Greece (the East) and one located in Rome (the West).[2] However, the Church essentially remained one body until 1054, when it split into the Orthodox Church in the East and the Roman Catholic Church in the West. The reasons for the split are complex, but they include geography, culture, language, politics, and religious issues.[1]

The Roman Catholic Church claims the apostle Peter as its first Pope after Christ selected him as the guardian of the keys of heaven and earth and as the chief apostle.[3] With this, St. Peter became the 'representative' or 'vicar' of Jesus here on earth. It is believed that the power of St. Peter is passed to each of his successors that assume the role of Bishop of Rome (the Pope).[4] As of 2013, there have been a total of 266 men to occupy this position.[5]

Roman Catholicism has the largest membership of all religions.[5] Approximately half of all Christians are Roman Catholics.[6]

Religious Representatives[3, 4, 7]

- **Pope** (the Bishop of Rome): He is supreme authority in all matters of faith and discipline.
- **Cardinal** (acts as advisor to the Pope): Heads or holds membership in various commissions that oversee the administration of the Church. Cardinals elect successors to the Pope and hold authority until the office is filled.
- **Archbishop**: A distinguished Bishop who has authority in an archdiocese (a large territory that is divided into dioceses).
- **Bishop**: Has authority in a diocese (district or territory) and is responsible for all regulations.
- **Priest**: (May be addressed as 'Father'): Celebrates Mass; administers sacraments with the exception of Confirmation and Holy Orders.
- **Deacon**: Distributes Holy Communion, baptizes, and can officiate at weddings.
- **Sister**: A Catholic woman who has taken religious vows and engages primarily in education, philanthropy, and charitable work.
- **Brother:** A Catholic man who has taken religious vows and engages primarily in education, philanthropy, and charitable work.

Religious Beliefs[1, 3, 8]

- The Holy Bible
- Acceptance of the Nicene Creed, the Apostles Creed, the Athanasian Creed, Creed of Pius IV.

- **The Holy Trinity:** There is one God, who has revealed Himself to mankind in three different ways: as God the Father, as Jesus Christ the Son, and as the Holy Spirit that continues God's work on earth.
- The Church is the teaching authority, the divinely appointed custodian of the Bible, and is the final authority on what is meant in any specific passage.
- The Church serves as a sacramental agent. It provides assistance and guidance for humans to live above human nature through providing the sacraments to accomplish this goal.
- The message of Christ is both a belief and a way of life.
- Special honor is given to the Virgin Mary because of her role as the mother of Jesus.

Special Religious Observations

- All Sundays observed as holy days.
- **January 1:** Solemnity of Mary, Mother of God.
- **Lenten Season:** Occurs in the spring of the year and is one of the most sacred periods of the Catholic liturgical year. For Catholics, it is a season for reflection, penitence, prayer, and rededication. The last week of the Lenten Season is called Holy Week and begins with Palm Sunday, the Sunday before Easter. The season covers forty days (Sundays are not included in the official forty days because they are always celebrated as holy days) and commemorates the forty day period of fasting and prayer by Jesus in the wilderness. The Season commences with Ash Wednesday and ends officially on Holy Thursday, the day before Good Friday. However, acts of penance and sacrifice are traditionally continued through Holy Saturday, the day following Good Friday and preceding Easter Sunday. On Ash Wednesday, some individuals attend religious services and their foreheads are marked with palm ash in the shape of a cross as a symbol of penance and a reminder of the mortality of man. If caring for the individual as a patient, the ash should not be removed, but allowed to wear off unless the patient/family deems otherwise. Various levels of fasting and sacrifice are practiced during the Lenten Season. Explore specific practices with the patient.

- **Ascension Thursday** (forty days after Easter): The Lord's Bodily Ascension into Heaven
- **August 15**: Feast of the Assumption
- **November 1**: All Saints Day
- **December 8**: Feast of the Immaculate Conception
- **December 25**: Christmas

Recognized sacraments (rites considered to have been established by Christ as a channel for grace):

- Baptism
- **Reconciliation**: Confession or Penance
- **Holy Communion**: Eucharist
- Confirmation
- Matrimony
- Holy Orders
- **Anointing of the Sick** (formerly *Extreme Unction*): During illness, the *Sacrament of the Sick* (formerly known as the Last Rites) is performed. It includes anointing of the sick, communion (if possible based on the sick individual's condition), and a blessing by a priest. May include prayers for the sick individual and members of the family. **A private, quiet, environment should be provided unless an emergency situation exists. An abbreviated form of the rite will be performed during emergency situations, which will not interfere with the necessary activities of health care personnel.**[9]

Health Beliefs/Practices

- God does not cause suffering, but allows suffering to exist for the potential of furthering human growth.[7]

- Fasting advocated for healthy individuals between the ages of 18 and 62 years old on *Ash Wednesday, Good Friday,* and the *Fridays of Lent.* Sick persons are not bound to this practice.

- Leave any items of religious significance in place. Remove them from the individual's body only if unavoidable since these items will bring comfort. Religious statues and other objects may be found in the home. Leave close to the individual.

- The Catholic Church subscribes to the *principle of totality* (medical treatments allowed as long as they are used for the good of the whole person).

- **Circumcision**: Permitted

- **Amniocentesis**: Permitted as long as it does not injure the fetus or is not used for the purpose of determining findings that persuade the couple in any way toward a decision to terminate a pregnancy.

- **Birth Control**: The church only supports abstinence, the temperature method, and the ovulation method as means of birth control. Hormonal treatments that prevent ovulation may be used to regulate the menstrual cycle.

- **Elective Pregnancy Termination**: Prohibited. Indirect pregnancy termination may be morally acceptable in some instances such as tubal pregnancy or removal of the uterus during pregnancy because of cancer.[10]

Death

- The soul is immortal; therefore, the deceased person does not cease to exist or lose identity. The dead will be resurrected.[11]
- Souls are detained in *Purgatory*, a condition of cleansing, transition, and adaptation before entering heaven. Individuals can pray for the welfare of souls in Purgatory.[4, 11]
- **Baptism**: Baptism is necessary for salvation. It is a serious matter for one to die without having been baptized. **During emergencies and in the absence of a priest, any baptized Christian may, and should, perform the baptism**. Any viable fetus should be baptized. If in doubt about the viability of a fetus, perform the baptism. It is not necessary to baptize non-viable fetuses or products of abortion unless requested by the family. The person performing the baptism should pour or sprinkle water (any available type) three times over the head of the individual while saying, "I baptize you in the name of the Father, and of the Son, and of the Holy Spirit." Notify the priest immediately after performing the baptism.[4, 12]
- **Autopsy:** Generally, acceptable
- **Organ Donation**: Permitted as long as the anticipated benefit to the recipient is proportionate to the harm done to the donor. The loss of the donor's organ should not deprive the donor of life itself or of the functional integrity of the body.[9]
- **Cremation**: Acceptable

---

1 Smith, H. (1991). *The world's religions: Our great wisdom traditions.* New York, NY: HarperCollins Publishers.

2 Smart, N. (1989). *The world's religions: Old traditions and modern transformations.* London, England: Cambridge University Press.

3 Mead, F., Hill, S., & Atwood, C.D. (2010). *Handbook of denominations in the United States.* (13th ed.). Nashville, TN: Abingdon Press.

4 McCollister, J. (1983). *The Christian book of why.* Middle Village, NY: Jonathan David Publishers, Inc.

5 *Catholic Encyclopedia.* (2013). Retrieved from http://www.newadvent.org/cathen/12272b.htm

6 Toropov, B. & Buckles, L. (2011). *The complete idiot's guide to the world's religions.* (4th ed.). New York: Alpha Books.

7 Cleary, R. (1998). Roman Catholicism. In C. Johnson and M. McGee (Eds.), *How different religions view death and afterlife* (pp. 193-204). Philadelphia, PA: The Charles Press, Publishers.

[8] Hendricks, D. (1975). What is a Catholic? In L. Rosten (Ed.)., *Religions in America* (pp. 39-67). New York, NY: Simon and Schuster.

[9] Andrews, M. & Boyle, J. (2012). *Transcultural concepts in nursing care* (6th ed.). Philadelphia, PA: Lippincott.

[10] Brannigan, M. & Boss, J. (2001). *Healthcare ethics in a diverse society.* Mountain View, CA: Mayfield Publishing Company.

[11] Johnson, K. (1994). *Why do Catholics do that? A guide to the teachings and practices of the Catholic Church.* New York: Ballantine Books.

[12] Carroll, P. & Shiraishi, C. (1995). The Catholic patient in the emergency department. *Journal of Emergency Nursing, 21*(6), 513-514.

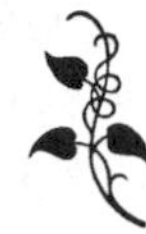

CHRISTIAN SCIENTISTS

Background

Christian Science is a religious system of therapy and metaphysics founded by Mary Baker Eddy (1821–1910). It is one of the few religious faiths to have its origins in the United States.[1, 2] *The Mother Church, The First Church of Christ, Scientist* is located in Boston, Massachusetts. In recent years, membership has continued on a downward spiral. There are no official membership statistics published by the Mother Church; however, worldwide membership is estimated at approximately 100,000 members in 1,600 congregations worldwide.[3, 4, 6]

Religious Representatives

- No specific religious titles are used. There is no clergy or priesthood. Religious services are conducted by Readers who read from the religious texts.[7]

Religious Beliefs

- **Religious Texts**: The Holy Bible, Science and Health with Key to the Scriptures by Mary Baker Eddy.[7] The Christian Science Hymnal is important in the life of a Christian Scientist since the words of the hymns are quite meaningful and comforting. During illness, the patient/family may want to sing or read from the Hymnal, as well as read from religious texts.

- God is viewed as the *Divine Principle*, *Mind*, *Soul*, *Spirit*, *Life*, *Truth*, and *Love*. He is superior to any other method of healing. Jesus is viewed as the ultimate Christian Scientist because He overcame sin, sickness, and death through his perception of the fullness of the Spirit and the nothingness of the body.

- Christian Science teaches that man was created in the image of God and must, therefore, be wholly spiritual. This spiritual man must be as incapable of evil as his Maker. Health, happiness, and wealth are the rewards for those that give up negative, limited thinking and accept their spiritual selfhood. It is believed that mind, not matter, constitutes what is real. Therefore, the body is a reflection of one's thoughts and is entirely 'mental' in nature. God is reflected in one's soul and there lies one's identity.[8] An individual's mind conceives and controls all things, including illness. 'Illness' is not real, only a perception of the Mortal Mind.[5,9]

- Health is not a physical condition, but a spiritual reality. True health is eternal. Disease is a delusion of the non-spiritual mind and can be overcome by prayer. Prayer is not focused on appealing to God for specific results. It is focused on bringing about thoughts that are in congruence with God's, the Divine Mind. Once an individual gains the knowledge and understanding that everything is God's reflection, illness and disease, manifestations of the physical and material world, cease to exist and are only illusions.[5,9,10,11]

Special/Religious Observations

- Church services are held on Sunday. Wednesday evenings are dedicated to gatherings of members to share their experiences with each other about the healing nature of Christian Science in their lives. There are no outward observances of sacraments.[5,7,11]

- There are no formal holy days or celebrations. Twice per year, during regular Sunday services, the congregation is invited to kneel to commemorate the joyous morning meal beside the Lake of Galilee that was attended by the risen Christ. Christmas and Easter are not observed.[2, 5]

Health Beliefs/Practices

- Illness has a mental origin; prayer is the antidote to any illness. Children who are ill are seen as cured by the parents bringing their own spiritual lives together through prayer. Healing practices are most often done in the home. When an individual experiences healing of an 'illness,' it is said that the individual has 'demonstrated' over the illness.[9, 11]

- The Church approves members as 'practitioners' after completing special training in prayer and consecration. They must demonstrate the ability to facilitate spiritual understanding in the destruction of human discord. These persons may be consulted when an individual's prayers have not produced improvements in an illness. The practitioner then offers prayer on behalf of the individual.[5, 10]

- Private Christian Science nursing homes are available to adult members. They are unlicensed by government agencies and accredited by the Commission for Accreditation of Christian Science Nursing Organizations & Facilities. Non-licensed 'nurses' provide basic care such as feeding, bathing, etc. They assist in providing an environment that decreases the likelihood of outside intrusions of the mind, thereby facilitating an environment for healing. No technology or medications are used. Training is not based on mainstream nursing curricula.[5, 10]

- Tobacco and alcohol are discouraged because they are seen as drugs.

- No dietary restrictions.

- Members are encouraged to obey all public health laws and to comply with compulsory immunization schedules. Members may use the services of physicians/midwives for delivering babies, dentists, and optometrists. Bones may be set by physicians, but treatment is generally limited to application of a cast rather than surgery. Pain medications may be used for the alleviation of severe pain.[5, 11, 12, 13]

- **Elective Pregnancy Termination**: Generally not acceptable.
- **Amniocentesis**: Not likely to seek this type of testing.
- **Birth Control**: No restrictions.[10]
- **Blood and Blood Products**: Generally not used. Likely to consent if needed for a child.
- **Circumcision**: Individual choice.
- **Organ Donation**: Not likely to act as donors.

Death

- Death is not God's will; God is life. Life is eternal, changeless, and spiritual. Therefore, death is an illusion of the Mortal Mind and must be opposed through prayer.[14]
- The words 'passed on' may be used instead of 'death' or 'died' because this event does not mark the termination of an individual's life. Death is seen as another phase of the belief that life is material. The immortal life lives on in a new state of consciousness.[10, 14]
- Outward signs of grief may be minimal.[5]
- **Autopsy**: Acceptable if required by law.
- Burial is based on individual preferences.

---

1 Simmons, J. (1995). Christian Science and American culture. In T. Miller (Ed.), *America's alternative religions* (pp. 61-68). Albany, NY: State University of New York Press.

2 Edwards, L. (2001). *Beliefs: A Brief guide to ideas, theologies, mysteries, and movements.* Louisville, KY: Westminster John Knox Press.

3 About the Church (2013). *The Christian Science Board of Directors.* Retrieved from http://christianscience.com/church-of-christ-scientist/about-the-church-of-christ-scientist

4 Paulson, M. (2009, January). *Church struggles to keep its voice: Christian Science refocuses mission. Boston Globe.* Retrieved from http://www.boston.com/news/local/massachusetts/articles/2009/01/05/church_struggles_to_keep_its_voice/

5 Fraser, C. (1999). *God's perfect child: Living and dying in the Christian Science Church.* New York, NY: Henry Holt and Company.

[6] Christian Way, Inc. (2004). *Questions about Christian Scientists.* Retrieved from http://www.christianway.org

[7] Robinson, B. (2007). *The Church of Christ, Scientist (Christian Science).* Retrieved from http://religioustolerance.org

[8] Hildner, J. (2008). Who am I? *The Christian Science Journal, 126*(2), 36-42.

[9] Corey, A. (1945). *Christian Science class instruction.* Santa Clarita, CA: The Bookmark.

[10] Stokes, J. (1975). What is a Christian Scientist? In L. Rosten (Ed.). *Religions of America* (pp. 69-81). New York, NY: Simon and Schuster.

[11] Schoepflin, R. (2003). *Christian Science on trial: Religious healing in America.* Baltimore, MD: The Johns Hopkins University Press.

[12] Gevits, N. (1991). Christian Science healing and the health care of children. *Perspectives in Biology and Medicine, 34*(3), 421-438.

[13] May, L. (1995). Challenging medical authority: The refusal of treatment by Christian Scientists. *Hastings Center Report, 25(*1), 15-21.

[14] Folis, E. (1991). Christian Science. In: *How different religions view death and afterlife* (2nd ed.). Johnson, C. & McGee, M. (Eds.), 64-75. Philadelphia, PA: Charles Press, Publishers.

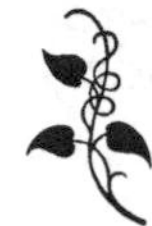

THE CHURCH OF JESUS CHRIST OF LATTER-DAY SAINTS

Commonly known as 'Latter-Day Saints (LDS)' or 'Mormons'

Many people erroneously refer to The Church of Jesus Christ of Latter-Day Saints and its members as the 'Mormon Church' or as 'Mormons'. These nicknames are associated with the church's belief in the "Book of Mormon." The word "Mormon" should only be used within the context of the Book of Mormon.[1]

Background

The Church of Jesus Christ of Latter-Day Saints was organized on April 6, 1830 in Fayette, New York by Joseph Smith, Jr.[2] The members of the church experienced hostility and persecutions throughout the years as they established new congregations and settlements. In 1847, the first wagons entered Salt Lake City, Utah, under the leadership of Brigham Young, who succeeded Joseph Smith, Jr. following his death in 1844.[3] Since that time, church growth has been phenomenal. As of the end of 2010, there were more than 28,600 congregations worldwide, with a membership in excess of fourteen million. The geographical base of the church is in Utah where approximately 60 percent of the population is Latter-Day Saints.[4]

Religious Representatives

- There is no professional clergy in the church. All members are given the opportunity to participate in accomplishing the church's needs. Any worthy practicing male may rise to the level of priesthood after the age of twelve.[5,6,7,8] There are two levels of priesthood:
  - **Aaronic** (also called Levitical): A preparatory priesthood. Adult men joining the church may be approved to enter the priesthood at this level.
    - **Deacon** (12 years of age and older): Serves in an auxiliary capacity to senior members.
    - **Teacher** (14 years of age and older): Serves in auxiliary capacity to senior members. Performs all deacon functions, prepares sacraments, and participates in home spiritual teaching sessions.
    - **Priest** (16 years of age and older): Assists elders, visits homes of members, teaches, baptizes, administers the sacrament, ordains deacons and teachers into the priesthood.
    - **Bishop:** Presides over a ward. May be designated to preside over the Aaronic priesthood in a ward.
  - **Melchizedek** (also called the Holy Priesthood after the Order of the Son of God).
    - **Elder** (18 years of age and older): Marks full adult status. Administers divine ordinances within the parameters defined by the organizational structure and discipline of the church. Gives blessings and prayers for healing.
    - **High Priest:** Generally middle aged, mature men, holding most of the leading office in the church.
    - **Patriarch:** Generally at least 55 years of age, married, and ordained High Priests who are authorized to provide special blessings to Church members.
    - **Seventy**: Generally middle-aged, mature men. They are elders who are called to be traveling missionaries.
    - **Apostle**: Married and granted the authority to perform all duties of the priesthood. They are seen as special witnesses of Jesus Christ worldwide.
- Membership is divided in 'wards' (approximately 200 to 1,800 members each. Several wards comprise a 'stake,' which is made up of approximately 2,000 to 10,000 members.

Stakes are presided over by a male whose title is *Stake President.* An *area* is the largest administrative unit of the Church as a whole.

- Additionally, there are several quorums in each of the priesthoods, comprised of persons at the same level of priesthood. Quorum membership is seen as a sacred honor. The Quorum of the Twelve Apostles is second in governing power in the Church, next to the First Presidency, the highest governing body. The First Presidency is also known as the Quorum of the Presidency and consists of the First President and his two counselors. The highest office in the church is the First President. The male holding the title of *First President* is considered a *Prophet* (**Thomas S. Monson** currently holds this office).[1,2,5,9]

- Women do not serve in the priesthood. However, they control the Relief Society, which has a structure similar to the priesthood. Its purpose is to assist the sick, the poor, and others who are in need of assistance.[1,5]

Religious Beliefs

- **The King James Bible**: Old and New Testaments.

- **The Book of Mormon** (another Testament of Jesus Christ): Revealed and translated from the original gold plates by Joseph Smith, Jr. It is used equally with the Bible and is seen as divinely inspired text.

- **The Doctrine and Covenants** (defines church beliefs): Contains later revelations from God recorded by Joseph Smith, Jr., Brigham Young, and other prophets.

- **The Pearl of Great Price**: Contains the *Thirteen Articles of Faith*, additional revelations from God, some revisions to the King James Bible.

- Other texts are used, but have not been deemed scriptures.

- The LDS Church is viewed as neither Catholic nor Protestant, but Christian. It is seen as a restoration of the original Church of Jesus Christ.[1]

- Belief is the *Godhead* comprised of three distinct, divine beings: *Elohim* (God the Father who is all-powerful, all-knowing, the ultimate authority, and the spiritual father of all mankind), *Jehovah* (Jesus), and the *Holy Ghost/Spirit*. Of the three divine beings, only the

Holy Ghost/Spirit has never existed as a physical body. Some of the functions of the Holy Ghost/Spirit include delivering comfort and peace to the troubled, bringing understanding through faith, and purifying the human heart.[5,10]

Special/Religious Observations

- In the United States, Sunday is recognized as the Sabbath. In other countries, the Sabbath may be recognized on a different day of the week.
- **Sacrament of the Lord's Supper**: Occurs weekly on Sundays.
- **Fasting Sunday**: Generally occurs on the first Sunday of the month. Members abstain from food and drink (including water) for two consecutive meals. Money that would have been spent for these two meals is donated to the church for the care of the needy.[1,11] Children and persons who are ill or pregnant are not expected to fast.
- In addition to regular family devotionals, etc., Monday evenings are generally designated for *Family Home Evening*. It is a time for putting aside work and other activities to focus completely on family togetherness and spiritual enrichment.[12]
- **Blessing of Infants**: Generally occurs on the first Sunday of the month after a child is born. The child is named during this ceremony.
- **Blessing of the Sick**: May be given to sick members.
- **Baptism**: Generally occurs at the age of accountability (eight years of age).
- Special religious 'endowments' (sacred ordinances) occur only in temple ceremonies. After members have completed endowment ceremonies at the temple, the temple garments are given to the member and are generally worn next to the skin all of the time henceforth, with few exceptions.[2] The garments remind the wearer of the commitments that have been made to God. The garment is frequently two pieces in younger persons, resembling a T-shirt with knee-length bottoms. One-piece garments may be worn by older adults and resemble long underwear. The garments should be left in place if at all possible. They have sacred meaning and should be given to the family if necessary to be removed for medical treatment. Assure that the garments are not placed among facility laundry or separated from the patient and lost. Ask permission to remove for bathing. Fold and place in a clean bag. Assist with

putting on clean garments. Garments should never be placed on the floor or allowed to touch the floor, as this is considered disrespectful.[5,10]

- **July 24th**: Celebration of the religious heritage of the church's people. The celebrations may differ based on locale.[9]
- **General Conferences**: Occurs in April and October each year. Generally held on the first Saturday and Sunday of these months.
- The traditional holidays Easter, Thanksgiving, and Christmas are observed.

Health Beliefs

- Dietary habits are based on the *Word of Wisdom*, which contains a health code revealed to Joseph Smith, Jr. The body should be kept pure mentally, physically, and spiritually as it is considered sacred, the spirit's tabernacle. Coffee, tea, alcoholic beverages, tobacco, illegal drugs, and/or overuse of prescription drugs are prohibited. Herbal supplements may be used. Explore what supplements are used and for what purpose.[11,13]
- When sick, members are likely to receive anointing, blessings, and laying-on of hands from religious leaders. Generally, a small amount of consecrated olive oil is used for these purposes. Requests may also be made for anointing and blessing prior to surgery or before CPR is discontinued. Provide privacy.[10]
- Members are encouraged to seek medical treatment from competent health care providers. Likely to comply with medical appointments and to have regular medical checkups that lead to early detection of illness and disease.
- **Blood/Blood Products**: Acceptable

Male-Female/Kinship/Social Relationships

- Very family-oriented. Modesty is valued. Tend to have larger families, which include many extended family members. Expect large numbers of visitors, including religious leaders and church members during hospitalizations.[10]

- Motherhood is considered the highest calling for women. Fathers are considered the head of the household and are the ultimate decision-makers. However, men and women are considered equal in God's eyes. It is considered a sacred duty for spouses to care for each other and for their children. Health care decisions will be made jointly.[5,14,15]

- Young persons of the church, especially males, often serve two-year terms as missionaries for the church, live together, and are instructed to stay together at all times. When in health care facilities, allow to stay together if at all possible. During emergency situations, the 'mission president' should be notified.[10]

- Family relations can continue through eternity, if an individual is deemed worthy. Spouses and children can be 'sealed' through special temple covenants so that their relationships are eternally connected.[1,12]

Birth/Children

- Childbirth is often seen as a spiritual experience. Each child is viewed as a blessing from God. Children are believed to live with the Heavenly Father in a pre-mortal existence prior to birth. Every person is born to receive his or her physical body, gain experiences, and live in such a way that they will be worthy to return to live again with God.[3,5,12,16,17]

- Likely to obtain prenatal care to provide optimal care for the unborn child. Parents are likely to be extremely distraught if a spontaneous abortion or perinatal loss occurs.

- Labor is seen as a natural process, occurring at nine months gestation. May prefer an obstetrician of the same faith.[14]

- Husband likely to want to remain with the wife during labor. Blessings may be offered to the mother by her husband if he is a member of the priesthood. Parents may want their children, if any, to be present during the delivery.[14,16]

- A birth blessing given by the child's father shortly after birth and naming of the infant may be desired if the baby is premature or sick. This provides comfort for the family, allows the infant to be recognized as an official member of the family, and is an acknowledgement of God. Additional blessings may be offered while the infant is in the hospital.[14]

- **Breastfeeding**: Strongly supported.

- **Circumcision**: Acceptable.
- **Postpartum Period of Confinement**: Six weeks to six months. Parents are generally well supported by family and church members.
- **Corporal Punishment of Children**: Not supported.
- **Birth Control**: Personal choice, but procreation is strongly supported by the church.
- Families may be very distressed if pregnancy occurs outside of wedlock. The infant is likely to be placed for adoption if marriage does not occur. Unmarried mothers may need strong support because of extreme grief.[14]
- **Amniocentesis**: No restrictions. However, if genetic defects are detected, elective pregnancy termination will be refused unless the mother's life is in danger.
- **Artificial Insemination/In-Vitro Fertilization**: Acceptable, if the sperm is from the husband or egg is from the wife. Artificial insemination of unmarried women is not supported.[11]
- **Elective Pregnancy Termination**: Opposed except in cases of rape, incest, or danger to the health of the mother.

Dietary Considerations

- May limit intake of meats. Generally, a healthy diet is consumed as the body is believed to be the temple of God.[5]
- Drinks containing caffeine are refused by most. Herbal teas may be acceptable. Alcoholic beverages are not permitted.

Death

- Members are encouraged to look upon death as a blessing and a part of eternal existence in another world.[10, 12]

- No baptism is required at the time immediately preceding death. At the time of death, the spirit leaves the body, goes to a spirit world, and awaits resurrection and judgment. The spirit world is a place of joy and peace. Intellect, consciousness, affection, and the ability to be receptive to truth continue into the next world. One can continue to grow in one of three levels of the spiritual kingdom of glory: the *telestial* kingdom, the *terrestrial* kingdom, and the *celestial* kingdom, where individuals receive the fullness of God's glory. Persons who do not know Christ can learn about Him while in these spiritual kingdoms. Those individuals who have willfully chosen to sin against God and defy faith are doomed to become *sons of perdition* and live in darkness forever.[12, 18]

- Persons who die before the age of eight immediately return to God.

- **Prolongation of Life**: Discouraged when death is inevitable.

- **Suicide**: The fate of the person can only be judged by God.

- **Organ Transplants/Donations**: Individual choice.

- **Autopsy**: Acceptable if supported by the family.

- **Cremation**: Not encouraged, but not prohibited.

---

1 Intellectual Reserve, Inc. (2010). The Church of Jesus Christ of Latter-Day Saints: Mormon: *The people, the Church, the prophet*. Retrieved from http://classic.lds.org/topic/mormon

2 O'Dea, T. (1957). *The Mormons*. Chicago, IL: The University of Chicago Press.

3 Brown, K., Cannon, D., & Jackson, R. (1994). *Historical atlas of Mormonism*. New York, NY: Simon & Schuster, Inc.

4 Temples of the Church of Jesus Christ of Latter-Day Saints: Statistics. (2012). Retrieved from http://www.ldschurchtemples.com/statistics/

5 Williams, D. (2003). *The idiot's guide to understanding Mormonism*. New York, NY: Alpha Books.

6 Evans, R. (1975). What is a Mormon? In L. Rosten (Ed.). *Religions of America* (pp. 186-199). New York, NY: Simon & Schuster.

7 Bushman, R. (1984). *Joseph Smith and the beginnings of Mormonism*. Chicago, IL: University of Illinois Press.

8 Ostling, R. & Ostling, J. (1999). *Mormon America: The power and the promise*. HarperCollins Publishers: New York, NY.

9 Shipps, J. (1985). *Mormonism: The story of a new religious tradition*. Chicago, IL: University of Illinois Press.

10 Mullen, R. (1966). *The Latter-Day Saints: The Mormons yesterday and today*. Garden City, NY: Doubleday & Company, Inc.

[11] Andrews, M. & Boyles, J. (2012). *Transcultural concepts in nursing care* (6th ed.). Philadelphia, PA: Lippincott Williams & Wilkins.

[12] Millet, R. (1998). *The Mormon faith: A new look at Christianity.* Salt Lake City, UT: Deseret Book Company.

[13] Cramer, C. & Cramer, A.A. (1995). Caring for the Latter-Day Saint patient. *Journal of Emergency Nursing, 21*(6), 503-504.

[14] Conley, L. (1990). Childbearing and childrearing practices in Mormonism. *Neonatal Network, 9*(2), 41-48.

[15] Shah, M. (2004). *Transcultural aspects of perinatal health care: A resource guide.* Binghamton, NY: National Perinatal Association.

[16] Callister, L., Semenic, S., & Foster, J. (1999). Cultural and spiritual meanings of childbirth: Orthodox Jewish and Mormon women. *Journal of Holistic Nursing, 17*(3), 280-295.

[17] Marshall, E., Olsen, S., Mandleco, B., Dyches, T., Allred, K., & Sansom, N. (2003). "This is a spiritual experience: Perspectives of Latter-Day Saint families living with a child with disabilities. *Qualitative Health Research, 13*(1), 57-76.

[18] Eyre, R. (1991). The Church of Jesus Christ of Latter-Day Saints. In C. Johnson and McGee (Eds.). *How different religious view death and afterlife* (pp. 129-155). Philadelphia, PA: The Charles Publishers.

EASTERN ORTHODOXY

Background

Eastern Orthodoxy is one of three major branches of Christianity. The original Christian Church began approximately two thousand years ago in Palestine. Early Christians believed that even though Christ had left the earth (after His crucifixion), He was continuing His mission through a new physical body—the Church—of which He remained the head. The Holy Spirit was the soul of the Church.[1]

The message of Christianity was carried to places such as Greece and Rome. With the Roman Conquest of the Greek East, a firm Graeco-Roman civilization was formed. The Roman Empire was eventually divided and essentially had two capitals – one located in Greece (the East) and one located in Rome (the West).[1]

The term 'Orthodox' was created from two Greek words—*orthos*, meaning "rightly or correct" and *doxa*, meaning "belief." Hence, Orthodox Christians see themselves as those who "rightly believe in God" or as those who have the "right belief." Orthodox members often point out three distinctive characteristics of their church: "its changelessness, its determination to remain loyal to the past, and its sense of living continuity with the ancient church manifested in faith and worship."[2]

Eastern Orthodox Churches are self-governing and are classified as either autocephalous or autonomous. Autocephalous Churches have a full governing hierarchy including a Church head who does not report to any other higher Church authority. Autonomous Churches are self-governing, but the Church head is determined by the Mother Church. Worldwide, there are more than three hundred million members of the various autocephalous and autonomous Orthodox Churches in countries including, but not limited to: Greece, Russia, Albania, Romania, Bulgaria, Finland, Poland, Serbia, Georgia, Japan, and North America. All churches with the term 'Orthodox' in the name are not a part of Eastern Orthodoxy. Churches based on Eastern Orthodoxy in various countries agree on religious doctrines even though language and culture varies. In the United States and Canada, the Greek Orthodox Church has the largest membership.[3,4,5,6,7,8]

Religious Representatives[2,5,9]

- **Patriarch/Archbishop**: President of a synod (ecclesiastical council) of bishops.
- **Bishop**: Has received the highest of sacred orders. Two or three other bishops ordain new bishops. A bishop is considered a successor to the Apostles. Generally, a bishop is the leader of a diocese (district).
- **Priest**: Leader of an Orthodox Church whose responsibilities include conducting services, administering sacraments and other activities related to the preservation of the faith.
- **Deacon**: Assists the bishop and/or priest with church services and ministries. Deacons do not perform sacraments.

Religious Beliefs[2,10,11]

- Sunday is generally the day of worship. However, the Sabbath or feast day begins at sundown the night before.
- **The Holy Bible**: The Greek translation of the Old Testament is used (the Septuagint).

- **Holy Tradition**: Refers to the entire systems of doctrine, church government, art, and worship that have been passed down from the ancient church. It includes the following:
  - Books of the Bible.
  - The Nicene Creed.
  - The decrees of the Ecumenical Councils.
  - Writings of the Fathers (those great religious masters in Christian instruction who transmitted and disseminated the right doctrine and teachings of the Apostles).
  - The Canons (define church organization, sacramental and disciplinary practices).
  - The Service Books (contain the hymns and services of the Orthodox Church).
  - The Holy Icons (sacred images of extraordinary religious persons who have achieved divinity through grace). Frequently, icons are images of persons who have achieved sainthood, but may also be representations of other religious persons or events such as the Virgin Mary or the Nativity. Icons are not worshipped in the Orthodox Church, but they are honored, treated with reverence, and seen as windows into the spiritual world. Icons serve as models for persons to imitate and reveal heavenly possibilities for those who view them. Icons are produced within very formal rules of composition and are produced by persons known as iconographers. Iconographers are pious persons that have been trained by holy fathers; therefore, traditionally, iconographers are often monks or nuns.
- **The Holy Trinity**: There is one God, who has revealed Himself to mankind in three different ways – as God the Father, as Jesus Christ the Son, and as the Holy Spirit that continues God's work on earth.[3]
- The human person is composed of three inseparable elements: the body, the soul, and the spirit. The body is the physical aspect, the soul gives life to the physical body, and the spirit is the 'breath' from God.[12]
- Special honor is given to the Blessed Virgin Mary for her position as the Mother of God (also called *Theotokos*, *Aeiparthenos* (Ever Virgin), and *Panagia* (All Holy).[2]

Special Celebrations/Religious Observations

- A number of sacraments (rites considered to have been established by Christ as a channel for grace) are recognized in the Orthodox Church. All are not equal in importance. Some of the more frequently practiced sacraments include:
  - **Baptism** (by immersion unless the person is too ill to tolerate immersion).
  - **Chrismation** (Confirmation): Involves baptism of a child, anointing with holy oil, and the Eucharist.
  - **Holy Eucharist** (Holy Communion): The most important sacrament.
  - **Repentance** (Confession): There are two types in the Orthodox Church—private confession by prayer and sacramental confession (before a priest).
  - **Ordination.**
  - **Marriage** (Holy Matrimony).
  - **Holy Unction:** Consists of anointment of various parts of the body with special sanctified oil. The sacrament may be administered to any baptized person, can be repeated, and is generally administered to those who are sick with the hope of assisting with healing. Unlike the Roman Catholic Church, the Orthodox Church does not have a sacrament that is administered specifically during extreme crisis or when one is dying.[7, 10]
- Some Orthodox Churches use both the Julian and Gregorian calendars. The Julian calendar is thirteen days behind the Gregorian calendar, so celebration dates may be different based on which calendar is followed. The church liturgical calendar begins on September 1st.
- **Easter** (Pascha): The most important celebration in the Orthodox Church.
- **Twelve Great Feasts**: Some dates are movable based on the date of Easter. The purpose of these feasts is to move Orthodox members toward greater devotion and commitment to the Lord.
- The feasts are divided into two groups: *The Feasts of the Mother of God* and *The Feasts of Our Lord*.[13]

The Feasts of the Mother of God

- The Birth of the Theotokos (Virgin Mary) – September 8th.
- The Entry of the Theotokus into the Temple – November 21st.
- The Meeting of Our Lord (The Presentation of Christ in the Temple) – February 2nd.
- The Annunciation (The announcement of the conception of Christ) – March 25th.
- The Dormition of the Theotokos (The Repose of the Virgin Mary) – August 15th.

The Feasts of Our Lord

- The Exaltation of the Cross (The Elevation of the Life-Giving Cross) – September 14th.
- Christmas – December 25th.
- Theophany (Commemorates the manifestation of Christ to the Gentiles in Magi) – January 6th.
- Palm Sunday – One week before Easter.
- The Ascension of Our Lord – Forty days after Easter.
- Pentecost – Fifty days after Easter.
- The Transfiguration of Our Lord – August 6th.

Health Beliefs

- There is a special devotion to the Saint whose name one receives at baptism. Icons of the Saint may be found in the home or room and provide special comfort for the person who is ill. Daily morning and evening prayers may be recited before the icons. Often, persons will face the East during prayer since it is believed that Christ will come again from the East.[2, 11]

- The body and the soul are of equal importance. God and the physician are perceived as healers and not in conflict with each other.[14]

- Caring for the body and preventive care is a Christian responsibility.

- Sickness is an evil to overcome. It can be seen as an opportunity for growth in the real purpose of life and is to be faced with courage and fortitude. Suffering in some form is inevitably a part of everyone's life.[14]

- May be stoic in the face of pain and discomfort. Offer pain medication even if the patient does not ask.

Kinship/Social Factors

- Individuals are viewed as a part of the larger family of the church.

- Christians have an obligation to visit and care for those who are ill.

Birth/Children

- The birth of a child is viewed as a blessing.

- Some mothers may practice a lying-in period of forty days during which she is to rest and recover from birth. Relatives and friends assist in caring for the mother.[14]

- Pre-baptismal prayers or short services may be offered on the first day after birth, the eighth day and the 40th day. The *Forty-Day Blessing* (churching) involves a brief service of purification and formally brings the baby into the church. Among some Orthodox, this is the first time that the mother and baby are allowed to enter the church after birth.[11]

- At baptism, infants are often given the name of a Saint. This serves as a symbol of entry into the unity of the earthly and heavenly Church. The Saint is viewed as a role model and protector of life.[2, 11]

- **Amniocentesis**: Acceptable.

- **Circumcision**: Acceptable.
- **Elective Pregnancy Termination**: Not permitted unless the mother's life is endangered.[15]
- **Birth Control**: Acceptable.

Dietary Considerations

- Fasting is practiced as a method of disciplining the body and overcoming passions. Some of the major fasting periods are:[11, 13, 16]
  - Each Wednesday and Friday throughout the year, in memory of the betrayal and crucifixion of the Lord, respectively, except during Easter and Pentecost week and between Christmas and Epiphany.
  - **The Christmas Fast** (Forty Days): November 15th to December 24th.
  - **Great Feast of Lent:** Begins seven weeks before Easter.
  - **Holy Apostles Lent:** Monday after the week following Pentecost through June 28th.
  - **Fast before the Transfiguration of Christ:** August 1st through August 6th.
  - **Fast before the Feast of the Dormition of the Theotokos:** August 7th through August 15th.
  - **Fast on the Exaltation of the Holy Cross:** September 14th.
  - **The Beheading of St. John the Baptist:** August 29th.
  - **The Eve of the Epiphany:** January 5th.
- There are various levels of fasting in the Orthodox Church. Ask specifically about fasting practices to determine appropriate treatment regimens.[14]
  - **Severe fasting:** Complete avoidance of all food. Has been abandoned among most Orthodox adherents, with the exception of the period of midnight to the reception of the Holy Communion.

- **Strict fasting:** Also called "dry eating" – shellfish, fruit, vegetables, bread, legumes, vegetable oil/margarine are permitted.
- **Moderate fasting:** Some foods, particularly meat, are given up.

- Pregnant women, those giving birth during fasting periods, the very young, and the elderly are not required to fast.

Death

- The priest should be called if death is imminent. Holy Communion may be administered if the person is conscious. If the person is unconscious, the priest may anoint the person.[14]
- The soul does not sleep after death, only the body. Orthodox adherents believe that immediately after death, one is judged and experiences a 'foretaste' of heaven or hell (called Particular or Intermediate Judgment). The state of the soul during the period of Particular or Intermediate Judgment is fixed and unchangeable. There can be no repentance after death. At the Second Coming of Christ, the individual will experience punishment or reward in its fullness forever.[5,9,13]
- **Preparation of the Body**: Immediately following death, some Orthodox may want to prepare the body of the deceased by performing a ritual wash and dressing the person in a white shroud known as a savanon.[14] Provide privacy and adequate time for preparation.
- **Euthanasia**: Not permitted.
- **Suicide**: Prevents a church funeral unless there is medical documentation of psychological problems that contributed to the suicide.[17]
- **Organ Donation/Transplants**: Acceptable.
- **Autopsy**: Acceptable.
- **Disposition of the Body**: Cremation is forbidden because it prevents the resurrection.[17]
- Burial does not have to occur within twenty-four hours.

- The period of mourning is forty days. Memorial services are conducted at forty days, six months, and one year after death.

Other Considerations

- **Baptism**: Generally, a priest performs baptism. However, during emergencies, baptism may be performed by a deacon or any baptized Christian man or woman.[2]

- **Blood Transfusions**: Permitted.

---

1 Smith, H. (1991). *The world's religions: Our great wisdom traditions.* New York, NY: HarperCollins Publishers.

2 Ware, T. (1993). *The Orthodox Church.* New York, NY: Penguin Books.

3 Keene, M. (1993). *Believers in one God: Judaism, Christianity, Islam.* Great Britain: Cambridge University Press.

4 Mead, F. & Hill, S., & Atwood, C.D. (2010). *Handbook of denominations in the United States* (13th ed.). Nashville, TN: Abingdon Press.

5 Matlins, S. & Magida, A. (2010). *How to be a perfect stranger* (3rd ed.). Skylight Paths Publishing: Woodstock: VT.

6 Edwards, L. (2001). *A brief guide to beliefs: Ideas, theologies, mysteries, and movements.* Westminster John Knox Press: Louisville.

7 BBC Religions. (2013). *Eastern Orthodox Church.* Retrieved from http://www.bbc.co.uk/religion/religions/christianity/subdivisions/easternorthodox_1.shtml

8 Kindatch, A. (2010). *Results of 2010 census of Orthodox Christian Churches in the USA.* Retrieved from http://www.hartfordinstitute.org/research/orthodoxindex.html

9 Pollock, R. (2002). *The everything world's religions book.* Adams Media Corporation: Avon, MA.

10 Clendenin, D. (1995). *Handbook of denominations in the United States* (10th ed.). Nashville, TN: Abingdon Press.

11 Rouvelas, M. (1993). *A guide to Greek traditions and customs in America.* Bethesda, MD: Nea Attiki Press.

12 Ware, K. (1996). *The Orthodox way.* New York, NY: St. Vladimir's Seminary Press.

13 Coniaris, A. (1982). *Introducing the Orthodox Church: Its faith and life.* Minneapolis, MN: Light and Life Publishing Company.

14 Harakas, S. (1996). *Health and medicine in the Eastern Orthodox Tradition.* Minneapolis, MN: Light and Life Publishing Company.

15 Constantelos, D. (1990). *Understanding the Greek Orthodox Church: Its faith, history and practice.* Brookline, MA: Hellenic College Press.

[16] Lazarou, C. & Matalas, A. (2010). A critical review of current evidence, perspectives, and research implications of diet-related traditions of the Eastern Christian Orthodox Church on dietary intakes and health consequences. *International Journal of Food Sciences and Nutrition, 61*(7), 739-758.

[17] Harakas, S. (1988). *The Orthodox Church: 455 questions and answers.* Minneapolis, MN: Light and Life Publishing Company.

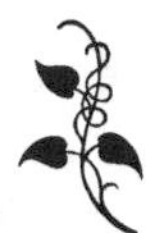

FOLK AND HERBAL TREATMENTS

There are thousands of folk and herbal treatments. This information is not intended for use as medical advice for the treatment of any disorder. Health care providers should consistently assess the use of folk and herbal treatments with patients and how the treatment plan will be impacted by continued use. Appropriate members of the treatment team should be alerted and consulted as appropriate. A number of resources are available to health care providers for more comprehensive reference information.

Treatment	Common Medicinal Uses
Aloe Vera (*Savila* - Spanish)	**Internally**: Laxative, asthma, diabetes. **Topically**: Burns, cuts, abrasions. **Precautions**: Aloe taken internally is thought to lower blood sugar. May stimulate uterine contractions.
Alum Powder	**Externally**: Reduction of swelling in gums, bleeding gums.
Anise (*Yerba aniz* - Spanish)	**Internally**: *Susto*, laxative, digestive problems, colic, sedative, expectorant, promotion of lactation. **Precautions**: Caution use during pregnancy. Larger doses may interfere with effectiveness of birth control pills, anticoagulants, and MAOI therapy.

Treatment	Common Medicinal Uses
Apple Cider Vinegar	**Internally**: Hypertension, weight loss, headache. **Topically**: Skin irritations, sprains.
Asafetida	**Internally**: "Heart trouble," coughs, asthma, bronchitis. Dissolved in liquor–few drops diluted in sugar water to relieve colic in babies. **Other**: Small piece hung around children's necks to keep away colds.
Baking Soda	**Internally**: Indigestion. **Topically**: Burns.
Basil (*albacar* - Spanish)	**Internally**: Tea–*susto*, insomnia, promotion of menstruation, infections. **Other**: Used to ward off evil spirits. **Precautions**: Caution use during pregnancy; caution use in diabetics–may lower blood sugar.
Blackberry	**Internally**: Tea–diarrhea; Juice–mouth sores, coughs, indigestion.
Black Cohosh	**Internally**: Menopause symptoms, PMS, dysmenorrhea, arthritis, osteoporosis, sore throat, sedative. **Topically**: Rattlesnake bites. **Precautions**: Large doses may cause miscarriage/premature birth. Should be discontinued at least two weeks prior to surgery because of hypotensive reactions to anesthetics. May lower blood pressure. Monitor patients closely taking anti-hypertensive drugs.
Black Salve/Ointment (Ichthammol Ointment)	**Topically**: Applied to draw splinters to the skin surface, bee stings, insect bites, boils. **Precautions**: Not for ingestion.

Treatment	Common Medicinal Uses
Boric Acid Powder (dissolved in water)	The eye is "bathed" and some of the solution is placed in the eye for treatment of eye infections, eye irritations, styes.
Buttermilk	**Topically**: Skin ailments.
Cabbage (green)	**Topically**: Raw leaves applied for painful joints, breast engorgement. **Internally**: Juice taken for gastric ulcers, constipation.
Camphor Block	**Internally**: Dissolved in liquor–upset stomach, stomach pain, and diarrhea.
Camphorated Oil (rubbed on the chest and back)	Chest colds and/or congestion.
Castor Oil	Dryness of hair, breaking hair. Drops are used in the eyes for eye irritations. Soreness, general healing after having a baby, laxative, wart removal. Applied to umbilical cords to promote healing.
Catnip	**Internally**: Tea–given to infants for "hives"
Cayenne Pepper	Mixed with vinegar–circulation problems, stiffness
Chamomile (*manzanilla* - Spanish)	**Internally**: Tea–upset stomachs, diarrhea, and eye irritations, insomnia, *susto.*
Cinnamon	Type 2 Diabetes, rheumatism, GI problems, cholesterol management. **Caution**: May cause skin irritation in some individuals.
Cobwebs	**Topically**: To stop bleeding of wounds.
Cod Liver Oil	Colds, prevention of colds.
Copper Bracelets/ Bands	Rheumatism, arthritis.

Treatment	Common Medicinal Uses
Corn Silk	**Internally**: Tea–urinary disorders, diuretic, diabetes, hypertension. **Precautions**: Diuretic effects may lead to hypokalemia, reduced blood glucose levels, and interference with anticoagulation therapy.
Damiana	**Internally**: Menstrual cramps, chickenpox, headaches, bed-wetting, sexual problems. **Inhalation**: Leaves may be smoked to produce euphoria and relaxation. **Precautions**: May lower blood sugar.
Echinacea	**Internally**: Colds, boost immune system, infections. **Topically**: Burns, skin ulcers, eczema.
Epsom Salts	**Internally**: Laxative, gas. **Topically**: Dissolved in water–sore muscles, sprains.
Eucalyptus	**Internally**: Colds, asthma, bronchitis, tuberculosis. **Topically**: As a poultice for colds and coughs. **Precautions**: Children–Application of eucalyptus oil to a large area of a child's skin may cause toxicity, including seizures. Hypoglycemic properties.

Treatment	Common Medicinal Uses
Fenugreek	**Internally**: Gastric problems, loss of appetite, promotion of lactation, kidney problems, impotence. **Topically**: Mouth ulcers, inflammation, boils, cellulitis, leg ulcers, eczema. **Precautions**: Lowers blood sugar, anticoagulant properties. Ingestion causes odor similar to maple syrup in some individuals. The newborns of women who have ingested fenugreek close to delivery may have an odor similar to maple syrup sometimes leading health care providers to suspect maple syrup disease.
Garlic (*ajo* - Spanish)	**Internally**: Antibiotic purposes, high blood pressure, digestive problems, insomnia. **Topically**: Earache, insect bites.
Ginger	**Internally**: Morning sickness, upset stomach, motion sickness, arthritis, diarrhea. **Topically**: Burns. **Precautions**: May increase insulin levels, anticoagulant effects in some individuals.
Ginkgo	**Internally**: Circulation problems, tinnitus, memory problems, PMS. **Topically**: Scabies, skin lesions. **Precautions**: Anticoagulant effects in some individuals. Ingestion of ginkgo seeds by children may cause seizures; in adults, ingestion of more than 8-10 seeds/day may lead to adverse effects, including seizures. Avoid using ginkgo when taking drugs that lower the seizure threshold; may antagonize the effects of anticonvulsants.

Treatment	Common Medicinal Uses
Ginseng (American)	**Internally**: Arthritis, back/leg pains, builds blood after childbirth, stress, increase stamina and concentration, relief of symptoms of aging. **Precautions**: Anti-hypertensive effects in some individuals, may lower blood sugar, may increase effects of caffeine and stimulant drugs, may interfere with anti-psychotic drugs, may decrease blood coagulation.
Ginseng (Panax)	**Internally**: Indigestion, vomiting in pregnancy, fever, expectorant, hot flashes, menstrual problems, stress, headaches, stimulation of immune system, improve concentration and memory, diuretic, anemia, diabetes, impotence, to slow the aging process. **Precautions**: May cause insomnia, may lower blood sugar, may interfere with platelet aggregation, may potentiate effects of caffeine and other stimulants.
Ginseng (Siberian)	**Internally**: Stress, blood pressure problems, insomnia, prevention of colds and flu. **Precautions**: May inhibit platelet aggregation. May have lower blood sugar: estrogenic effects.

Treatment	Common Medicinal Uses
Goldenseal	**Internally**: Infections, gallbladder problems, colds, build immune system, dysmenorrhea, diuretic. **Topically**: Used as a mouthwash for sore gums and mouth. Used topically for skin rashes/ulcers/infections, ringworm, herpes blisters. **Other**: Eyewash for eye infections and inflammation. Ear solution for tinnitus and earache. **Precautions**: May raise blood pressure in some individuals, contraindicated during pregnancy and lactation as a possible contributor to neonatal jaundice: may stimulate uterine contractions. May increase or interfere with effects of some cardiac drugs such as beta-blockers, calcium channel blockers, and Digoxin. May increase sedative effects of CNS depressants.
Honey	**Internally**: Insomnia, sore throats (taken with lemon), asthma, gastric ulcers, illness prevention. **Topically**: Burns, skin ulcers, wounds. **Precautions**: Contraindicated in children less than one year of age.
Kava Kava (Used ceremonially among some cultural groups—particularly among Pacific Islanders)	**Internally**: Anxiety, stress, insomnia, restlessness, migraines, UTI. **Topically**: Used as a mouthwash for toothache. Used for skin diseases and as an analgesic. **Precautions**: Sedative effect in some individuals, may interfere with cholesterol metabolism.
Kerosene / Coal Oil	**Internally**: Taken on sugar–chest colds/congestion, coughs. **Topically**: Placed directly on abrasions, cuts, insect bites, etc. to remove pain and discomfort. **Precautions: Highly flammable; can be toxic.**

Treatment	Common Medicinal Uses
Milkweed Juice	**Internally**: Arthritis, asthma, coughs. **Topically**: Warts. **Precautions**: Contains digitalis-type glycosides. Not to be taken internally with taking Digitalis.
Mugmort / Mexican Mugmort (*estafiate* – Spanish)	**Internally**: Colic, nausea, gas, seizures, stress. Caution use during pregnancy as it is believed to cause uterine contractions. **Topically**: Used in conjunction with moxibustion treatments. **Precautions**: Contraindicated during pregnancy since it is thought to cause uterine contractions. May interfere with effects of anticoagulants.
Nutmeg	**Internally**: Tea or powder dissolved in water – digestive disorders, incontinence, aphrodisiac, impotence, menstrual pain. **Topically**: Oil – muscular pain, toothache, rubbed on genitals as sexual stimulant. **Precautions**: Nutmeg contains the chemical, Myristica Fragrans. Large quantities can be toxic leading to hallucinations or even death. Is sometimes smoked or snorted for a hallucinogenic high.
Oil of Cloves	Toothache.
Onions	Prepared in various ways for infections, colds, and fever.
Orange Leaf Tea (*te de naranjo* – Spanish)	**Internally**: Tea–as a sedative, menstrual cramps, nervousness.
Oswego Tea (*oregano* – Spanish)	**Internally**: Tea–digestive orders, PMS, promotion of menstrual flow, colds, flu. **Precautions**: Caution use during pregnancy.
Peach Tree Leaves	Bruised and made into a poultice; placed on the forehead to reduce fever.

Treatment	Common Medicinal Uses
Peppermint Leaves	**Internally**: Tea–indigestion, colic, *susto*, dysmenorrheal.
Peppermint Oil	**Internally**: GI problems, respiratory problems, and nausea/ vomiting during pregnancy, dysmenorrheal. **Topically**: Headache, toothache, itching.
Pokeweed	**Internally**: Tea–for rheumatism and arthritis, laxative. **Topically**: Boiled–liquid used to bathe infected parts of the body. **Precautions**: All parts of the plant can be toxic when ingested raw. **Caution parents to keep all parts of the plant away from children.**
Potato	Made into a poultice–boils, carbuncles.
Rectified Turpentine (Several drops on sugar)	Chest colds/congestion, coughs.
Ruda (Spanish for *ruta graveolens* or *rue*) (Similar substances: Azarcon, Greta, Azoque, Maria Luisa)	**Topically**: Earache. **Internally**: Used internally to induce menstruation or abortion. Also used for upset stomach and postpartum pain, treatment of *empacho* in Mexico. **Precautions**: Highly toxic in large doses that may lead to liver and kidney damage. Especially toxic in children. Likely to contain lead.
Sage	**Internally**: Tea–colds, diabetes, sore throat, dysmenorrhea, diarrhea, digestive disorders. **Topically**: Bath–purification, skin problems, cold sores, gingivitis. **Precautions**: May cause uterine contractions, may decrease blood sugar levels.

Treatment	Common Medicinal Uses
Sloans Liniment	**Internally**: Several drops on sugar for flatus **Topically**: Muscle aches.
Soot	To stop bleeding of wounds.
Spearmint (*Yerba buena* - Spanish)	**Internally**: Colic, upset stomach, stomach cancer, intestinal parasites, menstrual cramps, nervousness, colds, sore throat. **Topically**: Arthritis, muscle pain, skin irritations.
St. John's Wort	**Internally**: Anxiety, depression, nervousness, cancer, heart palpitations. **Topically**: Oily preparations–burns, wounds, insect bites, warts, skin diseases, hemorrhoids. **Precautions**: May interfere with MAOI therapy.
Sweet Oil (several drops)	Earaches.
Tea Bag (wet)	Styles, eye infections, eye swelling. **Precautions**: Infections can be reintroduced into eye if tea bags are reused.
Tobacco / Snuff "juice"	Insect bites and stings
Toothpaste	Burns, acne.

Treatment	Common Medicinal Uses
Urine (human and certain animals)	Viewed as an antibacterial, antifungal, and antiviral. **Topically**: Earaches, sore throat, massaged for pain, skin moisturizer, wounds, skin disorders. **Internally**: Cancer, infections, fertility problems, diabetes.
Vapo-Rub Ointment	**Internally**: Small amount of the ointment is swallowed for colds and congestion. **Topically**: Chest and nose congestion, muscle pain, headache. **Inhalation**: Via vaporizer, rubbing on skin above upper lip.
Wormwood	**Internally**: Tea–intestinal worms, *empacho*, diarrhea, colic, gout, arthritis, stimulate menstruation. **Topically**: Wounds, insect bites. **Precautions**: Contraindicated during pregnancy and for individuals with gastric ulcers.

1 Spector, R. (2009). *Cultural diversity in health and illness* (7th ed.). Upper Saddle River, NJ: Pearson Prentice Hall.

2 Crellin, J. & Philpott, J. (1990). *Trying to give ease.* Durham, NC: Duke University Press.

3 Schirmer, G. (1998). Alternative medicine. Bedford, MA: Med 2000, Inc.

4 Thacker, E. (2012). *The vinegar book* II (2nd ed.).. Hartville, OH: James Direct, Inc.

5 Null, G. (1998). *Secrets of the White Buffalo: Native American healing remedies, rites and rituals.* Upper Saddle River, NJ: Prentice Hall.

6 Kloss, J. (1988). *Back to Eden* (2nd ed.). Loma Linda, CA: Back to Eden Books Publishing Company.

7 Higgs, R., Manning, A. & Miller, J. (1995). *Appalachia inside out: Culture and custom.* Knoxville, TN: The University of Tennessee Press.

8 Thompson, J. (2002). Cultural aspects of treating Mexican patients. *Clinician Reviews, 12*(5), 56-62.

9 Natural Medicines Comprehensive Database. (2013). Retrieved from http://www.naturaldatabase.com

10 Fetrow, C. & Avila, J. (2001). *Professional's handbook of complementary & alternative medicines* (2nd ed.). Springhouse, PA: Springhouse Corporation.

11 DerMarderosian, A. (Ed.). (1999). *A guide to popular natural products.* St. Louis, MO: Facts and Comparisons.

12 DeStefano, A. (2001). *Latino folk medicines.* New York, NY: Ballantine Books.

13 Fugh-Berman, A. (2003). *The 5-minute herb & dietary supplement consult.* Philadelphia, PA: Lippincott Williams & Wilkins.

[14] Abramson, R. & Haskell, J. (Eds.). (2006). *Encyclopedia of Appalachia*. Knoxville, TN: The University of Tennessee Press.

[15] Braunstein, M. (2010). *Urine therapy*. Retrieved from http://www.heartlandhealing.com/pages/archive/urine_therapy/index.html

[16] Dhama, K., Chauhan, R.S. & Lokesh, S. (2005). Anti-cancer activity of cow urine: Current status and future directions. *International Journal of Cow Science, 1*(2), 1-25.

[17] U.S. Food and Drug Administration. (2011, March 18). *Import alert 66-20: Azoque, greta, azarcon, and similar Mexican folk remedies*. Retrieved from http://www.accessdata.fda.gov/cms_ia/importalert_179.html

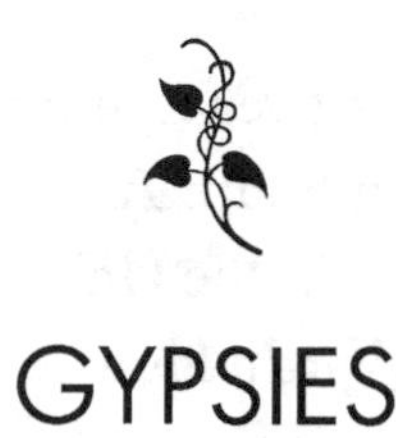

GYPSIES

"Also known as Rom, Roma, or Romani"

Although the term 'Gypsy' is often used in reference to members of this ethnic group, it is disliked by most persons within the group. The term *Rom* or *Roma* is acceptable by many groups. The term *Romani* is acceptable by all groups. Romani (plural *Romanies*) does not imply an origin from Romania. In the United Kingdom, the word *Travellers* is often used in reference to the Romani.

There are many divisions and subgroups among the Romani; specific cultural practices and beliefs will vary. Traditionally, Romani have lived mostly separate and apart from the larger society, associating with non-Romani only to the extent needed to sustain their lives. In some areas of the world, that isolation is slowly changing. Among larger subgroups in the United States are those whose origins are in England/Scotland (Romnichals), Eastern Europe (Rom who are further subdivided into Kalderesh, Machvaya, Lovari, Churari), Romania (Ludar), and Germany (Sinti).[1,2,3,4,5]

Background

Romanies originated in Northern India. After leaving India, the migrants divided into two groups and have since migrated to countries all over the world. The group that migrated south through Persia and Armenia are the ancestors of European Gypsies. They eventually came to call themselves the Rom or Roma.[6,7] When the group entered Western Europe, they represented themselves as Egyptians, from which the word 'Gypsy' was derived.[8] Throughout the majority of their existence, they suffered severe discrimination and persecution. The greatest atrocity occurred in Nazi Germany, where approximately one million Gypsies were killed in gas chambers and were subjected to various forms of genocide.[9] The group has been a nomadic one, moving to new locations as needed to sustain their existence and unique identity. The earliest evidence of the presence of the Romani in the United States was 1695 in Virginia.[7]

Worldwide, there are approximately twelve million Roma. The largest populations are found in Europe and in both North and South America.[1,10] Although census data is unreliable, an estimated one million Roma live in the United States. The largest groups of Romani are found in larger cities such as Fort Worth, Houston, Seattle, and Atlanta. Smaller groups reside in rural areas throughout the United States.[10]

Each Romani has four loyalties–his or her tribe/nation/Rom group (*natsia*), *kumpania*, *vista,* and his or her extended family. Worldwide, there are at least thirteen Romani nations. *Kumpanias* are groups of extended families that occupy a specific geographic area and travel together. The extended families may or may not belong to the same nation. Each kumpania has a leader who represents the group in dealing with outsiders and other Romani groups. The leader is known as the *Rom barto/shato m*eaning "big man." Kumpanias are further divided into vistas, which are groups of extended, patrilineal families who work together as an economic unit. A vista may consist of as many as two hundred families.[4,11] A Romani's personal extended family may include three or four generations who reside together.[12] Romanies often practice a nomadic way of life, moving frequently from one place to another.

The Romani have their own system of law and justice and pay little attention to the majority of the laws of the mainstream justice system. Infractions to their group laws are handled by a group of two to five adult males who have been selected based on their status and reputation within the group. This group of men composes what is known as a *kris* and determine the punishment for infractions.[11]

Most Romani do not register with military agencies. Many have no birth certificates or marriage licenses. Because of discrimination and stereotyping, a Romani may claim to be of another ethnic group such as Mexican, Native American, etc.[1,13]

Very few studies related to Romani health status have been conducted. Because of continued persecution, prejudice, discrimination, and the group's suspicions of non-Romani, mortality and morbidity rates are much higher than in the general population. Poverty, poor nutritional status, infectious diseases, and avoidance of health care facilities lead to increased rates of infant mortality, chronic disease, and premature death.[2] There is a high rate of illiteracy among the Romani; younger Romani are more likely to be literate.

Language

- Romany and/or the language of the country of residence. Dialects vary widely among groups.[1,7,10]

Worldview/Religious Beliefs

- The Romani should remain a separate people. Although there is much diversity among Romani groups, unique Romani lifeways are dictated by a strict set of rules collectively known as *Romaniya.* Abiding by these rules and avoiding shame because of pollution leads to spiritual balance. Interaction with non-Romanies drains an individual of spiritual energy, which must be restored by spending time within the all-Romani environment. Non-Romani are sometimes referred to as the *gaje* or *gadje.* Romani assimilation occurs only to the extent to support survival within a society. This separation from non-Romani groups is governed by the belief in the condition of *marime.* These beliefs define almost everything and everyone as *wuzho* (pure) or *marime* (impure or shameful). A severe state of 'pollution' can lead to total exclusion from the Romani community; therefore, it is important that Romani avoid close contact with non-Romani.[1,8,11,14]

- One God is worshiped and is call *Del.* Del is recognized as the Creator and is associated with the principle of good. *O'Bengh* is recognized as the devil and is associated with the principle of evil. There is a constant struggle between Del and O'Bengh for dominance over an individual's life. Romanies may adopt some of the religious practices of the dominant religion of their place of residence. However, core Rom beliefs and practices remain dominant in their lifeways.[1,15,16]

- The world is viewed from a dual perspective (i.e., Del vs. O'Bengh, pure/clean vs. polluted, two stages of life, children/old age vs. adulthood, Romani and non-Romani). Old age is defined by the inability to no longer bear children.[1,14]

- Small shrines may be maintained in the home with icons of Jesus, various saints, candles, holy water, and pictures of dead relatives. These saints are particularly comforting and important to Romani women. Special celebrations dedicated to patron saints and pilgrimages to places known for healing are not uncommon among Romanies.[15,17]

- There are strong beliefs in supernatural powers and ancestor spirits (the *mulè*). Ancestor spirits will remain pleased and provide protection to those that maintain a state of cleanliness. However, if the ancestors are displeased, they are capable of punishing an individual through giving a warning called a *prikaza*.[17] The warning may range from a very minor accident to severe illness and death. Based on these beliefs, Romanies generally believe that nothing happens by chance. Special amulets may be carried or worn to prevent illnesses.[1,15]

- Living things are to be killed only for food.[7]

Health Beliefs/Practices

- Health is influenced by fate and luck. Attributes of a good life are directly related to living a clean and moral family life.[7] Traveling is associated with health and good luck; staying in one place is associated with sickness and bad luck.[3,8]

- The dominant health belief is associated with the concept of *marime*, which has the dual meaning of pollution/uncleanliness and rejection. This concept is of a moral and ritual nature. It provides the primary division of Romanies from non-Romanies. According to this concept, the human body is divided at the waist into two halves. The upper half is seen as pure and clean, while the lower half is considered dirty (marime) and a source of pollution because of the genital and anal areas. The feet are also considered impure. Both males and females must abide by marime rules, beginning at puberty. Violation of these rules can be grounds for exclusion of the offender and his or her entire family from Romani society. Offenses are handled by the *kris*, who determines the punishment. All non-Romani are considered marime and are seen as a source of impurity and disease. Public restrooms, offices, and prolonged stays in hospitals are considered potential sources of disease. There is very little modesty regarding the upper body. Body fluids from the upper body such as saliva, tears, and vomitus are considered clean. Blood from blood vessels is also considered clean. The head is considered the most important area of the body to keep clean and is believed to be the seat of power, particularly for men.[7,8,13,14]

- If it is necessary for a health care provider to visit the home of a Romani, one may find that the home is divided into marime and wuzho areas. Furniture may be covered in plastic and at least one chair is reserved for seating non-Romani visitors. Generally, a non-Romani will not be allowed in the back of the home as it is considered a 'clean' area not to be polluted by a non-Romani.[14]

- When hospitalized, provide separate soaps, washbasins, washcloths, and towels for upper and lower body. If ambulatory, a Romani will likely prefer to shower since sitting in water would make the water unclean. Disposable covers for the toilet seat are desirable.[14,15,18]

- Clothing from the upper and lower body should be placed in separate bags and never washed together. Men's and women's clothing cannot be washed together.

- Folk medicines and treatments are commonly used. Generally, there is a female elder who is revered for her wisdom and skill in treating illness. She may be referred to as *drabarni*. The drabarni will treat 'natural' illnesses such as rashes, vomiting, cardiac problems, etc.

- Some illnesses, such as sexually transmitted diseases are attributed to excessive contact with non-Romani people. Sexually transmitted diseases and AIDS must be treated by a non-Romani physician. Family members will likely not visit an individual with such diagnosis and risks. Usually, the person with AIDS is banished from the family. This exclusion is cause for great emotional distress for the patient.[1,19]

- Generally, Romanies only come to hospitals for childbirth or acute/critical health problems that cannot be cured by the drabarni. Excluding childbirth, the hospital is generally seen as a place where people come to die.[19,20]

- Surgery and general anesthesia are feared because the person under general anesthesia is believed to undergo a "little death." Family members will desire to be at the bedside to assist the patient in coming out of anesthesia.[13]

- The color red is associated with good health and happiness.[18]

- Adherence to medication regimes may be influenced by the color, shape, and origin of the medication. Medications prescribed by private physicians are valued more than those prescribed by non-private physicians. Large, dark-colored capsules are thought to be powerful, while small, light-colored pills are thought to be much less effective.[13]

- An overweight person is often considered healthy and fortunate. Thin persons are considered ill or too poor to buy adequate food and are pitied.[3,13,21]

Expression of Pain

- Likely to be expressive.

Male-Female/Kinship/Social Relationships

- A Romani usually carries more than one name–one used within the Romani community and one or more used when among non-Romani and on administrative documents. The name used among non-Romani can change several times during the course of an individual's lifetime.[14,22]

- Adult men are called *rom*. Adult women are called *romni*. Other terms may be used among the various divisions. Married women wear head scarfs. The scarf is called a *diklo*.[12,19]

- Economically, families share expenses. Medical bills are many times paid in cash.[16]

- During hospitalization, massive numbers of relatives, friends, etc. are likely to visit and possibly "camp out" at the health care facility. Allow liberal visitation since it is quite disturbing for a Rom to be alone. A larger, private room is desirable to accommodate visitation from family and friends. It may be helpful if the room is located at the end of a hallway to decrease disruption to other patients. Prayers and chants may be offered.[9,11]

- Romanies are generally distrustful of non-Romanies. Many times, it is extremely difficult to establish trust with the group, which may impair obtaining accurate information.

- Elders have high status and respect from others in the family because it is believed that they have more knowledge and experience. They also obtain a 'clean' status during their senior years. Decision-making, informed consent, etc., are generally the responsibility of the oldest dominant male in the extended family. The oldest dominant female will be included in decision-making.[11, 12, 18]

- It is very unlikely that elders will be admitted into nursing homes, extended care facilities, etc. Family members care for elders.
- Teen marriages are common. The young couple frequently lives with the husband's parents until they have several children of their own. In many instances, the youngest son is obligated to care for his parents until their death.[8, 12]
- Unmarried males and females sleep separately. During menstruation, girls may not sleep with girls who have not reached puberty, but must sleep alone.[8]
- Dress and behaviors are in accordance with marime laws. Women must have the lower half of the body covered, generally to the mid-calf. The skirt of a female must not touch an adult male in public. Protect the modesty of both men and women. Cover legs with a blanket while sitting if the legs are not covered by a gown or robe. Provide same-sex caregivers if at all possible.[1, 14, 15]
- Sexual intercourse and sleeping in the same bed is prohibited between couples during menstruation, seven days after the last day of menstruation, and after childbirth for approximately six to eight weeks (length of time may vary among various Romani groups).[7, 14]
- Topics of a sexual nature or concerning bodily functions should not be discussed in the presence of mixed-gender groups.[1, 14]

Birth/Children

- Children are loved, believed to bring good luck and prestige to the couple. All family members participate in childrearing. Families generally have several children. Infertile women are seen as being "out of balance."[11, 13, 14]
- Check for immunization status of children. Children who are not attending school may have not received immunizations.[21]

- Boys may be preferred to girls because a son is likely to stay with his parents after marriage and help to care for them when they are old.

- The first grandson may be raised by the paternal grandparents.[19]

- Children frequently attend public schools up to ten or eleven years of age. Generally, they are then removed from public schools to be fully educated in the activities of Romani adults. There is a fear of Romani children being influenced by other children in the public schools.[11] It may be extremely difficult to intervene in the practice of early removal of children from public school systems because of frequent changes in family residence. This practice is changing, and more Romanies are seeking formal education for their children.[15,23]

- Prenatal care and Pap smears may be avoided because of vaginal exams. Very careful, clear explanation will be required for consent.[4]

- During pregnancy, the woman is primarily cared for by other women. She is not allowed to cook for other Romani and may even use dishes that are hers alone. Husbands are allowed only limited time with pregnant wives. Among some groups, the wife cannot be seen by any man other than the husband before baptism of the newborn. Usually the father will not visit the wife and new baby between sunset and sunrise. Health care providers should not be surprised by the father's limited visitation and involvement with the wife and newborn following birth because of marime.[11,15]

- Births cannot take place in a Romani's home since the birth fluids, etc. are considered unclean, pollute the entire home, and must be destroyed. Women now frequently opt to deliver at a hospital so that all the "unclean" substances and articles associated with birth are left at the facility.

- Saliva may be placed on the shoulder of a woman in labor to ease the pain of childbirth.[8]

- Newborns are considered unclean until baptized six to eight weeks after birth. Baptism is frequently performed by immersing the baby under running water to wash away impurities.[15,24]

- Photographs of the baby are not permitted.

- Red ribbons may be placed on an infant/child's wrist or ankles to protect against the evil eye. The ribbons may be worn up to three years of age. The color red is seen as protective.[1]

- Mothers are likely to breastfeed. Green vegetables, tomatoes, and certain other foods may be avoided in an effort to prevent infant colic.[13]
- Family members may be restricted from going out at night, and windows/doors must be closed at night to protect the newborn from spirits.
- **Elective Pregnancy Termination/Birth Control**: Discouraged.

Death

- The death of a baby is considered bad luck for the parents. The grandparents will be responsible for burial of the baby in a place unknown to the parents, or the baby may be left at the hospital for disposal. The parents may choose not to participate in planning for the burial.[13]
- A dying Romani must never be left alone. This is important because of the need for compassion toward the dying and because of the fear that his or her spirit will be angered and cause unrest or illness for the surviving family and friends. It is desirable that relatives and friends have an opportunity to ask for forgiveness of any wrongdoing toward the dying person prior to death.[15,24]
- Families frequently choose to wash and dress the dying person prior to death since touching the body of the deceased person is discouraged because of fear of contamination. The nose may be plugged with ritually pure beeswax or pearls to ensure that no impurities enter.[8,24]
- Strong emotions may be shown when a young person dies (the exception may be with newborns). Death at an old age is considered natural, acceptable, and brings further prestige. However, it is acceptable behavior to liberally display grief after a family member dies. Suicide is seen as shameful.[12,13]
- In the past, Romanies have preferred to die outside. However, it is now permissible to die indoors, but the person should be next to an open window with a candle lit under the bed. This is said to allow the spirit to be shown the way to heaven. It is believed that the deceased will have those body parts returned that were lost during life. All possessions of

the deceased must be sold to non-Romanies or destroyed–generally by burning the items. Use of the deceased person's name will be avoided as a form of respect.[15,22,24]

- After a death, close relatives demonstrate their mourning and a state of pollution by not washing their face, body, and hands for three days. They also will not comb their hair, shave, or change clothing during these three days. On the third day, they wash themselves, change clothes, and present a more pleasant demeanor. Generally, the mourning period is twelve months.[8,24]
- Relatives may refuse to allow the deceased's body to be taken to the morgue and insist on keeping the body within view for fear of body mutilation and/or organ removal.[22]
- **Burial**: Generally occurs three days after the death.
- **Autopsies**: Not permitted.
- **Organ Donation**: Not permitted.[21,22]

Patient Teaching/Dietary Considerations

- Diet frequently high in salt, sugar, carbohydrates, and fat. High intake of strong coffee.
- Because being overweight may be associated with good health, the perception may serve as a barrier to nutrition counseling.[22]
- Generally, two meals are eaten per day with no lunch.[24]
- Garlic, onions, vinegar, and certain foods are considered good for health.
- Some Romanies fast on Friday as a cleansing act.[8]
- A Romani is more comfortable using disposable eating utensils, paper cups, etc. if hospitalized, or may choose to eat food with fingers to avoid touching non-disposable utensils. The family will likely want to bring food to a hospitalized family member since they cannot be assured that marime laws have been observed and the person(s) preparing the food may be non-Romani. Not likely to eat leftover food. In the absence of food brought by family, packaged food items will be preferred.[1,14]

- Principles of 'hot' and 'cold' apply to food.
- Many older Romanies cannot read. However, this does not mean that they are not intelligent. Younger Romani generally have some formal education. Teaching materials should be geared toward oral or visual approaches.

---

[1] Hancock, I. (2002). *We are the Romani people.* Great Britain: University of Hertfordshire Press

[2] Zeman, C., Depken, D., & Senchina, D. (2003). Roman health issues: A review of the literature and discussion. *Ethnicity and Health, 8*(3), 223-249.

[3] Miller, C. (2010). *The church of cheese: Gypsy ritual in the American heyday.* Boston, MA: GemmaMedia.

[4] Heimlich, E. (2012). *Gypsy Americans.* Retrieved from http://www.everyculture.com/multi/Du-Ha/Gypsy-Americans.html

[5] *Romani people.* (2005). Retrieved from http://www.nationmaster.com/encyclopedia/Romani-people#_note-2

[6] Moreau, R. (1995). *Walking in the paths of the gypsies.* Toronto: Key Porter Books.

[7] Sway, M. (1988). *Gypsy life in America: Familiar strangers.* Chicago: University of Illinois Press.

[8] Sutherland, A. (1975). *Gypsies: The hidden Americans.* Prospect Heights, IL: Waveland Press, Inc.

[9] Maas, P. (1975). *King of the gypsies.* New York, NY: The Viking Press.

[10] *The religion and culture of the Roma.* (2007). Retrieved from http://www.religioustolerance.org/roma2.htm/

[11] Bodner, A., & Leininger, M. (1992). Transcultural nursing care values, beliefs and practices of American (USA) gypsies. *Journal of Transcultural Nursing, 4*(1), 17-28.

[12] Nemeth, D. (2002). *The Gypsy-American: An ethnographic study.* Lewiston, NY: The Edwin Mellen Press.

[13] Sutherland, A. (1992). Gypsies and health care. *The Western Journal of Medicine, 157*(3), 276-280.

[14] Weyrauch, W. (Ed). (2001). *Gypsy law: Romani legal traditions and culture.* Los Angeles: University of California Press.

[15] Wallace, A. (2003). *The Gypsies.* San Diego, CA: Lucent Books.

[16] Kohn, B. (1972). *Gypsies.* New York, NY: The Bobbs-Merrill Company, Inc.

[17] Fraser, A. (1992). *The Gypsies.* Oxford, UK: Blackwell Publishers.

[18] Fonseca, I. (1995). *Bury me standing: The gypsies and their journey.* New York, NY: Vintage Books.

[19] Thomas, J. (1985). Gypsies and American medical care. *Annals of Internal Medicine, 102*(6), 842-845.

[20] Belgum, D. (1999). Dealing with cultural diversity: A hospital chaplain reflects on Gypsies and other such diversity. *Journal of Pastoral Care, 53*(2), 175-181.

[21] Vivian, C. & Dundes, L. (2004). The crossroads of culture and health among the Roma (Gypsies). *Journal of Nursing Scholarship, 36*(1), 86-91.

[22] Williams, P. (2003). *Gypsy world: The silence of the living and the voices of the dead.* Chicago, IL: The Chicago Press.

[23] Kates, G. & Gergely, V. (2011, April 7). For Roma, life in US has challenges. *Voice of America News.* Retrieved from ProQuest Central Database.

[24] Greenfield, H. (1977). *Gypsies.* New York, NY: Crown Publishers, Inc.

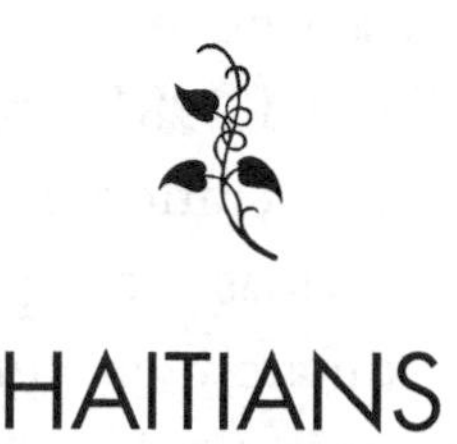

HAITIANS

"Behind every mountain, there is another mountain." Haitian proverb[1]

Background

The history of Haiti has included periods of both triumph and sorrow. Even through the sorrow, negative stereotypes, and environmental struggles, the people of Haiti have remained proud of their heritage.[2] The country of Haiti became the first independent Black republic and the second independent country in the Western Hemisphere in 1804 after a bloody slave revolt against France.[3] Haiti and the Dominican Republic share the island of Hispaniola, with Haiti occupying the western third of the island. The country is comparable in size to the state of Maryland and lies approximately 700 miles southeast of Florida between Cuba, Jamaica, and Puerto Rico.[4] Its capital is Port-au-Prince.

Haiti has been plagued by political upheaval, corruption, and natural disasters such as hurricanes, mudslides, flooding, and land erosion. In January 2010, a 7.0 magnitude earthquake struck Haiti. Estimates of fatalities varied from 100,000 to over 300,000, with over one million people displaced.[4] The results were further decline in the health of the Haitian people and the country. Currently, only approximately 28 percent of the land can support agricultural cultivation.[5]

Approximately nine million people live in what has been deemed the poorest country in the Western Hemisphere.[5] It is among the twenty-five poorest countries in the world.[4]

The majority of Haitians are descendants of the more than 500,000 West African slaves inhabiting the island at the time of the country's independence. Approximately five percent of Haitians are White or mulattos, descendants of African slaves and French colonists.[4,5]

Prior to 1979, the majority of people who left Haiti did so because of political reasons and were professionals, businessmen, or skilled craftsmen. They settled in French Canada (primarily Montreal), France, Africa, and the United States. Unskilled Haitians migrated to other Caribbean islands, primarily Cuba and the Dominican Republic.[6,7] After continued political corruption, and natural and man-made disasters, an estimated 80,000 Haitians left the island between 1979 and 1981. They were less prepared educationally and had few marketable skills. Out of desperation, many traveled by boat from the island, and became known in the United States as 'boat people,' a label that has persisted.[6,8] The United States is home to approximately one of every twenty Haitians worldwide. Currently, almost 75 percent of Haitians in the United States reside in two states: Florida and New York. Other states with larger Haitian populations include New Jersey, Massachusetts and Georgia.[6,9]

Health Risks

A number of Haitians with limited education and skills reside in low-income, overcrowded environments. Many have been subjected to harsh conditions in Haiti. Risk factors, particularly among new immigrants who have not received regular health care, include malnutrition, parasitic infections (including intestinal worms), Hepatitis A and E, leptospirosis, malaria, sickle cell anemia, and tuberculosis.[5,10,11,12]

Dental caries are common because of the lack of access to dental care in Haiti, poverty, and high sugar intake.[13,14] Haitians were once stigmatized as carriers of HIV/AIDS by the Centers for Disease Control (CDC). This was declared false in April, 1985. However, HIV/AIDS remains among the diseases of increased incidence among Haitians. Other diseases include hypertension, STDs, diabetes, heart disease, and cancer of the cervix, liver, and stomach.[15,16,17,18] Because Haitian refugees have been received with such negative support, stress-related physical and psychological illnesses must be included among risk factors for this population.[20,21,22] Additionally, migrant workers are at risk for accidents and diseases of overcrowding.[7]

Haiti's Current State[4, 5, 22, 23]

- Approximately 70-80 percent of the population resides in rural areas. Most have little or no access to medical care or dental care.

- Approximately 80 percent of the people live below the poverty line and about 54 percent live in the most severe state of poverty.

- Per capita income; $650 per year or less.[24] Estimates vary widely. The majority of wealth is distributed among a very small percentage of Haiti's population. Over half of the people have incomes of $1- $2 per day.

- Five physicians per 10,000 inhabitants; one hospital bed per 1,300 inhabitants. (The number of health care workers and hospitals available to rural inhabitants is significantly less.)

- Approximately 70 percent unemployment rate. Estimates vary widely.

- **Life Expectancy**: Overall 62.17 years; male–60.84 years, female–63.53 years.

- **Fertility Rate**: 3.07 children per woman.

- **Infant Mortality Rate**: 70 per 1,000 births.

- **Child Mortality Rate** (probability of dying less than 5 years of age): 165/1,000 live births.[25] The number one killer is diarrhea related to the lack of clean water for drinking.[26]

- **Literacy Rate**: Approximately 53 percent.

Language/Communication

- **French**: Only 10 to 15 percent of the population speaks French; mostly upper-class citizens, since knowledge of the French language is gained primarily through the school system.[8, 19] The ability to speak French fluently is associated with prestige.[27]

- **Haitian Kreyòl** (also referred to as *Kreyòl* and *Creole*): The language is a blend of 17th century French and West African dialects.[8] Kreyòl was granted official status by the

Haitian Constitution in 1987.[4] The majority of Haitians speak only Haitian Keryòl. Most Haitians that speak French also speak Kreyòl.[3, 28] Until recent years, Kreyòl was not a written language. Therefore, many Haitians have only shared information through spoken communication.[6, 16] Assure that professional interpreters are used to convey information related to health, treatments, etc.

- Hand gestures and voice intonations are frequently used to emphasize verbal language and may be pronounced during conversation.[16]

- Proverbs are an important part of conversation, are used frequently in everyday conversations, and to explain phenomena in Haitian life.[29]

- Direct eye contact, without staring, is important during interactions with adults. Patients may become uncomfortable when health care providers do not make direct eye contact.[16] However, children and Haitians who have had little or no contact with industrialized Western non-verbal behaviors may not make direct eye contact with people seen in authoritative positions.[17]

- Touch may be used to complement conversations to better connect with others and to display warmth and friendliness.[16, 30]

- Children may greet persons they know with a kiss on the cheek. Adult friends may be respectfully referred to as Auntie, Uncle, or Cousin.[30]

- Haitians may describe themselves in terms of the geographical area of Haiti from which they originated. *Capitol Haitians* - referencing origination from Port au Prince; *city Haitians* - originating from other cities in Haiti; *village Haitians* - originating from remote areas of Haiti, and *mountain Haitians* - originating from the mountainous areas of Haiti.[22] Explore further with the patient to gain more specific information.

- **Names**: Generally, Haitians have first, middle, and last names. Many names are of French origin. The first and middle names may be hyphenated. Nicknames are common among family and friends. However, health care providers should use formal greetings unless given permission by the patient/family. Married women are addressed as Mrs., followed by the husband's last name.[17]

Worldview/Religious Beliefs

- Religious affiliations among Haitians are 80 percent Catholic, 16 percent Protestant, and four percent other. Many Haitian Catholics, particularly those with limited access to Catholic priests and churches, practice some degree of *Vodou* in conjunction with Christianity or are affected by the religion in some manner (see Vodou in *Afro-Caribbean Religions*). Persons who are adherents of Vodou will likely be hesitant to admit or discuss their religious practices with health care providers for fear of ridicule and condemnation. Most of the Roman Catholic annual events are recognized by those that describe themselves as Catholic (see *Catholicism*).[4,5,10,31]

- Most devout Christians denounce Vodou, one of the most misunderstood religions in the world. The religion has been negatively portrayed in the media. However, the Christian God is central to the life of the Haitian, regardless of adherence to Christianity or Vodou. There is a strong reliance on the Christian God, prayer, and the Holy Bible.[7,15]

- **Bondyè** (pronounced 'bohn-dyay') is the Kreyòl word referring to God, the Supreme Being and Creator of all things. In French, the term *Le Bon Dieu* is sometimes used, meaning "The Good God." God may also be called *Gran Mèt* (Grand Master). Because God (Bondyè) is too busy to deal with the day-to-day needs and problems of His followers, He delegates the day-to-day management of these issues to cosmic, supernatural spirits known as *lwa* (pronounced 'L'wha'). The lwa participate in all aspects of daily life, and individuals must maintain positive relationships with them to maintain good health and good fortune in life.[32,33]

- Some Haitians believe that humans have two or more souls. The two major ones are *Gros Bon Ange* (The Big Good Angel) and *Ti Bon Ange* (Little Good Angel). The Gros Bon Ange is comparable to the Christian soul and is considered the life force of an individual. The Ti Bon Ange is seen as the guardian angel and is comparable to Western 'spirit.' This soul is thought to reside in the head.[34]

- The events of one's life are predetermined by God. Two phrases often heard are "Bondyè Bon" (God is Good) and "Si Bondyè Vie" (if God wants). One's future is in the hands of God.[17]

Health Beliefs/Practices

- Health-seeking behaviors vary widely among Haitians, based on level of acculturation, education, proximity of services, and socioeconomic level. The United States and Canada are fortunate to have a number of Haitians in professional health care careers. Haitians tend to seek services from Haitian professionals, if available.[17,28,35]

- Preventive health care/dental services may not be seen as valuable in that they may be viewed as having very little impact on one's present well-being. Among undocumented residents, lack of trust in the government and fear of discovery and deportation may contribute to presentation for medical care in advanced stages of disease/illness or when pain is experienced. Participation in preventive health care/dental services and application for government assistance programs may also be negatively impacted for the same reasons. Frequently, treatments are recommended by family or friends. Lay healers and prayer may be tried as a cure prior to seeking medical services.[16,26,28,30]

- Illnesses tend to be divided into natural and supernatural origins. Supernatural illnesses may result from a breach in rapport with one's spirit protector, God, or from a curse. A breach in rapport with one's spirit protector may lead to illness. Various healers and practitioners are consulted to treat an illness, based on its origin. Generally, diseases of natural origin are thought to be responsive to mainstream medicine and to home remedies. The 'germ theory' as a cause of illness may be foreign.[10,29,36] Explore the patient's thoughts regarding the origin of the illness.

- Cause and effect related to other illnesses such as cancer, as well as basic anatomical relationships may also be quite foreign to some Haitians. This will impact understanding of cancer sites, various types of cancer, and possible causes of cancer.[37] Use anatomical models and/or pictures to facilitate understanding. Seek to establish a trusting relationship with the patient, and use a sensitive, non-judgmental approach.

Name of Healer[1, 10, 16, 20, 34, 36]	Function
Doktè fey, medsen fey, docteur-feuille	Herbalist, leaf doctor. Consulted for common natural illnesses such as the common cold, diarrhea, and other gastric illnesses, worms, evil eye.
Matron, fam saj, accoucheuse, matwòn, fanmsaj diplome	**Midwife**: Manages prenatal, labor/delivery, and post-partum care for most women. Government-trained midwives' services are more expensive.
Docteur zo	**Bonesetter**: Uses massage, physical manipulation, poultices, and prayer to treat musculoskeletal problems. Also treats broken bones.
Pikirist (injectionist)	Administers herbal and Western medications by injection.
Docteur sangsue	**Blood-letter**: Treats illnesses using blood-letting techniques.
Hougan	**Vodou Priest**: Male specialist in serving the spirits. In rural areas, provides folk treatments for medical ailments, including HIV/AIDS and STDs. Treats supernatural illnesses.
Mambo	**Vodou Priestess**: Female specialist in serving the spirits. In rural areas, provides folk treatments for medical ailments, including HIV/AIDS and STDs. Treats supernatural illnesses.

- The condition of the blood plays a key role in the health of an individual. Disruptions in the quality, quantity, temperature, color, and concentration of one's blood can lead to illness. Strong emotions such as anger, shock, or fright can also affect the balance of one's blood and lead to illness. The flow of blood is thought to maintain equilibrium between hot and cold within the body. This balance can be negatively affected by environmental factors such as wind, rain, etc.

- Most illnesses, foods, medications, life cycles of individuals, and reproductive cycles of women are classified as 'hot' or 'cold.' Treatments are aimed at restoring the blood to a healthy balance through appropriate medications, diet, cleansing the blood/body, and/or cooling/warming the system. Because of these beliefs about the importance of blood, some Haitians may be very reluctant to submit to multiple blood tests and blood transfusions. Thoroughly explain the necessity of the test(s) and transfusion(s). Listed below are various conditions of the blood.

Term [10,29]	Meaning	Cause/Resulting Illness
Move san	Bad blood	Precipitated by fright, shock, or anger. Leads to skin eruptions, spoiled breast milk (lèt gate). Lèt gate leads to diarrhea and failure to thrive in the baby.
San boulvèse	Agitated blood	Leads to heavy or irregular menstrual periods.
San cho	Hot blood	Leads to fever, nervousness.
San épè	Thick blood	Precipitated by fright, shock, anger, or elevated blood pressure.
San fèb	Weak blood	Leads to physical or mental weakness.
San gate	Spoiled blood	Caused by venereal disease, fright, shock, or anger.
San jòn	Yellow blood	Caused by bile mixing with blood.
San klè	Thin blood	Leads to pallor, loss of consciousness.
San koupe	Cut off blood	Causes a girl never to begin menstrual cycles, to become anemic, and possibly die.
San nwa	Black blood	Is indicative of a terminal illness.
San pati	Departed blood	Leads to a missed menstrual cycle.
San pike	Spicy blood	Leads to itching.
San sal	Dirty blood	Caused by venereal disease.

- Some Haitians are reluctant to share personal information with persons other than family. Others may go to the other extreme and give very lengthy responses to health care providers.[24, 35]

- May not be concerned about diseases such as hypertension unless feeling ill. Therefore, adherence to medical regimens may be inconsistent. Stress the importance of taking medicines even after feeling better.[38, 39]

- The following items may be used for protection:[34]

  - **Kolye maldjòk**: Protective necklace against evil eye.

  - **Lepitèm**: Comb-like object worn in hair against headaches.

  - **Chemizèt twa paman**: Undershirt usually made of red, black, and white cloth worn to ward off evil and/or sickness.

  - Other protective amulets may be placed in the beds of patients when in the hospital. Protective items should be left in place. If it is absolutely necessary to remove the item, give careful explanation regarding reasons, keep the item in safekeeping, or give to family (with patient's permission).

- When completing assessments, always ask what treatments have been used for an illness. Family members or friends often share prescription medications, recommend herbal treatments, or obtain medications from Haiti where a prescription may not be required. Screen adults and children for immunization status.[3, 10]

- Questions asked by health care providers may be seen as a deficiency in knowledge on the part of the provider. It may be thought that the health care provider should know the answers. Generally, a physical exam, use of a stethoscope, rapid diagnosis, and a prescription will be expected.[40]

- Some Haitians may become quite anxious if clothes, hair, body fluids, etc. fall into the hands of unknown persons. Reassure the individual that clothes will be given to trusted family members or placed in safe keeping. Return hair that must be shaved to the patient or family. Explain methods of disposal of body fluids.[41]

- Expect and encourage family participation in care and in teaching. In Haiti, if an individual is hospitalized, daily care activities such as feeding, bathing, etc. are performed by family members.[35, 42]

- Injections may be thought to be more effective than oral medications.[28]

- Laxatives and enemas may be used as methods to cleanse the body during illness or as a measure to prevent illness.[28]

- Mental health services are extremely limited in Haiti. Mental illness may be ignored or attributed to supernatural causes.[43] A healer with supernatural healing skills may be consulted to achieve a complete cure. Mainstream psychiatric treatments may be seen as only palliative.[35]

- Some diseases are regarded as shameful leading to delayed medical care. These diseases include venereal disease, epilepsy, and hydrocele.[29]

- Carefully explain the need for surgery. Provide support and reassurance to the patient and family. Surgery is often seen as a procedure that may lead to death.[39]

- Explain the need to use wheelchairs for transportation, if policy demands. Riding in a wheelchair may be perceived as meaning the patient is extremely ill and is seen as a public display of weakness.[35, 39]

- Physical illnesses are expressed on a continuum of severity.[17] (See table below.)

Illness[17, 27, 29, 34, 39, 40]	Meaning
Kom pa bon ("I don't feel well.")	Generally, the person is not confined to bed; the illness is of short duration.
Da tan zan tan moin malad ("I feel sick from time to time.")	A statement of one's general state of health.
Moin an konvalésans ("I am convalescing.")	The person has been sick and is not getting better.

Illness[17, 27, 29, 34, 39, 40]	Meaning
Moin malad ("I am sick.")	Generally, the person is too ill to leave home; may be confined to bed and activity is decreased.
Moin malad anpil ("I am very sick.")	The person is confined to bed and feels very ill.
Moin pap réfè ("I am dying.")	The person is critically or terminally ill.
Biskèt tonbe (fallen breastbone or sternum)	Generally means that the person has a sore chest or has epigastric discomfort.
Depression	In Kreyòl, term is associated with physical exhaustion, extreme fatigue, or debility–not the psychological association that the term carries in French or English.
Eklampsi/èclampsie (toxemia of pregnancy, eclampsia)	Believed to be caused by anger during pregnancy causing blood to climb to the head.
Endispozisyon (indisposition)	May be described as shock, fainting spell and can be recurrent. Believed to be caused by unexpressed anger, shock, extreme emotional tension, or grief causing the blood to become too thick or rush toward the head. Is also associated with the condition and activity of blood during puberty, menstruation, and menopause. More common among females, teenagers, young adults, and the elderly. Heat is a common cause of indisposition among the elderly. Symptoms include extreme weakness, loss of consciousness, mental confusion, temporary blindness, and/or temporary deafness. Considered incurable by mainstream medicine.

Illness[17,27,29,34,39,40]	Meaning
Gaz (gas)	Believed to be caused by eating leftover foods, air entering the body through the ears (causes headaches) or mouth (causes stomach aches). Can lead to pain and anemia. Gaz can move to other parts of the body and cause pain in the shoulders, back, or extremities. Home remedies for gaz include garlic tea, mint, cloves, corn, and plantain.
Kriz (panic attack)	Characterized by hysteria.
Kriz de nè/maladi ner (emotional crisis)	Believed to be caused by blood rushing to the head as a result of intense emotion or grief. Manifested by seizures, alterations in consciousness, sudden collapse.
Lalouèt tonbe (fallen uvula)	Generally refers to acute respiratory distress or tonsillitis.
Maladi Bondyè, maladi péi	An illness of God or "country disease" (i.e., natural causes). Usually of short duration, caused by environmental agents such as food, air, imbalance between hot (*cho*) and cold (*fret*), bone displacement.
Maladi Satan	An illness of Satan (i.e., purposely sent upon one by an enemy, typically because of jealousy or revenge).
Mis tonbe (fallen coccyx)	Generally refers to lower back pain.
Pèdisyon	Refers to multiple female conditions including pelvic discomfort, menorrhagia, and false pregnancy. Also, refers to a condition in which a fetus is believed to be entrapped in the uterus and unable to develop because it is not receiving the blood necessary for development.
Sezisman (fright)	The blood becomes heated as a result of shock or emotional upset making it highly vulnerable to cold. The condition is thought to cause fever, diarrhea, or stroke.[44]
Tibèkiloz, tuberculose, poitrinaire (tuberculosis) – many other terms used	Carries very negative social stigma, leading persons to try to hide symptoms and to present late for treatment. Many Haitians do not believe that tuberculosis occurs in children.

Pain

- May have difficulty giving concrete descriptions of type and location of pain. Disease is thought to be able to travel, so the location of pain at any given time may be seen as unimportant.[10, 35]

- Pain may be caused by gaz moving to various parts of the body.[29]

- Pain is often referred to as *doule.*[17]

Male-Female/Kinship/Social Relationships

- In rural Haiti, clusters of extended family members live on small farming areas surrounding small villages. These clusters are called a *lakou.* This pattern of family living is reflective of the strong West African background of Haitians.[10]

- Among poor and rural Haitians, *plasaj* is a common conjugal relationship. The man is allowed to maintain several households with his common-law wives. He is expected to provide for each of the households. Under this system, the male can designate property to any of his children. If married, he can only designate property to children born within wedlock. Although not recognized by Haiti's government, it is considered a normal and proper union. Children born within the plasaj unions to different women often know each other as brothers and sisters and live without conflict. Children may carry either parent's last name.[4, 10, 13, 16]

- Gender roles tend to be well-defined with males providing for the family and females managing the home and caring for the children.[10]

- Strong intermediate and extended family connections. Godparents play important roles within the family.[7]

- Elderly family members and other elderly persons are highly respected, serving as advisors and counselors for the family unit. Multiple generations may live within the same household. Among traditional Haitians, it is considered an honor for an elderly parent to choose to live in one child's residence over another's.[4, 7, 16]

- Close family ties are maintained with relatives who remain in Haiti or other places. Allow time for health care decisions to be made. Families will often want to consult other family members (even if the family members are in Haiti), before making a decision.[4]

Birth/Children

- **Elective Pregnancy Termination**: Generally not supported.
- Infertility carries a negative social stigma. Women are expected to bear children.[29]
- The exact day and year of birth may not be known since no record is likely to be generated in settings outside of the hospital in Haiti. Even if born in a hospital, sometimes record-keeping may not be optimal and the birth may not be registered. The birth may be associated with a well-known event or holiday.[26]
- Children are considered gifts from God and provide some degree of security in old age. Parents are, therefore, obligated to do everything possible to assure that their children are cared for to the best of the parents' abilities.[4, 9, 15] However, in Haiti, over 200,000 children (more often girls) from very poor families are sent to work as *restaveks*, children who stay with families who are well-off financially and work as servants. In many cases, the parents are promised that the child will have food, shelter, and education, a better life than that child would be afforded at home. Frequently, the promises are not kept and the children are abused, subjected to long hours of work, and minimal to no educational opportunities. The children are often turned out to the streets at fifteen years of age, when Haitian law requires wages for work.[26]
- Pica during pregnancy is common and considered harmless.[43]
- Red fruits and vegetables are thought to be beneficial during pregnancy to build blood for the baby.[10]
- Foods to be avoided during pregnancy include very spicy foods, hot pepper.[45]
- May present late in the course of the pregnancy for prenatal care since pregnancy, labor, and birth are seen as normal parts of a woman's life cycle.[46]

- Provide careful explanation of the need for IV fluids during labor. This common practice in mainstream medicine may be seen as a sign that the mother is not doing well.[46]

- During labor, warm or hot tea (especially ginger tea) or hot milk may be desired. Hot liquids are thought to speed the labor process. Other actions thought to speed labor include firm abdominal massage using downward movements and walking. Sexual intercourse during the latter days of pregnancy is thought to dilate the birth canal, thereby speeding labor.[46]

- Labor pain or discomfort may be expressed through chanting, praying, moaning, crying, and combinations of all these. Touch is reassuring to a laboring woman.[46]

- In rural Haiti, mothers will generally bury the placenta and umbilical stump to prevent harm to the child.[47] In some instances, a Haitian mother may ask to take her placenta home for burial.

- May want sponge baths instead of showers during the first week(s) post-partum.[46]

- The mother's bones are considered to be 'open' during the first two to three days following birth. Mothers may not want to get out of bed because bed rest is seen as essential to allow the bones to 'close.' Wearing an abdominal binder or girdle is thought to assist the bones in closing and to help the abdominal muscles return to their pre-pregnancy state. Binders may be worn after a miscarriage, as well as after a term pregnancy.[43]

- The lying-in or period of seclusion after birth varies from two to forty days. Mothers and babies are considered very vulnerable to chilling during the post-partum period. Exposure to cold air is thought to lead to hemorrhage, cold in the womb or vagina, and/or delay in the uterus returning to its normal position/status. The mother and baby must be kept warm during this period. If the baby must be brought back for checkups, a relative may bring the baby. If the baby cannot go home with the mother because of illness or prematurity, the mother may not visit as regularly during this time. Assess the reason for the mother not visiting before concluding that there are issues with maternal-infant bonding.[10,43,46]

- The mother takes a very active part in her post-partum care, including the following:

  - Vapor baths, using orange leaves in steaming water. A cloth is draped over the woman's head and shoulders during the vapor bath.[43]

- Teas made from various leaves and herbs to cleanse and heal the body.[43, 46]
- **Three Baths**: A series of baths taken by the mother after birth to cleanse the body and become healthy again. For the first three days following birth, hot bath water is prepared using special leaves, roots, and herbs. Hot baths are thought to assist in purging the uterus and tightening the woman's vagina. Hot tea made from the same ingredients is ingested. Over the next three days, warm water is used for the second series of baths. In rural areas, the water is warmed in the sun for the baths and for ingestion. At the end of two weeks to forty days, the mother will take a third bath. At this time, the mother takes a bath in cold water, is allowed to drink cold water/beverages, and resume normal activities. In addition, she may take a laxative to "clean her insides."[43, 46]
- The post-partum period is considered a 'cold' state. Foods to be avoided include tomatoes, lima beans, okra, certain kinds of fish, eggplant, milk, cold drinks, bananas, and foods that are white in color unless colored with a food that is non-white (e.g., coffee added to milk). Some Haitian women link eating tomatoes and foods white in color to increased vaginal discharge.[43, 46]
- During menstruation, cold water may be avoided. Eating and drinking citrus foods may also be avoided because of the acid content.[46]

- May place a bellyband on the newborn for the first two to three months of age to assist in developing a strong body and a good sense of balance.[43]
- Oils, nutmeg, charcoal, and other substances may be placed on the baby's umbilical cord stump to speed healing and to avoid the baby "catching umbilical cold."[29, 46]
- Purgatives (sometimes called a *lok*) are often given to newborns to clean the baby's insides of first stools. A common purgative for newborns is made with a base of red oil from a plant known as *maskreti* in Haitian Kreyòl. Various other ingredients are added such as sugar, castor oil, garlic, boiled water, salt, and nutmeg. Caution mothers that rapid dehydration of the newborn may result from this practice.[43, 46]
- The nose of the newborn may be gently pinched several times a day in an effort to narrow the nostrils. Narrow nostrils are considered more attractive by many Haitians.[29]

- Provide careful explanation if a child's hair must be cut for treatment purposes. Avoid the head as a site for IV administration. Many Haitians do not cut a child's hair prior to one year of age.[29]

- **Circumcisions**: Often not done.[29]

- A mother may stop breast-feeding if the infant develops diarrhea, fearing her breast milk is 'spoiled.' Provide reassurance that breast milk is not the source of the infant's diarrhea.[29]

- Children may routinely be given various teas and purgatives to prevent/cure illnesses and rid the body of impurities. Health care providers should routinely assess the type and frequency of home remedies for children.[45]

- Some parents may believe that illness can be inflicted upon children by the evil eye and spells. Children may also be taught not to accept food from persons that are strangers for fear that harm may come to the child. Bead necklaces, bracelets, red ribbons around the wrist, and cloths may be placed on children for protection.[15, 29, 45]

- Malnutrition and parasitosis is widespread in Haiti. Screen newly-immigrated children for vitamin deficiencies and other symptoms of malnutrition. Stool specimens may be indicated to analyze for intestinal parasites.[14, 42]

- Screen children for history of immunizations since many children do not receive them in Haiti. Vitamin deficiency is a common cause of vision problems in Haiti.[42]

- Children are taught obedience and to refrain from questioning their elders. Children asking questions related to intimate subjects may be considered disrespectful.[27] Do not ask children to interpret such matters to elders.

- Children may be the recipients of corporal punishment for failure to show respect to adults or for misbehaving.[7]

- Potty training and self-feeding may seem unimportant to mothers until the child is able to speak in phrases and respond to commands appropriately, indicating that the child is then ready for training toward independence.[15]

Patient Teaching/Dietary Considerations

- Traditional Haitian foods are reflective of West African, French, and Caribbean influences. Foods frequently eaten include beans, rice, pigeon peas, black mushrooms, avocado, fried plantain, corn, chicken, conch (called *lambi* in Kreyòl), beef, pork, goat, sweet potatoes, orange/papaya juice, pumpkin, sugar cane, and cassava bread. Foods are frequently marinated in spicy Creole sauce.[7]

- Most foods are classified as having hot or cold properties and as being heavy or light. Generally, light foods are eaten in the evening and heavy foods during the daytime to provide needed energy.[10]

- Haitians may believe that certain foods are harmful to the body at different stages of one's life. The food must be in harmony with one's life cycle (e.g., certain foods are better or worse for babies, teenagers, women who are menstruating, etc.).[21]

- A common belief is that the male needs the best portion of a meal to help him to maintain physical strength and as a way to keep him in the household. This belief may contribute to nutritional deficiencies among women and children within poor families.[21]

- Being plump or overweight may be equated with beauty, and good physical and emotional well-being. Treatment for being overweight may be impeded by this belief.[10]

- Leftovers may be avoided because they are believed to produce *gaz* (gas), which leads to pain and anemia.[27]

- Lactose intolerance is common among Haitians.

- **Access Literacy Level:** For Haitians who are less educated, and because Kreyòl is primarily an oral language, teaching may be more effective through demonstrations, videos, and lectures rather than written materials.[7]

- New immigrants with limited education may have little or no exposure to technology. Explore familiarity with technological equipment. This includes familiarity with voicemail, electronic answering systems, etc. if the patient/family will have a need to use following discharge. Provide thorough explanations, including pictures or diagrams to reinforce instructions.

- The concept of time may be associated with events such as 'when the sun goes down or comes up.' Assess the patient's concept of time and adjust discharge instructions accordingly. If 'clock time' is used during teaching, ask about the presence of a clock in the home.[22]

- Follow-ups may be difficult for undocumented Haitians since many will give false identification or use different hospitals and physicians for treatment.[39]

- Church connections are strong in Haitian communities. Form collaborative relationships with ministers to facilitate accessing persons for health promotion activities.[47]

Death

- The relationship with family members does not end when death occurs. The dead continue to be important to the social integrity of the entire family. Dead family members are believed to affect the living family, even though they live in a different plane. Dead family members may be seen as being able to advise the living family members through dreams and through rebirth as new members of the community.[10]

- **Le Gros Bon Ange** (the Big Good Angel): Sometimes thought to be comparable to the Christian soul. Is thought to leave the body after death, ascend into the cosmos, and return to God.[49]

- Autopsies and organ donation may be refused because of the belief that the body should stay intact for burial.[17]

- Organ transplants may be refused because of the belief that the donor's spirit/personality will be shifted to the receiving individual as a result of the transplant. A religious representative may be helpful in providing support during the decision-making process.[17]

- Specific death rituals are based primarily on the person's religious beliefs (e.g., Catholic, Protestant, Vodou, or a combination of these religions.)

- Death arrangements generally fall to a male relative of the deceased, preferably the oldest son or cousin.[39]

Significant Haitian Holidays/Celebrations[4, 50]

- **January 1**: Independence Day - Haiti's independence was proclaimed.
- **January 2**: Forefathers' Day.
- **Carnaval**: Three days before Ash Wednesday.
- Ash Wednesday.
- Good Friday.
- Easter Sunday.
- **April 14**: Pan American Day.
- **May 1**: Agriculture and Labor Day.
- **May 18**: Flag Day.
- **Haitian Mother's Day**: The last Sunday in May.
- **June**: **Corpus Christi** (The Thursday following Trinity Sunday).
- **July 16: Saut D'Eau Pilgrimate**: Pilgrims travel to bathe in a sacred waterfall and to visit a church built on a spot where the Virgin Mary reportedly appeared in a palm tree in 1884. Both Catholic and Vodou adherents may participate in the pilgrimage to cleanse themselves.
- **July 25: Festival of Plaine du Nord** (a village southwest of Cap Haitien). This is the day of Saint James. Pilgrims wear red and blue costumes. Ceremonies and sacrifices take place, and some pilgrims bathe in the mud.
- **July 26: Feast of Saint Anne:** Celebrated in Limonade, southeast of Cap Haitien, to honor Erzulie, a Vodou spirit.
- Assumption Day.
- **October 17**: Anniversary of Jean-Jacques Dessalines' death.

- **November 1**: All Saints Day.
- **November 2**: All Souls Day.
- **November 18**: Anniversary of the Victory of Vertières (the last battle against the French).
- **December 5**: Anniversary of the discovery of Haiti.
- **Christmas Day.**

---

1 Fitzgerald, D. & Simon, T. (2001). Telling the stories of people with AIDS in rural Haiti. *AIDS Patient Care and STDs, 16*(6), 301-309.

2 Santana, M. & Dancy, B. (2000). The stigma of being named "AIDS Carriers" on Haitian-American women. *Health Care for Women International, 21*(3), 161-171.

3 Wucker, Michele (1999). *Why the cocks fight: Dominicans, Haitians, and the struggle for Hispaniola.* New York, NY: Hill & Wang.

4 United States Geological Survey. (2011). *Magnitude 7.0 – Haiti region.* Retrieved from http://earthquake.usgs.gov/earthquakes/recenteqsww/Quakes/us2010rja6.php#summary

5 CIA – The World Factbook. (2011). *Haiti.* Retrieved from https://www.cia.gov/library/publications/the-world-factbook/geos/ha.html
Miller, N. L. (2000). Haitian ethnomedical systems and biomedical practitioners: Directions for clinicians. *Journal of Transcultural Nursing, 11*(3), 204-211.

6 Cantanese, A. (1999). *Haitians: Migration and diaspora.* Boulder, CO: Westview Press.

7 Stepick, A. (1998). *Pride against prejudice: Haitians in the United States.* Boston, MA: Allyn and Bacon.

8 Heinl, R., Heinl, N. & Heinl, M. (1996). *Written in blood.* New York, NY: University Press of America, Inc.

9 Terrazas, A. (2010). *U.S. in focus: Haitian immigrants in the United States.* Retrieved from http://www.migrationinformation.org/USfocus/display.cfm?id=214

10 Miller, N. L. (2000). Haitian ethnomedical systems and biomedical practitioners: Directions for clinicians. *Journal of Transcultural Nursing, 11(*3), 204-211.

11 Ungar, B. (1986). Intestinal parasites in a migrant farmworker population. *Archives of Internal Medicine, 146*(3), 513-515.

12 Yangco, B. (1984). A survey of filariasis among refugees in south Florida. *American Journal of Tropical Medicine and Hygiene, 33*(2), 246-51.

13 Chierici, R. (1991). *Demele: "Making it": Migration and adaptation among Haitian boat people in the United States.* New York, NY: AMS Press, Inc.

14 Bentivegna, J. (1991). *The neglected and abused: A physician's year in Haiti.* Rocky Hill, CT: Michelle Publishing Company.

15 DeSantis, L. & Thomas, J. (1992). Health education and the immigrant Haitian mother: Cultural insights for community health nurses. *Health Values, 17*(6), 3-16.

16 Holcomb, L., Parsons, L., Giger, J., & Davidhizar, R. (1996). Haitian Americans: Implications for nursing care. *Journal of Community Health Nursing 13*(4), 249-260.

[17] Colin, J. & Paperwalla, G. (2013). People of Haitian Heritage. In L. Purnell. *Transcultural health care: A culturally competent approach.* (4th ed.) (pp. 269-309). Philadelphia, PA: F. A. Davis Company.
[18] Fruchter, R., Remy, J., Burnett, W. & Boyce, J. (1986). Cervical cancer in immigrant Caribbean women. American Journal of Public Health, 76(7), 797-799.
[19] Pierre, J. & Fournier, A. (1999). Human immunodeficiency virus infection in Haiti. *Journal of the National Medical Association, 91(*3), 165-170.
[20] Portes, A. & Grosfoguel, R. (1994*). Caribbean diasporas: Migration and ethnic communities.* Annals of the American Academy of Political and Social Science (Vol. 533, 48-69).
[21] Leguerre, M. (1984). *American odyssey: Haitians in New York City.* New York, NY: Cornell University Press.
[22] Potocky, M., Dodge, K. & Greene, M. (2007). Bridging cultural chasms between providers and HIV-positive Haitians in Palm Beach County, Florida. *Journal of Health Care for the Poor and Underserved, 18*(3 Supplement), 105-117.
[23] Junod, S. (2000). Diethylene glycol deaths in Haiti. *Public Health Reports, 115*(1), 78-86.
[24] World Bank Group. (2011). *Countries and economies: Haiti.* Retrieved from http://web.worldbank.org/WBSITE/EXTERNAL/DATASTATISTICS/0,,contentMDK:20535285~menuPK:1192694~pagePK:64133150~piPK:64133175~theSitePK:239419,00.html
[25] Countdown to 2015. (2010). *Maternal, newborn, & child survival: Haiti.* Retrieved from http://www.countdown2015mnch.org/documents/2012Report/2012/2012_Haiti.pdf
[26] Kovats-Bernat, J. (2006). *Sleeping rough.* Gainesville, FL: University Press of Florida.
[27] Lassiter, S. (1998). *Cultures of color in America: A guide to family, religion, and health.* Westport, CT: Greenwood Press.
[28] Prudent, N. & David, M. (1997). Health beliefs and approaches for care in Haitian immigrants in the United States. *Society for General Internal Medicine Forum, 20*(3), 2-9.
[29] Freeman, B. (1998). *Third-world folk beliefs and practices: Haitian medical anthropology.* Port-au-Prince: La Presse Evangélique.
[30] Cosgray, R. (2008). Haitian Americans. In J. Giger & R. Davidhizar. *Transcultural nursing: Assessment & intervention* (5th ed.) (pp. 563-591). St. Louis, MO: Mosby.
[31] DeSantis, L. (1993). Haitian immigrant concepts of health. *Health Values, 17*(6), 3-16.
[32] Fleurant, G. (1996). *Dancing spirits: Rhythms and rituals of Haitian vodon, the rada rite.* Westport, CT: Greenwood.
[33] Turlington, S. (2002). *The complete idiot's guide to voodoo.* Indianapolis, IN: AlphaBooks.
[34] Brodwin, P. (1996). *Medicine and morality in Haiti.* Great Britain: Cambridge University Press.
[35] Gustafson, M. (1989). Western voodoo: Providing mental health care to Haitian refugees. *Journal of Psychosocial Nursing and Mental Health Services, 27(*12), 22-25.
[36] Laguerre, M. (1984). *Afro-Caribbean folk medicine.* South Hadley, MA: Bergin & Garvey Publishers, Inc.
[37] Meade, C., Menard, J., Thervil, C. & Rivera, M. (2009). Addressing cancer disparities through community engagement: Improving breast health among Haitian women. *Oncology Nursing Forum, 36*(6), 716-722.
[38] Shipp, M. (2001). Awareness status and prevalence of hypertension in a group of urban Haitians: Findings of a population-based survey. *Ethnicity and Disease, 11*(3), 419-430.
[39] Preston, R., Materson, B., Yohan, M. & Anapol, H. (1996). Hypertension in Haitians: Results of a pilot survey of a public teaching hospital multispecialty clinic. *Journal of Human Hypertension, 19*(11), 743-745.

[40] Laguerre, M. (1981). In A. Harwood (Ed.). *Ethnicity and medical care.* (pp. 172-210). Cambridge, MA: Harvard University Press.

[41] Philippe, J. (1979). Indispositino in Haiti. *Social Science and Medicine, 13B*(2), 129-133.

[42] Stobinski, J. (1999). A perioperative nurse's experience in Haiti. *AORN Journal, 69*(2), 346-357.

[43] Chelala, C. (1994). Letter from Haiti: Fighting for survival. *British Medical Journal, 309*(6953), 525-526.

[44] Nicolas, G., DeSilva, A., Grey, K., & Gonzalez-Eastep, D. (2006). Using a multicultural lens to understand illnesses among Haitians living in America. *Professional Psychology: Research and Practice, 37*(6), 716-722.

[45] Dempsey, P. & Geese, T. (1983). The childbearing Haitian refugee – cultural applications to clinical nursing. *Public Health Reports, 98*(3), 261-267.

[46] Harris, K. (1987). Beliefs and practices among Haitian American women in relation to childbearing. *Journal of Nurse Midwifery, 32*(3), 149-155.

[47] Mooney, M. (2009). *Faith makes us live: Surviving and thriving in the Haitian Diaspora.* Los Angeles, CA: University of California Press.

[48] DeSantis, L. & Thomas, J. (1990). The immigrant Haitian mother: Transcultural nursing perspectives on preventive health for children. *Journal of Transcultural Nursing, 2*(1), 2-15.

[49] Trouillot, M. (1991). The ways and nature of the Zombi. *Journal of American Folklore, 104*(414), 466-493.

[50] Doggett, S. & Gordon, L. (1999). *Dominican Republic & Haiti.* Melbourne Evangélique, Port-au-Prince: Lonely Planet Publications.

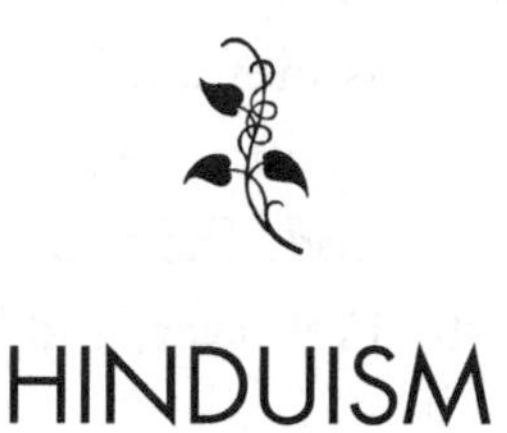

HINDUISM

Background

Hinduism is the world's oldest living faith, the third largest religion, and embodies the spirit of religious harmony. Hinduism acknowledges that only one God exists, but teaches that God may be realized through differing spiritual paths.[1,2,3,4]

The origins of Hinduism are somewhat unclear. Unlike many other religions, Hinduism cannot be traced to any one founder or historic event. Historians believe that the beginning of the religion dates back to 2,000 BC in northwest India near the Indus river.[5,6] The religion spread along trade routes in India to other countries in the East.[1] Hinduism has no set creed, doctrines, or religious organization, but emphasizes a way of living. There is much diversity in the beliefs and practices of its followers.[7] The caste system has been legally abolished, but the practices within Hinduism remain affected by this system because of beliefs concerning reincarnation.

Today, more than 80 percent of India's people are Hindu. There are sizeable populations in Thailand, Malaysia, Canada, Britain, and the United States. Worldwide, there are over 950 million Hindus.[1,6]

Religious Representatives

- Priests are the only religious representatives.

Religious Beliefs

- Hundreds of diverse sects, so practices may differ. However, Hindus affirm God (Nirguna Brahman) is the highest power and is eternal. He is present in all living beings, and it is possible to worship Him in a variety of ways. The numerous deities in Hinduism are seen as aspects or manifestations of God. The triune of God in Hinduism is manifested as Brahmā, the Creator; Vishnu, the Preserver; and Shiva, the Destroyer or Liberator.[8, 9]
- *Om/Aum* is the most sacred word in Hinduism. It is non-denominational and a non-personal word and, therefore, is used as a visual symbol of God by all Hindu sects. The word is frequently mentioned in the *Vedas* and other Hindu scriptures.[3, 9]
- There are four stages of an individual's life:[3, 9]
  - **Brahmacharya**: Covers the period prior to marriage. The individual is seen as a student and in a period of education and character development.
  - **Gārhasthya**: The period during which an individual is working in the world and establishes a family household.
  - **Vānaprasthya**: The stage of retiring from worldly attachments.
  - **Pravrajya**: The period of waiting for death and release of the spirit to unite with Brahmān.
- There are many rituals/practices based on the occasion and/or purpose. Important events in a Hindu's life such as childbirth, marriage, and cremation are sanctified through a religious sacrament known as *samskāra*.[3, 10, 11]
- The religion supports the belief in reincarnation according to the law of *Karma*. The belief is that rebirth is dependent on moral behavior in an individual's previous existence. An individual experiences multiple rebirths to purify the soul. The goal of one's present

existence is to be released from the cycle of rebirth and death, thereby achieving *moksha* where the soul becomes one with God. Brahām is the universal soul, the ultimate intelligence. It is believed that all people are caught up in a cosmic system of everlasting *becoming* and *perishing*. All things proceed from and return to Brahmān. In simpler terms, there is the belief in one God who energizes the entire universe. Hindus believe in the existence of other superhuman powers (devas) that serve different functions in controlling nature and other life events. However, Brahmān is the Supreme. There are four aims of living:

- **Artha**: Material prosperity.
- **Kāma**: Satisfaction of desires.
- **Dharma**: Performing the moral and ethical duties of one's place in life.
- **Moksha**: Obtaining release from the cycle of rebirths that every soul is subject to.

- Hindus strive to fulfill his or her duty toward family, traditions, and devotion to the gods.[2,3,7,12,13,14]
- The five daily duties are:[2,10]
  - **Yoga and Meditation**: Yoga is aimed at decreasing one's distraction by the senses, allowing the individual to be more focused on the inner spirit.
  - Worship and reverence for a deity.
  - Respect for elders and ancestors.
  - Extending hospitality to the needy and to holy men.
  - Respect and kindness for all living creatures.
- Generally, a Hindu will wear some distinctive mark (pundra) on the forehead and may carry some symbol of his or her religion.
- Shrines dedicated to a specific deity may be found in the home for private worship.

Religious Texts

- Sacred scriptures of the *Vedas* or *Divine Truth*. The word Veda means knowledge. These are the oldest of the Hindu texts and are arranged in four collections. The roots of Hindu wisdom and teaching are contained in these scriptures. Each of the Vedas contains supplementary texts which contributed to the development of Hindu beliefs.[3,15]

- **Smriti** (remembering): These writings provide information about kings and gods, the activities of a particular deity, and guides to proper conduct.[15]

Special/Religious Observations

Most special events are based on the lunar calendar. The dates may vary from year to year. Ways to celebrate the special days vary among communities.[4,14,16]

- **Caturmasya**: A four-month period of practicing varying degrees of self-denial to minimize gratification of the senses, generally occurring July through November.

- **Diwali** (Festival of Light): The New Year festival, taking place in September through October and is a five-day festival. It is the beginning of the new Hindu year.

- **Dussehara** (Celebrated during September or October for ten days.) The festival is focused on the worship of the goddesses Durga, Lakshmi, and Saraswati.

- **Holi** (Occurs in February or March): Celebration is symbolic of destroying all the evils of the world.

- **Kumbh Mela** (Festival held every twelve years): Hindus make a pilgrimage to the holy city of Allahabad, located on the banks of the Ganges River to bathe in the water. It is believed that bathing in the river will wash away their sins.

- **Makara Samkranti** (Winter Solstice Festival occurring in mid-January): The day is spent in prayer.

- **Navarātri** (Nine-day Durgā festival, occurs September through October): Some persons fast for the full nine days of the celebration.

- **Purnima**: Day of the full moon.

- **Rām Navamī** (Birthday of Rama): Fasting accompanies this celebration.
- **Shiva Rātri** (Celebrates the birth of Lord Shiva; occurs February through March): Fasting accompanies this celebration.
- **Krishna Janmāsthtamī** (Birthday of Lord Krishna): Occurs August through September.

Health Beliefs/Practices

- There are strong beliefs in astrology. The movement of the planets has a major influence on human life. Illness may be attributed to supernatural causes.[11,12]
- Pain and suffering may be seen as the result of sinful acts/deeds in this or previous lives. This belief may impact the individual's self-report of pain levels. Meditation may be used as an intervention to manage pain instead of pain medications.[9]
- Males have a responsibility to look after females. Males may not leave females in the presence of an unfamiliar male. Provide same-sex caregivers. Gown patient in a manner that protects modesty.[10]
- Family members, especially elders, have a strong influence on decisions. Determine who will make treatment decisions.
- Protective jewelry or sacred strings may be worn. Provide careful explanation to patient and/or family if absolutely necessary to remove these objects. Give to relatives for safekeeping.[11]
- The concept of purity is important to Hindu life, leading many Hindus to be meticulous about personal cleanliness. Showers are preferred to baths since the individual would not want to be sitting in dirty water. Nasal flushing is not uncommon, and the tongue may be cleaned prior to eating. Bodily discharges may be considered impure. Females are considered temporarily impure or polluted when menstruating and following childbirth. The left hand is generally used for toileting hygiene and other unclean tasks. Genitals may be cleaned following toileting. The right had is generally used for eating and other clean tasks. Be cognizant of this when considering IV placement. Assist with cleanliness practices as needed.[10,11,17]

- Individuals will have specific times for prayer and meditation, generally after bathing in the early morning and in the early evening. They may have a desire to keep religious statues or pictures close by. Prayer for recovery from illness is generally unacceptable. Use flexibility in planning care to accommodate prayer and meditation; provide privacy.

- There are three body humors: *wind* (vata), *bile* (pitta) and *phlegm* (kapha). Hot and cold theory applies to foods and equilibrium within the body. Imbalances are believed to cause illness.[11]

- Shoes are often removed prior to entering the Hindu home to avoid bringing dirt into the home. For home health visits, inquire about the necessity of removing shoes prior to entering the home.[11]

Birth/Children

- The fetus is considered a person from the time of conception. The moment of conception marks the rebirth of an individual who has lived multiple lives previously. Frequent prayers during pregnancy are necessary for the development of a healthy child.[11]

- There are no religious requirements for a fetus delivered at less than seven months gestation. The soul is thought to enter the body at seven months gestation and, therefore, requires appropriate death and funeral rites.[11]

- **Elective Pregnancy Termination**: No restrictions. However, individual attitudes vary. Some Hindus believe that pregnancy termination sends the soul back to the cycle of rebirth.[11,13]

- **Amniocentesis**: Acceptable.

- **Birth Control**: No restrictions.

- **Circumcision**: Acceptable. No special rituals.

Dietary Considerations

- Many Hindus are strict vegetarians and connect this dietary choice to spirituality. The type of food eaten is also thought to impact not only the person's body, but the mind and emotions as well. Foods are divided into three main categories based on its potential effects on the mind and body. *Sattwic* foods have the most desirable effects and maximum benefits. *Rajasic* foods produce unrest, pain, and disease. These may include highly spiced foods, foods with strong smells, highly caffeinated foods, and meat. *Tamasic* foods are the least desirable foods and have the most negative effects on the body. They include leftovers, stale foods, fermented foods, etc.[11,18,19]

- Fasting is common. It may be practiced on specific days of the week, on some holidays, and in conjunction with special prayers. Food intake on fasting days may vary from complete abstinence to one meal per day. Consider this when providing education about disease processes that may be affected by fasting, such as diabetes. The sick and infirm are not required to fast.[11,17]

- Eating beef is prohibited. Cows are considered sacred; they are thought to symbolize fertility, represent life and the sustenance of life. The animal is considered to possess qualities that Hindus can strive to gain because the cow takes little for itself, existing on grass and grain. However, it is the most generous animal, giving back to man such things as milk, bones for soup, leather for shoes, etc. Other meat is not eaten because it involves harming a living creature, or in the case of pork, the pig is seen as a scavenger and, therefore, the meat is considered unclean. Chicken and fish may be acceptable to some Hindus. However, food prepared in a medical facility may not be accepted because it may have come in contact with a forbidden food. The hospitalized individual may desire food to be brought from home.[11]

- Hindus may refuse medication by capsule. Cows and pigs are a source for the manufacture of some capsules.

Death

- Because of the diversity among Hindus, death rituals will vary based on factors such as acculturation, socioeconomic status, geographical region, etc.

- Family members may be reluctant to have a diagnosis of terminal illness disclosed to the dying relative. To do so may be seen as hastening the family member's death and destroying hope.[9]

- Dying patients may choose to fast to ensure that the body is pure at the time of death. Fasting may also be done in an effort to decrease the likelihood of vomiting and incontinence. Vomiting and/or incontinence may be viewed as signs of a "bad death." Keep the patient clean and dry.[9]

- Alleviation of unnecessary suffering during the dying process is desirable. However, the desire for an unclouded mind during death is important. Seek medications and non-pharmacological measures that will accomplish this goal.

- **Suicide**: Strongly condemned. The belief is that taking one's life prematurely results in forces of karma that lead to much more pain and suffering than would have been encountered if one had not committed suicide.[3]

- The physical body dies, but the soul has no beginning or end. The person may pass into another reincarnation.[20]

- Although death rituals vary, if death occurs in the home, the family may want to place the dying person's body on a clean sheet and/or mat on the floor with the head pointing north (toward Mount Kailasha in the Himalayas, the home of Lord Siva/Shiva). This symbolizes closeness to Mother Earth and freedom from physical constraints. It is also believed to facilitate the departure of the soul.[9,11,16]

- Expect that family members will want to stay in close attendance with the dying Hindu. It is viewed as a family responsibility and of great importance to hear/acknowledge the last words of a dying relative. The last words of the dying relative may give some comfort to family members that the individual's soul will have a 'good' journey into the next world. It is desirable that God be in the thoughts of the dying person at the time of death. Prayers may be offered, as well as other death rites to facilitate the appropriate transmigration of the soul. If friends live close by, it will be a religious duty to pay respects to the family. Allow privacy and adequate time.[9,11,21]

- Consult family members about their beliefs regarding non-family members touching the body after death. Religious rites will be performed. The oldest son has a sacred duty to perform death rites for the father. A close male family member will be selected to perform these duties if it is impossible for the eldest son to do so. The family will want to wash the family member's body following death (symbolizes cleansing of the soul). Threads tied to the body by a priest or any jewelry should be left in place. The priest may pour a small amount of sacred water in the mouth of the dead person as part of religious rites of death.[8, 22]

- **Autopsy**: Generally acceptable only if legally necessary because of the belief that an incomplete body will interfere with reincarnation of the individual's soul.
- **Organ Donation**: Acceptable.
- Cremation is generally the disposition of choice for adults and is preferably completed within twenty-four hours following death. Cremation is seen as a method of purifying the dead and expediting the travel of the soul from this world to the next. Children are generally buried because their personalities are not fully formed and, therefore, do not need the purification provided through cremation.[9, 22, 23]

Miscellaneous

- **Blood and Blood Products**: Acceptable.

---

[1] Central Intelligence Agency. (2011). *The world factbook: World.* Retrieved from https://www.cia.gov/library/publications/the-world-factbook/geos/xx.html

[2] Keene, M. (1993). *Seekers after truth: Buddhism, Sikhism.* Great Britain: Cambridge University Press.

[3] Bhaskarananda, S. (2002). *The essentials of Hinduism: A comprehensive overview of the world's oldest religion.* Seattle, WA: Viveka Press.

[4] Meredith, S. & Hickman, C. (2001). *The Usborne Internet-linked encyclopedia of word religions.* London: Usborne Publishing Ltd.

[5] Burke, T. (1996). *The major religions: An introduction with texts.* Cambridge: Blackwell Publishers.

[6] Toropov, B. & Buckles, L. (2011). *The complete idiot's guide to the world's religions* (4th ed.).New York, NY: Alpha Books.

[7] Goring, R. & Whaling, F. (Eds.). (1994). *Larousse dictionary of beliefs and religions.* New York, NY: Larousse Kingfisher Chambers, Inc.

[8] Pearson, A. (1998). Hinduism. In C. Johnson & M. McGee (Eds.). *How different religions view death and afterlife* (pp. 109-131). Philadelphia, PA: The Charles Press, Publishers.

[9] Gatrad, R., Choudhury, P., Brown, E. & Sheikh, A. (2003). Palliative care for Hindus. *International Journal of Palliative Nursing, 9*(10), 442-448.

[10] Kinsley, D. (1993) *Hinduism: A cultural perspective.* Englewood Cliffs, NJ: Prentice Hall.

[11] Jootum, D. (2002). Nursing with dignity–Part 7–Hinduism. *Nursing Times, 98*(15), 38-40.

[12] Flood, G. (1996). *An introduction to Hinduism.* Melbourne, Australia: Cambridge University Press.

[13] Coward, H. & Sidhu, T. (2000). Bioethics for clinicians: Hinduism and Sikhism. *Canadian Medical Association Journal, 163*(9), 1167-1170.
[14] Johnsen, L. (2002). *The complete idiot's guide to Hinduism*. Indianapolis, IN: Alpha Books.
[15] Littleton, C. (1996). *The sacred East.* London, England: Duncan Baird Publishers.
[16] Warrier, S. & Walshe, J. (2001). *Dates and meanings of religious and other multi-ethnic festival: 2002-2005.* New York, NY: Foulsham Educational.
[17] Wilkins, A. & Mailoo, V. J. (2010). Care of the older person: A Hindu perspective. *Nursing & Residential Care, 12*(5), 249-251.
[18] Jayaram, V. (2010). *Hinduism and food.* Retrieved from http://www.hinduwebsite.com/hinduism/h_food.asp
[19] ElGindy, G. (2005, Fall). Hindu dietary practices: Feeding the body, mind, and soul. *Minority Nurse.* Retrieved from http://www.minoritynurse.com/dietic/hindu-dietary-practices-feeding-body-mind-and-soul
[20] Magida, A. (2003). *How to be a perfect stranger: A guide to etiquette in other people's religious ceremonies.* Woodstock, VT: Jewish Lights Publishing.
[21] Doorenbos, A. (2003). Hospice access for Asian Indian immigrants. *Journal of Hospice and Palliative Nursing, 5*(1), 27-33.
[22] Laungani, P. (2001). Hindu deaths in India–Part 1. *International Journal of Health Promotion and Education, 39*(3), 88-96.
[23] Clements, P., Vigil, G., Manno, M., Henry, G., Wilks, J., Das, S., & Foster, W. (2003). Cultural perspectives of death, grief, and bereavement. *Journal of Psychosocial Nursing, 41*(7), 18.

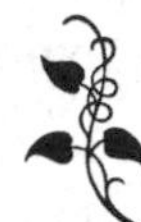

HISPANICS AND LATINOS

Background

The terms *Hispanic* and *Latino* are often used interchangeably. However, the term Hispanic **does not** denote race, and only considers that the individual is of Spanish-speaking origin or descent. The term was first used in the United States to categorize groups of people for census purposes. The term Latino denotes a person of Latin American origin. All persons from Latin America do not speak Spanish and all persons from Spanish-speaking countries are not Latinos. For instance, persons from Spain are not Latinos. Many Hispanics/Latinos prefer not to be grouped under this umbrella term, but to be identified based on their specific country of origin (e.g., Mexican, Cuban, etc).[1]

More than 50 million persons in the United States are of Hispanic/Latino origin. They are the fastest growing population in the United States and, collectively, the largest ethnic group. The number of Hispanics/Latinos is expected to constitute 30 percent of the total population by 2050. Mexicans comprise approximately 63 percent of Hispanics/Latinos living in the United States; followed by Central/South Americans (14 percent), Puerto Ricans (9.2 percent), Cubans (3.5 percent), and other groups.[2] A common belief is that Hispanics/Latinos are culturally the same. To the contrary, there is a tremendous diversity among and within the groups.

Health risks among Hispanics/Latinos include hypertension, obesity, diabetes and its sequelae (particularly among Mexicans and Puerto Ricans), cirrhosis, cervical cancer, HIV/AIDS, and accidents/homicides. A large percentage of migrant workers are Hispanics/Latinos. Health care services such as those available through the Community and Migrant Health Programs have been established in the United States to assist with meeting the health care needs of migrant workers. However, because of decreased funding to these facilities and other economic factors, migrant workers face health risks that are seen less often in the general Hispanic population. These include poverty, substandard living conditions, isolation, violence, poor access to or lack of medical treatment, exposure to toxic chemicals such as pesticides, over-exposure to sun and its related effects, substance abuse, nutrition deficiencies, tuberculosis, asthma, dental disease, infectious/parasitic diseases, and occupational/agricultural/farm injuries. Child labor laws in the United States related to farm and agricultural work differ in some ways from requirements for other jobs in mainstream society. Also, child labor laws are often relaxed or ignored, particularly in rural areas. Consequently, children of migrant workers are particularly at risk for serious and sometimes, life-threatening injuries when they accompany parents to work and are left unattended, when they work with parents or relatives, or work alone as migrant workers. Urinary tract infections are more prevalent because of long hours spent in fields without ready access to bathroom facilities and poor hygienic conditions.[3, 4, 5, 6]

Mercury and lead may be contained in substances used for folk treatments, folk rituals, and in amulets. Exposure to lead among young children may be environmentally related, especially among migrant children in substandard living conditions. Children are particularly vulnerable to the effects of mercury and lead exposure. Exposure to pesticides/insecticides is another risk factor among children of migrant workers often because the toxic substances are brought home on adult clothing.[5, 7, 8, 9]

Language

- Spanish is the first language of many Hispanics/Latinos. However, French, Portuguese, Dutch, English, and regional dialects may be first languages. Native Central and South American Indians may speak their tribal language only, such as *Maya*, *Quechua*, *Aymara*, *Guarani*, etc. Other languages include *Mixteco*, *Zapoteco*, *Trique*, *Quiché*, *Kanjobal*, and *Tarascan*. Persons who speak these languages in the United States reside most often in rural areas of Florida, Colorado, California, and Texas.[6]

- Hispanics/Latinos are frequently expressive in communicating. Their comfortable social distance is about half the distance as that of many United States Americans.[10]

Worldview/Religious Beliefs

- The majority of Hispanics/Latinos are Roman Catholic. There are growing numbers of individuals who are followers of other Christian religions. African-based religions such as Santeria, Voodoo, Macumba, and Condomble may be practiced solely or in conjunction with Christianity.[11,12]

- Individuals often believe that they have limited control over what happens in their life. Good things may be seen as rewards from God, bad things/illnesses as punishment by God.[13]

- There are common beliefs in the supernatural, including the evil eye. A *brujo(a)* is a person believed to use magical powers that affect health such as hexes and curses. *Brujos* are believed to be able to cast or cure illnesses resulting from magic.[5]

- Important values include:

  - **Compadrazgo**: A traditional fictive kinship relationship is often formed with individuals outside the family, which promotes a sense of belonging and community. Health care providers may recognize compadrazgo as a cultural strength, which promotes health and provides support during illness.[14]

  - **Familismo**: The family is the center of activity. It includes extended family, friends, godparents, etc.

  - **Machismo**: Males are head of the household and responsible for protecting and providing for the family. Other machismo values include courage, fearlessness, pride, honor, and leadership. Machismo has been erroneously interpreted as being exclusively aggressive and associated with sexual prowess, which are traits not valued in the Hispanic/Latino culture.[15]

  - **Marianismo**: Females are caretakers of the home and children. They strive for the purity of the Virgin Mary. This is a complementary role to machismo, maintaining a balance of power in the home.[10,15]

- **Personalismo/Confianza**: Refers to identifying with and establishing a personal relationship with another individual. It is important that health care providers establish a trusting relationship. This means taking personal interest in the family, spending time with family, etc.

- **Respeto**: Involves giving respect, particularly to elders. Health care providers will be approached with this same respect. Anticipate that questions may not be asked and lack of understanding of the treatment plan may not be acknowledged out of a sense of respect. Acknowledge elders when entering a room. Because of this strong value, nodding the head may not necessarily indicate agreement or understanding. Individuals may not give eye contact out of respect to the health care provider.[9]

- **Simpatia**: Involves being agreeable instead of confrontational. Health care providers should present themselves in a warm and caring manner, acknowledging the presence of family members during interactions.[9]

Health Beliefs/Practices

- Illness can be caused by physical, psychological, spiritual imbalances and/or disharmony with nature.

- Hot and cold principles apply. Foods, medicines, illnesses, etc. that are considered hot or cold will vary among groups.

- Illness is God's will, and recovery is in His hands. All persons must endure a certain amount of suffering and must bear it with dignity and courage. This belief may interfere with preventive care and long-term treatment plans. Stress and relate the importance of preventive care and adherence to treatment plans to being as healthy as possible to be able to fulfill one's family role.

- Susceptibility to illness is related to age. Babies and children are considered weaker than adults.

- Preventive care may not be practiced. Folk or self-treatments are frequently tried prior to presentation to mainstream medical facilities. In Mexico and some other countries, prescriptions are not required for a number of medications, including injectable medicines.

Needles may be shared, including in treatment of children. Likely to seek mainstream medical care when health is in crisis.[5,9,16]

- Hispanics/Latinos will often consult traditional folk healers prior to presenting to mainstream medical sources. *Curanderismo* is a health care system widely used among Hispanics/Latinos throughout Mexico, Puerto Rico, Central, and South America. It blends African, Native American, and Spanish healing approaches. It focuses on a holistic approach to bringing individuals back into harmony with all aspects of self and nature, believing that the mind, body, and spirit cannot be treated as separate entities. The word 'curanderismo' is derived from the Spanish word *curar*, meaning "to heal." Folk healers' names may differ in various regions, but healing techniques and principles are similar. Healers may be female or male and are often known as a *curandera* or *curandero*, respectively. A *curandero total* is skilled in the use of all the healing tools within curanderismo. Curanderos are broadly categorized as follows:[17,18,19,20]

  - **Hierbero** (herbalist): Herbs are not only ingested, but are also used for cleansing baths and other rituals. Herbalists are extremely skilled in herbal use and view plants as spiritually powerful.

  - **Sobadora**: Specializes in the use of massage for healing.

  - **Partera**: Provides midwifery care. Parteras care for the obstetrical and spiritual needs of their patients.

  - **Consejera** (counselor): Consejeras counsel individuals on a wide variety of problems, including marital problems, problems with children, matters of self-esteem, etc.

  - **Espiritualista**: Thought to have special powers to serve as a medium linking to the spiritual world through trances. The espiritualista is able to communicate with the spirits who provide protection and advice for those persons who still deal with the problems of their earthly life. Espiritualistas often perform special rites and may use candles, prayer, and offerings during healing sessions.

  - **Huesero**: Uses folk practices similar to those of a chiropractor.

  - **Santguadoro/Santguadora**: Puerto Rican folk healer.

- Folk healers are commonly consulted for many reasons. Folk illnesses limited to the Hispanic/Latino population that folk healers are commonly consulted for treatment include:

  - *Empacho* is a commonly reported illness among Mexicans. It is believed to be caused by undigested or uncooked food that sticks to the wall of the stomach or intestine. It is not limited to certain age groups. Symptoms include vomiting, loss of appetite, bloating, or constipation. Treatment includes massaging the back or stomach, pinching the skin on the back, and herbal teas. A tea made from wormwood is a cerebral stimulant that may lead to psychosis and death. Diarrhea following treatment is considered to be a sign of curing. Lead and mercury poisoning is a risk related to common folk treatments for empacho using lead salts commonly purchased in Mexican pottery supply, hardware, and drug stores. These include *greta* (lead oxide), *azarcon* (lead tetroxide), and *albayalde* (lead carbonate). *Asoque* (elemental mercury) and *anil* (laundry bluing) may be used also. Provide appropriate testing for toxicity, particularly among children.[9, 21, 22]

  - **Susto** (soul loss): A culture-bound illness believed to be caused by severe fright or shock. The illness can affect persons of all ages. Symptoms can be vague, but include complaints of personality changes, anorexia, lethargy, insomnia, headaches.[5, 23]

  - **Bilis** (rage): Gastric discomfort caused by hypersecretion of bile, secondary to high levels of anger. Symptoms include vomiting, diarrhea, migraine headaches, and dizziness.[17]

  - **Mal Aire** (bad air): Caused by exposure to night air. It is thought to result in cold-like symptoms, earaches in children, and facial paralysis in adults. Caution parents about the hazard of overheating infants who are wrapped tightly in blankets in an effort to prevent exposure.[17]

  - **Nervios** (nerves): Describes a broad range of psychological disorders ranging from simple everyday blues to more severe disorders.[24]

  - **Caida de mollera** (fallen fontanel): Commonly seen in infants who are dehydrated. The folk belief is that the sunken fontanel is caused by separating the nipple from the infant's mouth too quickly, falling, or being dropped, riding on a bumpy road, rocking the baby too fast, etc. The resulting symptoms include vomiting, diarrhea, fever, sunken or 'runny' eyes, and/or irritability. Based on the belief that the condition is a mechanical one, folk treatments include:[25, 26]

- Applying upward pressure with the finger to the infant's hard palate.
- Sucking on the fontanel to create a vacuum and draw the fontanel back to its original position, holding the baby upside down and dipping the top of the head in water.
- Applying a poultice to the fontanel, which is thought to "pull" the fontanel up as it dries.

- Cupping may be used as a method of treating illnesses, leaving reddened or slightly bruised areas on the skin. Inquire about the origin of such areas on the skin so as not to confuse them with signs of physical abuse.[5]

- May wear protective strings (red is a common color in children), charms with images of the Virgin Mary, or a crucifix. These should be left on the patient and should not be removed unless absolutely necessary for medical purposes. Provide careful explanation and rationale to the patient/family. Give to the family for safekeeping. Altars and other religious symbols are often found in and around homes.

- Mental illness carries a stigma within some Latino families. Families may attempt to hide or deny the illness until no longer able to manage the individual. A variety of folk treatments may be tried before the individual presents for mainstream medical treatment. Assessment of the presence or history of mental illness within families may be more successful if family members are asked about specific symptoms that may have been exhibited instead of asking if there is a history of mental illness.[24]

- Psychological and mental distress may be expressed somatically through symptoms such as general lethargy, headaches, and abdominal discomforts. It is important to validate the individual's physical symptoms prior to assessment of psychological symptoms. Explore patient's perspective on the origin of symptoms.[24]

Expression of Pain

- Expressive. However, this expressiveness is a culturally acceptable response and is not necessarily synonymous with the severity of pain or of the individual's ability to tolerate pain.[27]

Male-Female/Kinship/Social Relationships

- High respect for authority and the elderly.
- Males are often authority figures and generally act as spokesperson for family decisions. However, the extended family will have a part in decision-making.
- Family is highly valued. Important for family members to stay with the sick individual and participate in care as much as possible. It is not unusual for a large number of family members to accompany an individual to a health care facility.[9]
- There may be multiple generations and/or friends, extended family members living within the same household.[28] Families provide financial and emotional support to each other.
- Provide same-sex caregivers, if at all possible.
- It is inappropriate for the Hispanic male to discuss 'private' body parts or sexual subjects with his mother and other females.
- Modesty is highly valued. The area between the waist and the knees is viewed as particularly private.
- The progress of male and elderly patients with self-care activities may be impeded by the expectation that female family members and children carry out activities for them.

Birth/Children

- Children are highly valued. Teenage marriages are common. Women may become very disturbed if pregnancy does not occur soon after marriage. Typically, there are several births. Children often live at home until marriage.
- Pregnancy is considered a 'hot' condition. Therefore, foods and conditions that are classified as 'hot' will be avoided. Prenatal vitamins and iron tablets may be avoided because they are considered to have hot properties.[25, 29]
- May seek prenatal care late during pregnancy since pregnancy is considered a 'normal' condition.

- Unborn babies can be 'marked' by the mother's actions during pregnancy, such as food cravings causing birthmarks on the infant.[30]

- Expressive of discomfort during labor. Mexicans may often repeat "aye yie yie" during labor, which may serve as a form of "folk Lamaze." Repeating these words several times in succession requires long, slow, deep breaths and is, therefore, a method of relieving pain in this culture.[31] Generally, among Mexicans, the laboring woman's mother provides support during labor.

- Some men may consider it inappropriate to assist during delivery. Some husbands may not want to see the wife or child until after the delivery and after they have been cleaned up and dressed.

- Approximately 70 percent of Hispanic infants have Mongolian spots. These should not be confused with bruises. They are most often found in the lumbosacral and gluteal areas, but are not limited to these areas. They begin to fade during the first two years of life, but may persist into adolescence.[32]

- During menstruation and following delivery, females may not want to walk barefoot, wash the hair, and take showers or baths. Sponge baths may be substituted for hygiene maintenance. They may observe the practice of having a "lying-in" period (several weeks) following birth. Cold liquids, 'cold' foods such as vegetables, citrus fruits, bananas, tomatoes, and pork may be avoided. Exercise may be limited or avoided. The woman will want to rest and stay warm. If the baby must stay in the hospital after the mother's discharge, she may refrain from accompanying the father to the hospital to visit the baby during the lying-in period.

- May be resistant to early breastfeeding, believing that colostrum is "bad milk." For this reason, the mother may insist on bottle-feeding the infant until her "real milk" comes in. Should be provided with privacy while breastfeeding.

- A coin applied next to the infant's umbilical cord, then wrapped with a bellyband, is common in an effort to prevent the navel from protruding after it is healed. Health care workers who are concerned about infection should instruct the mother to clean the coin with alcohol before application and to keep the belly band clean.[31]

- Children are highly valued and viewed as a gift from God. Relatives and friends are strongly involved in child rearing.

- The godparent (*padrino* or *madrina*) may be heavily involved in the care of children during hospitalization. The godparent is viewed as a co-parent.[33]

- Girls may be taught at an early age not to completely undress and that touching the genital area is "bad."

Death

- The family may not be supportive of a terminally ill relative being told a grim prognosis. It is believed that, if the person is told, it prevents enjoyment of whatever life is left.[34]

- When talking with parents about Sudden Infant Death Syndrome, avoid using the acronym SIDS. The Spanish acronym for AIDS is *SIDA*. The family may confuse the cause of the infant's death.[35]

- Puerto Ricans may believe that a person's spirit will not be free to enter the next life if that person has died leaving something unsaid. Family members should be allowed as much interaction as possible with the dying relative. *El Ataque de nervios* may be seen among Puerto Ricans associated with grief. It is accepted as a way to discharge grief and is displayed by seizure-like behavior, displays of aggression, hyperkinetic episodes, and sometimes stupor.[36]

- Hispanic males are generally raised to lim it expressions of suffering. Other family members may openly express feelings of anguish and grief.

Patient Teaching/Dietary Considerations

- Hot foods may be avoided during pregnancy since it is considered a hot condition.

- Usual diet is high in salt, sugar, starches, and fat.

- Rice, beans, and fruit are popular foods. Dietary preferences vary among Hispanic groups.

- In the Puerto Rican population, lactating women may drink malt beer with the belief that it increases the amount of milk.[33]

- Being overweight may be seen as a sign of good health and well-being.[10]
- Use caution when using the written word *once* in instructions for medications, treatments, etc. *Once* in Spanish means eleven (11) in English.[11]
- At social gatherings, declining food may be seen as impolite and socially unacceptable increasing the possibility of overeating.[23]
- It is common that families eat meals together; therefore, including the family in dietary teaching is useful and can improve nutrition for the entire family.[23]
- Type 2 Diabetes is perceived as a serious illness, which can cause a premature death and the fear of identity loss related to having the disease. Patient educators should explore with the patient how having diabetes changes how they feel about themselves, how they are perceived by others, and their role in society.[23]

---

1 U.S. Census Bureau. (2011, March). *The Hispanic population: 2010.* (C2010BR-04). Retrieved from http://www.census.gov/prod/cen2010/briefs/c2010br-04.pdf

2 U.S. Census Bureau. (2010, July 15). *Profile America facts for features: Hispanic heritage month 2010: Sept. 15- Oct. 15.* Retrieved from http://www.census.gov/newsroom/releases/archives/facts_for_features_special_editions/cb10-ff17.html

3 Benabe, J. & Rios, E. (2004). Kidney disease in the Hispanic population: Facing the growing challenge. *Journal of the National Medical Association, 96*(6), 789-98.

4 Reynolds, D. (2004). Cervical cancer in Hispanic/Latino women. *Clinical Journal of Oncology Nursing, 8*(2), 146-150.

5 American Academy of Pediatrics & Migrant Clinicians Network (2000). *Guidelines for the care of migrant farmworkers' children.* Elk Grove Village, IL & Austin, TX: American Academy of Pediatrics and the Migrant Clinicians Network.

6 Aquirre-Molina, M., Molina, C., & Zambrana, R. (2001). *Health issues in the Latino community.* San Francisco, CA: Jossey-Bass.

7 Riley, D., Newby, C., Leal-Almeraz, T. & Thomas, V. (2001). Assessing elemental mercury vapor exposure from cultural and religious practices. *Environmental Health Perspectives, 109*(8), 779-87.

8 Forman, J., Moline, J., Cernichiari, E., Sayegh, S., Torres, J., Landrigan, M.,…Ladrigan, P. (2000). A cluster of pediatric metallic mercury exposure cases treated with meso02,3-dimercaptoduccinic acid (DSMA). *Environmental Health Perspectives, 108*(6), 575-77.

9 Lasseter, J. & Baldwin, J. (2004). Health care barriers for Latino children and provision of culturally competent care. *Journal of Pediatric Nursing,* 19(3), 184-92.

10 Clark, J. & Hoffman, C. (1998). Suggestions for meeting the health and nutrition education needs of Hispanic and immigrant families. *Topics in Clinical Nutrition, 13*(3), 73-82.

11 Nunez, L. (1992). *Santeria: A practical guide to Afro-Caribbean magic.* Woodstock, VT: Spring Publications, Inc.

[12] Voeks, R. (1997). *Sacred leaves of Candomble: African magic, medicine and religion in Brazil.* Austin, TX: University of Texas Press.

[13] Rehm, R. (1999). Religious faith in Mexican-American families dealing with chronic childhood illness. Image: *Journal of Nursing Scholarship, 31*(1), 33-38.

[14] Gill-Hopple, K. & Brage-Hudson, D. (2012). Compadrazgo: A literature review. *Journal of Transcultural Nursing, 23*(2), 117-123.

[15] Weaver, H. (2010). Social work practice with Latinos. In B. Thyer, J. Wodarski, L. Myers, & D. Harrison, *Cultural diversity and social work practice* (3rd ed.) (pp. 74-103). Springfield, IL: Charles C. Thomas, Publisher, Ltd.

[16] Zimmerman, S. (1997). Factors influencing Hispanic participation in prostate cancer screening. *Oncology Nursing Forum, 24*(3), 499-504.

[17] Avila, E. (1999). *Woman who glows in the dark.* New York, NY: Penguin Putnam, Inc.

[18] McClain, C. (1995). *Women as healers: Cross-cultural perspectives.* New Brunswick, NJ: Rutgers University Press.

[19] Graham, J.S. (n.d.), *Curanderismo: Handbook of Texas online.* Retrieved from http://www.tshaonline.org/handbook/online/articles/sdc01

[20] DeStefano, A. (2001). *Latino folk medicine.* New York, NY: Ballantine Books.

[21] Fishman, B., Bobo, L., Kosub, K. & Womeodu, J. (1993). Cultural issues in serving minority populations: Emphasis on Mexican Americans and African Americans. *The American Journal of the Medical Sciences, 306*(3), 160-166.

[22] Thompson, J. (2002). Cultural aspects of treating Mexican patients. *Clinician Reviews, 12*(5), 56-62.

[23] Caballero, A.E. (2011). Understanding the Hispanic/Lantino patient. *The American Journal of Medicine, 124*(10s), S10-S15.

[24] Lopez, A. & Carillo, E. (2001). *The Latino psychiatric patient: Assessment and treatment.* Washington, DC: American Psychiatric Publishing, Inc.

[25] DePacheco, M. & Hutti, M. (1998). Cultural beliefs and health care practices of childbearing Puerto Rican American women and Mexican American women: A review of the literature. *Mother Baby Journal, 3*(1), 14-23.

[26] Hansen, K. (1998). Folk remedies and child abuse: A review with emphasis on ciada de mollera and its relationship to shaken baby syndrome. *Child Abuse and Neglect, 22*(2), 117-127.

[27] Cavillo, E. & Flaskerud, J. (1991). Review of literature on culture and pain of adults with focus on Mexican Americans. *Journal of Transcultural Nursing, 2*(2), 16-23.

[28] Grothaus, K. (1996). Family dynamics and family therapy with Mexican Americans. *Journal of Psychosocial Nursing, 34*(2), 31-37.

[29] Torres, S. (1993). Nursing care of low-income battered Hispanic pregnant women. *AWHONN'S Clinical Issues, 4*(3), 416-423.

[30] Spicer, E. (1977). *Ethnic Medicine in the Southwest.* Tucson, AZ: University of Arizona Press.

[31] Galanti, G. (2008). *Caring for patients from different cultures: Case studies from American hospital.* (4th ed.). Philadelphia, PA: University of Pennsylvania Press.

[32] Dinulos, J. & Graham, E. (1998). Influence of culture and pigment on skin conditions in children. *Pediatrics in Review, 19*(8), 268-275.

[33] Giger, J.N. (2013). *Transcultural nursing: Assessment and intervention* (6th ed.). St. Louis: Mosby.

[34] Soto, A. & Villa, J. (1990). Una platica: Mexican American approaches to death and dying. In J. Parry, *Social work practice with the terminally ill: A transcultural perspective.* (pp. 113-127). Springfield, IL: Charles C. Thomas, Publisher.

[35] Lawson, L. (1990). Culturally sensitive support for grieving parents. *Maternal Child Nursing, 17*(4), 204-208.

[36] Andrews, M. & Boyle, J. (2012). *Transcultural concepts in nursing care* (6th ed.). Philadelphia, PA: Lippincott.

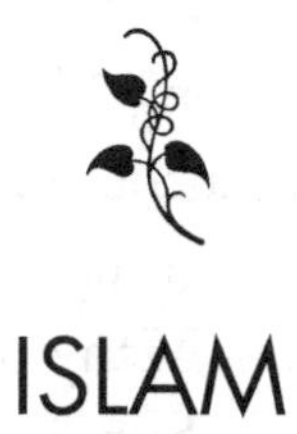

ISLAM

Background

Islam was founded during the seventh century in Arabia by the Prophet Muhammad (born Muhammad ibn Abdullah). Consequently, the religion is often erroneously called "Muhammadanism"[1, 2, 3, 4] In Mecca, Muhammad received divine revelations from God over a period of twenty-two years. These revelations were recorded in the Qur'án, meaning *The Recitation*. Muhammad, with approximately two-hundred followers, immigrated to Medina to serve as an arbitrator between feuding Arab tribes. This marked a turning point in enlarging his community of followers. The journey and the establishment of this new Islamic community-state on July 1, 622 CE, known as *hijra*, was adopted as the beginning of the Islamic calendar.[1, 2]

Islam quickly spread over parts of Africa, India, and Asia. It became the dominant religion in the Arab Middle East and continued to spread through many parts of the world.[5] Today, Islam is the second largest religion in the world with almost 1.6 billion followers. Estimates regarding the number of Muslims in the United States vary from approximately 2.6 million to as high as seven million. The Muslim population is projected to continue growing related to immigration and births.[6, 7, 8] Islam is one of the fastest growing religions in both North America and in the world. The cultural and ethnic diversity of Muslims varies widely.

The word 'Islam' is derived from an Arabic word meaning peace, submission, and obedience. Religiously, Islam means submission to the will of God and obedience to His law. The word *Allah* is the Arabic word for God. There is no gender or plural form. The Qur'án (also Koran, means *The Reading*) is viewed as the only authentic and complete book of Allah. Followers of Islam are called "Muslims." A Muslim is one who has submitted his or her life to the good will of God and is obedient to His law. Followers of Islam strive to totally reorganize their lives according to God's revealed guidance and the sayings of the Prophet Muhammad. Muslims work toward building human society on the same basis.[9,10]

Culture and geographic differences among Muslims may be reflected in some religious practices. However, there are two main branches of Islam: *Sunni* and *Shiite*. Approximately 85 percent of Muslims are Sunni. The two groups differ on the form of authority in Islam, but agree on the broad principles of Islam. Many of the Shiite followers are found in Iran, Iraq, and Syria. A very small group of both Sunni and Shi'ah Muslims seek to find a closer relationship with God and self-enlightenment through spiritual chanting, music, dancing, and meditation. They are called *Sufis*.[10,11,12,13]

The Nation of Islam, frequently called *Black Muslims*, is a controversial group that developed in the United States in 1930. This group believed that Elijah Muhammad, their second leader, was Allah's special spiritual messenger to Blacks. Religious texts used by this group include the Holy Bible and the Qur'án.[14,15] The group was reformed during the 1970s with a goal of moving closer to orthodox Sunni Islam in its beliefs and practices.[16] However, the group's support of black separatism strongly conflicts with orthodox Muslims' ideal of an all-embracing unity of humankind.[15,17]

Since the events of September 11, 2001, Muslims have been the target of markedly increased levels of discrimination, abuse, and violence. Stereotyping and profiling is more widespread. Recent studies suggest that Muslims may be at increased risk for psychological distress and illness secondary to the increase in negativity aimed at the group as a whole.[18,19]

Religious Representatives

- Islam lacks a hierarchical church structure. An *Imam* may lead prayer services, perform marriages, conduct funeral rites, and provide other spiritual support for the Muslim community.

Religious Beliefs

- **The Qur'án**: The Qur'án is written and recited in Arabic.
- **The Sunnah** or **Hadith**: Collections of the actions, practice, and sayings of Muhammad. Literally, Sunnah refers to a rule or mode of life. Hadith refers to a saying conveyed to man through hearing or revelation.[4]
- **Jihad** (striving): The Muslims daily striving to be pure in spirit and to resist evil.[20,21]
- There is no formal Sabbath in Islam. The thought is that prayer is a part of the everyday life of the Muslim. Muslims participate in congregational prayer at noon on Fridays, which takes the place of the early afternoon prayer.[4,9,21]
- There is only one God, who is the Creator of all things. He demands total obedience and worship.[22]
- The five pillars of Islam are:[16,22,23]
  - **Shahada**: The declaration of faith in Allah as the Supreme Being and that Muhammad is Allah's messenger.
  - **Salat** (formal prayer): A compulsory duty for Muslims.
  - **Zakat**: The spiritual obligation to give a percentage (at least 2.5 percent) of one's wealth.
  - **Saum/Sawm** (fasting): During the month of Ramadan.
  - **Hajj**: The pilgrimage to Mecca that is to be taken at least one time, if possible, during a Muslim's lifetime.
- Cleanliness is emphasized among Muslims. One must be ritually clean to take part in prayer and many other religious observations. Prayer (*salat*) and washing (*ablution* or *wudu*) is required five times a day. Ablution involves using clean water to cleanse the hands including the wrists, face, mouth, ears, nose, wiping the head with wet hands, cleansing feet to ankles. Prayer times are:[9,24,25]
  - Dawn to before sunrise (*Fajr/Fajar*)

- Midday – around noon (*Zuhr/Zohor*)
- Later afternoon but before sunset (*'Asr/Asar*)
- After sunset (*Maghrib*)
- At night (*'Isha*)

- During prayer, the individual must face toward Mecca (Saudi Arabia's Islamic holy city where the most sacred structure–*Kaaba*, is located). Prayer beads (*misbaha*) may be used to assist Muslims in maintaining their concentration during prayer. A prayer rug will be used to assure cleanliness. Plan care so that prayer time is not interrupted. Provide water for ritual washing if the individual is confined to bed or the patient may choose to perform dry ablution. A prayer rug or Qur'án brought by the patient/family should not be handled if there is blood or urine on an individual's hands or if ritually unclean. Generally, the Qur'án should be kept on a separate shelf and only handled by first covering it with a clean cloth. Nothing should be placed on the prayer rug or the Qur'án.[16, 22]
- The heads of men and women must be covered during worship.
- There is a belief in angels who bring revelations from God and communicate with the believer's soul.[4, 22]

Special/Religious Observations

- Religious holidays may occur at varying times of the year since the lunar calendar is used. There are many celebrations and observations throughout the lunar year in addition to the primary ones indicated.
- **Ramadan**: The ninth month of the Islamic lunar calendar. It celebrates the time during which the Prophet Muhammad received his first revelation of the Qur'án. It encompasses the period before *Eid al-Fitr*. The obligation to fast begins when a healthy individual reaches puberty. Fasting, including complete abstinence from food, drink, tobacco, and sex, from sunrise to sunset is required during the entire month. If a person is unable to fast during this period of time because of illness, pregnancy, up to forty days following childbirth, breastfeeding, menstruation, or travel, he or she is obligated to compensate by

fasting some other day. Persons who are very old, very young, or mentally challenged to the extent that he or she cannot understand the purpose of the fast may be excluded from fasting.[1,9,26,27]

- **Eid al-Fitr**: "End of the Fast" or "Feast of Fast Breaking."
- **Eid al-Adha**: "Feast of the Sacrifice"–Commemorates Abraham's willingness to sacrifice his son Ishmael in obedience to God.

Health Beliefs/Practices

- Preventive health care is important. Any steps necessary to preserve all aspects of health and well-being should be taken. The body is seen as belonging to God, with the individual only as caretaker. Only God has the power to determine the length of time an individual will live on earth. Therefore, treatment measures seen as not leading to a better quality or life or major health restoration may not be accepted.[24,28]
- *Tawiz/Taweez* (a black string or silver/gold chain attached to a pouch containing Islamic verses, prayers, symbols, etc.) may occasionally be found around the wrist, neck, or waist of a Muslim. It is sometimes placed on babies also by the parents; often on the wrist. The pouch is seen as protective and should be left undisturbed unless consent has been gained from the patient or family to remove it. The pouch should be protected from moisture.[29,30]
- Individuals may become ritually unclean as a result of various events that are considered polluting. Pollution may be acquired from external sources as a result of contact with a wet discharge from an animal or a human being (includes blood, pus, urine, feces, etc.). Menstruation (including five to six days following menstruation) and childbirth render a woman unclean. Pollution may also be acquired as a result of an action called *hadath*. Hadath is seen as major or minor. Major hadath may result from the emission of semen in males or orgasm in females. Minor hadath may result from sleeping, urinating, fainting, etc. Purification is obtained from washing. Washing is required with minor hadath; a complete bath is required with major hadath.[10,30]
- Allow to shower if condition permits vs. bed baths.[25]

- Many Muslims use water for cleansing after toileting. Providing a small disposable container that can be used for the purpose of cleansing is helpful.[30]

- The left hand is considered unclean and is used for unclean activities such as toileting activities. Food will not be handled with the left hand. Attempt to place intravenous lines to leave hands free. Secure IV tubing so that it will not drop into unclean areas such as while toileting.[10,31]

- May refuse to take medication in capsule form. Capsules are often made from pork sources. Insulin and vaccines derived from pork may be refused. Mouthwashes containing alcohol may also be refused.

- Though Muslims are exempt from fasting when ill, some will refuse medications including IV fluids while fasting. Medications may need to be rescheduled and/or dosages changed during fasting.[1,32]

- Medication to relieve physical or psychological pain is permitted as long as the intent of the medication is not to cause death. However, it is important for relatives to know if drugs are being used that impact cognitive ability and level of consciousness of the patient, particularly if close to death.[28,31,33]

- **Blood and Blood Products**: Acceptable as a treatment.

Kinship/Social Factors

- **Assalamu Alaikum**: "Peace be unto you" is an appropriate simple Muslim greeting to Muslims and will help to establish a positive bond.[29]

- Expect frequent visits from family and friends during illness.[29]

- Muslim men are responsible for looking after the well-being of the wife and female relatives.[18] Men may not leave a female relative alone with an unfamiliar male. If a male family member is not available, a close family member or friend should be allowed to stay.[33]

- **Hijab**: The word is derived from the Arabic word *hajaba*, meaning to conceal or hide from view. Hijab involves not only modesty in dress, but also morality in behavior, conduct, and attitude. Eye contact with members of the opposite gender will likely be avoided. Handshakes, hugs between unrelated persons of the opposite gender will likely be avoided.[34]

- Among men, hijab requires that the area between the navel and the knee be covered in front of everyone except the wife, that clothing is not tight or otherwise enticing. Gold and silk are not allowed for men. For women, the clothing should be of such that the body is covered except for the face and hands up to the wrist. It should be loose enough that the shape of her body is not revealed. For men and women, clothing should be thick enough that skin color is not shown. The degree to which women practice hijab in clothing varies from wearing traditional Western clothing to complete covering with a robe called a burqa.[9, 29, 34, 26]

- Provide longer, loose hospital gowns with long sleeves if available. Hospital-issued long-sleeved scrub jackets are available in most hospitals and can be worn over short-sleeved hospital gowns. If desired, allow patient to wear own clothing.

- Protect the high degree of modesty, particularly among Muslim women, by providing same-gender caregivers if at all possible. A strong emphasis is placed on avoiding *khalwa*–situations in which males and females are alone together with persons of the opposite gender who are not a spouse or approved kinship (*mahram*) as defined by the Qu'ran. This should be honored among all health care workers, including ancillary departments such as Lab, Environmental Services, etc.[33] Patients may not be willing to answer admission assessment questions of a personal/intimate nature. If no same-gender medical provider is available and the patient consents to examination by a person of the opposite gender, a designated family member/spouse should be permitted to stay with the patient and/or a second provider of the same gender as the patient should be present in the room during the exam. The medical provider should wear gloves to prevent skin-to-skin contact. Conduct as much of the exam as possible without removing clothing. Examinations of intimate body areas will likely be refused.

- Providers should knock prior to entering the patient's room and pause to allow patient to cover self before entering room. A sign placed on the door reminding personnel to knock is advisable.

- If the patient must go for procedures outside of the patient room, assure that coverage, including the head, remains covered unless otherwise directed by the patient. For females, surgical head coverings may be substituted for traditional head covering prior to the patient leaving the room with patient consent.

Birth/Children

- Medical practices often consist of multiple providers of both genders who rotate taking calls for deliveries. Discussion should take place early during pregnancy and agreement made as to the ability to provide a female provider during pregnancy, any hospitalizations during pregnancy, and at the time of delivery.

- Fathers may want to whisper a prayer in the newborn's ear immediately after birth, which places God at the center of the newborn and makes the baby an immediate member of the Islamic community.[16]

- Infants will usually receive their Islamic name at seven days after birth. In some cases the infant's hair will also be shaved or trimmed at seven days of age or after. There are a number of reasons for shaving the head. Among them are, to cleanse the child of any impurities, provide protection to the child from harm, and to celebrate the child as a blessing.[37,38,39]

- **Circumcision**: Frequently performed at seven days of life and is considered a form of purification. Parents may want newborn males circumcised prior to discharge from the hospital. The age of the child at the time of circumcision may vary, but it is usually performed by the age of ten.[10] It is obligatory for males. **Note**: Female genital mutilation (also called female circumcision) is sometimes seen among Muslims in some countries. The procedure is most often performed on newborn and young girls. However, this is a cultural practice and there is no religious basis for the practice. The practice is seen among non-Islamic religious groups as well. Occasionally, an immigrant may inquire about the procedure, not being aware of applicable laws. The procedure is illegal in the United States and punishable as a crime.[40]

- **Birth Control**: Mechanical forms of birth control such as diaphragms and condoms are acceptable. Tubal ligations and vasectomies are not acceptable.[37,41]

- **Fertility Issues**: Artificial insemination is permitted only if the husband's sperm is used. Donor sperm/ova, surrogacy, donated embryos, and adoption are not permitted. Fertility and infertility is based on God's will and plan.[33,41]

- **Elective Pregnancy Termination**: Not permitted. Therapeutic pregnancy termination is acceptable if the mother's life is endangered by continued pregnancy. Some Muslims support pregnancy termination in cases of rape or incest. Although not widely supported among Muslims, a few modern Islamic opinions support pregnancy termination as acceptable in the case of prenatal diagnosis of severe congenital anomalies.[1, 9, 41, 42]

Dietary Considerations

- Permissible foods are called *halal.* For meat to be considered halal, it must be slaughtered according to prescribed Islamic procedures. In the absence of halal foods, *kosher* foods are likely acceptable. Discuss with patient/family prior to substituting. Meats purchased from the usual meat sources served in most healthcare facilities are not halal. The following are among prohibited foods (known as *harem*).

- No pork/pork by-products, including foods containing fat from a pig. Gelatin-containing foods (often made from animal hide trimmings) are also prohibited. Foods such as biscuits, ice cream, soups, gravies, yogurt, cakes, etc. often contain animal-based gelatin or fat. Ingredients should be checked prior to serving. Wild birds/birds of prey are prohibited.[20]

- Glycerin is often derived from pork sources and may be found in many products such as toothpaste, lotions, shampoos, soaps, many over-the-counter medicines, etc. Plant-based glycerin is permissible.

- Meat whose method of slaughter is unknown or that contains the blood of the animal.

- **Alcohol or any other Intoxicants**: If prescribed liquid medicines contain alcohol, check with the pharmacist to determine if the medication is available without alcohol. If there are no other alternatives, the individual should be made aware and allowed to decide on taking the medication.

- Food prepared by the health care facility may be refused unless the patient or family can be assured that it has been prepared according to Muslim standards.[43]

- For diabetic Muslims who choose to fast during Ramadan, adjust insulin and other medications for control of blood sugar accordingly. Though Muslims are exempt from fasting when ill, some will refuse medications while fasting. Medications may need to be rescheduled and/or dosages changed during fasting.[1, 32, 44]

Death

- Based on the culture, families may prefer that a terminal prognosis not be shared with the patient, but with an immediate family member. Sharing such a prognosis with the patient may be seen as contributing to loss of hope.[28]

- Prolonging life by using life support machinery is unacceptable unless there is evidence that the person will be able to experience a reasonable quality of life. The standard of brain death is recognized by many Muslims. However, some argue that death occurs only when the heart stops and the soul departs. Explore family views thoroughly when withdrawal of mechanical support is under consideration.[29,33,41,42,45]

- Because one's body belongs to God, no one has the right to end life except God. Therefore, suicide and euthanasia are sinful and are thought to merit eternal suffering. Withdrawal of nutrition and/or hydration is prohibited.[11,25,31]

- Death is not an end of life, but the door to a higher form of life.[4] Muslims generally prefer to die at home. It is believed to be important for the individual to ask for forgiveness of violations against humans before asking for forgiveness from God for sins that have been committed and to re-declare his or her faith. If the person is unable to die at home, by religious recommendations, many visitors will come to the health care facility. Holy water (*zam zam*–obtained from wells of Mecca in Saudi Arabia) will be given in sips to the dying person close to the time of death, used to moisten the lips, or sprinkled on various parts of the individual's body, while reading from the Qur'án. The spiritual support of the Imam of the closest mosque should be requested if the patient has no family.[17,25,29]

- If death occurs in a health care facility, the presence of family is critical and should be allowed. The Muslim must confess sins before death. It is strongly desirable that only relatives and friends touch the body. If a non-Muslim must touch the body, disposable gloves should be used. The family will want to wash the body using water and certain additives such as leaves of the Lote tree, camphor, various perfumes, and/or other cleansing solutions. The deceased person's face is turned toward Mecca (Saudi Arabia, which is considered Islam's holiest city), then the body is draped. In the hospital, turning the deceased person's face to the right side is sufficient. Washing of the body may take up to an hour.

- Before ritual washings, legs and arms will be straightened, eyes and mouth closed (remove dentures). A piece of soft cloth may be secured under the lower jaw and tied over the top of the head to secure closure of the mouth if needed to prevent sagging. Unless an autopsy is required by law and prohibits removal, all tubes used in treatment will be removed. Prostheses, contact lenses, jewelry, etc. will also be removed and returned to family. Any open wounds, incisions, etc. will be packed to prevent drainage of body fluids. Clothes are to be removed by members of the same sex as the deceased and the body covered with a white sheet. The face of the deceased should not be exposed after the body has been shrouded.[1,25,29,46,47]

- Deaths of infants and children:
  - **Less than four months gestation:** No ritual washing. May be wrapped in white cloth. Baby will be buried. Parents may also want to bury placenta with baby.
  - **Stillbirth**: Consult parents. May do ritual washing. Will be shrouded. The baby must be named.
  - **Neonatal deaths and children up to age of puberty**: Newborns must be named. Washing and shrouding will be done.
  - **Children who have reached puberty**: Will be treated as adults for preparation of the body.[46,47,48]
- Refrain from hugging family members as a gesture of comfort.
- Burial is **required as soon as possible, generally within 24 hours**. Cremation is not permitted. To have a delayed burial because of autopsy may cause the family severe distress. There is also the risk of physical damage to the body, which is considered desecrating it, while moving it to the autopsy setting.[49]
- Muslim bodies are not embalmed.
- Females are encouraged **not** to attend burials, even in the case of the death of a child. Members of the immediate family may choose not to eat until after the funeral as a symbol of respect for the deceased. The period of mourning varies.
- **Autopsy**: Not permitted unless required by law.
- **Organ Donation**: Generally acceptable with very careful explanation.[31]

Other Considerations

- In the home, one room may be designated as a prayer room. The Qur'án may be kept in this room. It should never be placed on the floor nor should any object be placed on top of the book.[20]

- The health care provider may be asked to remove shoes prior to entering a Muslim individual's home to preserve environmental cleanliness. It is not unusual to find no wall decorations or pictures in Muslim homes. This is related to teachings prohibiting idolatry.[50]

- **Prayer Foot**: As a result of the positioning of the feet during prayer and the repeated localized pressure to the area, a callus may form on the upper outer surface of the foot. Suggest pressure-relieving methods or alternative positions for prayer when working with diabetic Muslims.[51]

- **Stomas**: Depending on the type of stoma, flatus and excreta may be discharged without control of timing which may interfere with ablutions and prayer. For individuals requiring surgery that will lead to the establishment of a stoma, careful support and consultation related to placement, care of the stoma, and guidance on how to continue to meet religious obligations may be needed.[52]

---

1 Aktar, A. (2003). Nursing with dignity: Islam. *Nursing Times, 98*(16), 40-42.

2 Esposito, J. (1998). *Islam: The straight path* (3rd ed.). New York, NY: Oxford University Press.

3 Smith, H. (1991). *The world's religions: Our great wisdom traditions.* New York, NY: HarperCollins Publishers.

4 Muhammad-Ali, M. (1990). *The religion of Islam* (6th ed.). Chelsea, MI: Book Crafters.

5 Smart, N. (1989). *The world's religions: Old traditions and modern transformations.* Melbourne, Australia: Cambridge University Press.

6 Council on American-Islamic Relations. (2012). *About Islam and American Muslims.* Retrieved from http://www.cair.com/aboutislam/islambasics.aspx

7 CIA World Factbook. (2012). *World and United States.* Retrieved from https://www.cia.gov/library

8 Pew Forum on Religion & Public Life. (2011). *The future of the global Muslim population.* Retrieved from http://features.pewforum.org/muslim-population-graphic/

9 Emerick, Y. (2011). *The complete idiot's guide to understanding Islam* (3rd ed.). New York, NY: Alpha Books.

10 Burke, T.P. (2004). *The major religions: An introduction with texts* (2nd ed.). Hoboken, NJ: Wiley-Blackwell Publishers.

11 Ott, B., Al-Khadhuri & Al-Junaibi, S. (2003). Preventing ethical dilemmas: Understanding Islamic health care practices. *Pediatric Nursing, 29*(3), 227-230.

[12] Fadiman, J. & Frager, J. (1997). *Essential Sufism*. Edison, NJ: Castle Books.
[13] Meredith, S. & Hickman, C. (2001). *The Usborne encyclopedia of world religions*. Tulsa, OK: EDC Publishing.
[14] McCloud, A. (1995). *African American Islam*. New York, NY: Routledge.
[15] Lincoln, C. (1994). *Black Muslims in America* (3rd ed.). Grand Rapids, MI: William B. Eerdmans Publishing Company.
[16] Robinson, D. (1997). *The simple guide to Islam*. Kent, England: Global Books, Ltd.
[17] Pinn, A. (1998). *Varieties of African American religious experience*. Minneapolis, MN: Fortress Press.
[18] Padela, A. I. & Heisler. (2010). The association of perceived abuse and discrimination after September 11, 2001, with psychological distress, level of happiness, and health status among Arab Americans. *American Journal of Public Health, 100*(2), 284-291.
[19] Rousseau, C., Hassan, G., Moreau, N., & Thombs, B.D. (2011). Perceived discrimination and its association with psychological distress among newly arrived immigrants before and after September 11, 2001. *American Journal of Public Health, 101*(5), 909-915.
[20] Masqood, R. (1994). *Teach yourself Islam*. Chicago, IL: NTC Publishing Group.
[21] Toropov, B. & Buckles, L. (2011). *The complete idiot's guide to the world's religions* (4th ed.). New York, NY: Alpha Books.
[22] Keene, M. (1993). *Believers in one God: Judaism, Christianity, Islam*. Great Britain: Cambridge University Press.
[23] Goring, R. & Whaling, F. (Eds.). (1994). *Larousse dictionary of beliefs and religions*. New York, NY: Larousse Kingfisher Chambers, Inc.
[24] Federation of Islamic Medical Associations. (2012). *Care of Muslim patients: A practical guide* (Version 1.2.0) [Mobile application software]. Retrieved from https://itunes.apple.com/us/app/care-muslim-patients-practical/id557157942?mt=8
[25] Salman, K., & Zoucha, R. (2010). Considering faith within culture when caring for the terminally ill Muslim patient and family. *Journal of Hospice and Palliative Nursing, 12*(3), 156-163.
[26] Zaidi, F. (2003). Fasting in Islam: Implications for midwifery practice. *British Journal of Midwifery, 11*(5), 289-292.
[27] Kridli, S. A. (2011). Health beliefs and practices of Muslim women during Ramadan. *MCN, 36*(4), 216-221.
[28] *Right to Die: Muslim views about end of life decisions*. Retrieved from http://www.people.virginia.edu/~aas/article/article3.htm
[29] Gatrad, A. & Sheikh, A. (2002). Palliative care for Muslims and issues before death. *International Journal of Palliative Nursing, 8*(11), 526-31).
[30] Sachedina, A. (n.d.). *Muslim beliefs and practices affecting health care*. Retrieved from http://people.virginia.edu/~aas/issues/care.htm
[31] Ross, H. (2001). Islamic tradition at the end of life. *Med Surg Nursing, 10*(2), 83-87.
[32] Taylor, A. (2003). Diabetes and fasting. *Practice Nurse, 25*(10), 34, 36-37.
[33] Brannigan, M. & Boss, J. (2001). *Healthcare ethics in a diverse society*. Mountain View, CA: Mayfield Publishing Company.
[34] *Institute of Islamic Information and Education*. (n.d.). Retrieved from http://www.iiie.net
[35] Roberts, K. (2002). Providing culturally sensitive care to the childbearing Islamic family. *Advances in Neonatal Care, 2*(4), 222-228.
[36] *Islam*. (n.d.). Retrieved from http://www.beliefnet.com

[37] Ramsey, D. (1986). The lifestyle of Afro-American Sunni Moslems in New York City. *Journal of the New York State Nurses Association, 17*(1), 21-30.
[38] Gatrad, A. & Sheikh, A. (2001). Muslim birth customs. *Archives of Disease in Childhood: Fetal & Neonatal, 84*(1), F6-F8. doi: 10.1136/fn.84.1.F6
[39] Joseph, S. (2005). *Encyclopedia of women & Islamic cultures: Family, body, sexuality and health.* (Vol. 3). Leiden, Netherlands: Brill Academic Publishers.
[40] AHA Foundation. (2012). *Female genital mutilation.* Retrieved from http://theahafoundation.org/issues/female-genital-mutilation/
[41] Sachedina, A. (2009). *Islamic biomedical ethics: Principles and application.* New York, NY: Oxford University Press, Inc.
[42] Daar, A. & Khitamy, A. (2001). Bioethics for clinicians: Islamic bioethics. *Canadian Medical Association Journal, 164(*1), 60-63.
[43] Kemp, C. & Bhungalia, S. (2002). Culture and the end of life: A review of major world religions. *Journal of Hospice and Palliative Nursing, 4(*4), 325-342.
[44] Wisher, A. M. (2012). Managing diabetes during the holy month of Ramadan. *Practice Nursing, 23*(3), 302-306.
[45] Abour, R., AlGhamdi, H.M.S., & Peters, L. (2012). Islam, brain death, and transplantation. *AACN Advanced Critical Care, 23*(4), 381-394.
[46] Gatrad, A. (1994). Muslim customs surrounding death, bereavement, postmortem examinations and organ transplants. *British Medical Journal, 309*(6953), 521-523
[47] Lundqvist, A., Nilstun, T., & Kykes, A. (2003). Neonatal end of life care in Sweden: Views of Muslim women. *Journal of Perinatal and Neonatal Nursing, 17*(1), 77-86.
[48] Siala, M.E. (n.d.). *Authentic step by step illustrated JANAZAH guide.* Retrieved from http://www.islamworld.net/resources/cache/264
[49] Rispler-Chaim, V. (1993). The ethics of postmortem examinations in contemporary Islam. *Journal of Medical Ethics, 19,* 164-168.
[50] Ohm, R. (2003). The African American experience in the Islamic faith. *Public Health Nursing, 20*(6), 478-486.
[51] Kaufman. B. & Hurst, N. (1999). Prayer foot: A potential cause of serious complication in diabetes. *Practical Diabetes International, 16*(5), 157-158.
[52] Black, P. (2012). Understanding religious beliefs of patients needing a stoma. *Gastrointestinal Nursing, 9*(10), 17-22.

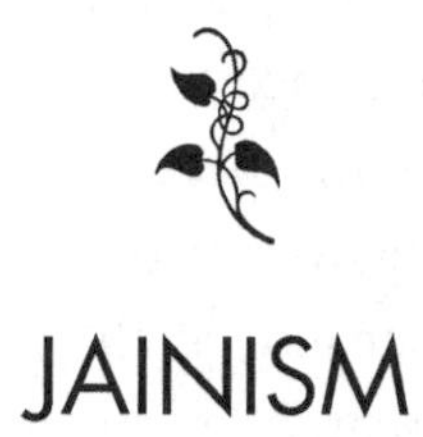

JAINISM

Background

Jainism originated in Eastern India and is one of the most ancient religions. Scholars and historians suggest that the current community of Jains was established around 598 BCE by Vardhamāna Mahāvīra, the last of the twenty-four Great Teachers of Jainism.[1,2] To Jains, there are continuous cosmic cycles (kalpas), each lasting billions of years. Therefore, there is no beginning or end to the universe and everything in it is eternal.[2,4] It is during these cosmic cycles that The Great Teachers, called *Tīrthaṅkaras* (Teer-TUN-daras), appear. They are part of a series of human teachers who appear in Jain history from time to time to preach about the way to achieve absolute freedom from the cycle of rebirth, *moksha*.[2]

Having discovered the path to enlightenment, the Sanskrit name, *jina*, meaning 'conqueror,' is ascribed to these teachers.[5,6] The term 'conqueror' does not refer to conquering others, but to conquering oneself and all of one's inner challenges. Followers of jinas are called Jains. As with previous Tīrthaṅkaras, Mahāvīra built the current *tirtha* or Jain community.[3,7] There are two major subdivisions of Jains: the Digambara and the Śvetāmbaras. There are further subdivisions within these two major groups.

Compared to many other religious groups, Jains are a relatively small group comprised of approximately five million adherents worldwide. At least four million still reside in India. Places outside of India with the largest Jain populations are the United States, Africa, United Kingdom, and Canada, respectively.[8,9] Although the Jain community is small, its tenet of non-violence has had powerful influences. It is believed that this principle may have strongly influenced the non-violent approaches adopted by Mahatma Gandhi and Martin Luther King, Jr.[2]

Religious Representatives

- **Monks/Nuns:** Monks and nuns make up a very small percentage of the Jain community and provide spiritual and moral guidance to lay Jains. They practice the strictest adherence to Jain principles and consequently believe they have the greatest chance of reaching *moksha*. Until 1980, monks and nuns were seen primarily in India because of restrictions on travel other than by walking. Because of the growing population of Jains outside of India, an additional order of Jain ascetics has been established. These spiritual leaders are allowed to use modern means of travel and to use flexibility with the usual monastic rules so that they can meet the needs of Jains around the world. They are known as *samans* and *samanīs*, male and female, respectively.[3] The two major Jain subdivisions differ primarily in the following two areas:[5, 6, 10]
    - Whether clothes should be worn or not.
    - Whether women can practice asceticism to the extent that liberation can be obtained.
- The Digambaras, meaning 'sky/space clad/clothed,' are more conservative and wear almost no clothing since they believe that nudity signifies a detachment from material things and a higher level of spiritual attainment. Nudity also signifies that the individual realizes that the soul is of ultimate importance, not the body.
- Digambara nuns are not allowed to go nude because of the fear of sexual assault and are not allowed in temples/monasteries. Therefore, they cannot achieve liberation unless they are reincarnated as a male in a future life.[3, 10]
- Digambara Jains may be seen using a small broom when walking to sweep away small insects that may be in their path. Stricter sub-sets of this group may also wear a mask (*muhpatti*) to prevent killing insects through inhalation.[3, 11]
- Monks and nuns are not allowed to cook because cooking would involve destruction of life found in the foods and water, so the lay community is depended upon for food.

Digambaras are provided food by lay Jains and eat only as much as they can hold in their hands.

- Śvetāmbaras wear simple robes, carry begging bowls for food/water from the lay Jain community, and may use a small broom protecting insects. Women are allowed to enter temples/ monasteries and are believed to be able to attain liberation.

- **Laymen/Laywomen:** Only nuns and monks practice nonviolence to the extent that has been described above. Lay Jains practice at varying levels, but continually strive to reach higher levels.[7]

Religious Beliefs/Philosophy

- Equality and respect for multiple viewpoints, including religious viewpoints, are stressed in Jainism.[7]

- There are many Jain scriptures and religious works containing the teachings of Mahāvīra and other *Tīrthaṅkaras*. Jains strive to achieve moksha through the *Three Jewels*. The Three Jewels include acquiring the right belief/faith (believing in the Jain creed), right knowledge (gaining the most knowledge about the Jain creed), and right conduct/action. Without achieving the first two Jewels, right conduct and action cannot be achieved.[6, 12]

- Five major vows are taken. Nuns and monks adhere to them **strictly**. For lay Jains, five lesser vows that reflect the major vows are written for a non-ascetic lifestyle that adheres to the Jain creed.

    1. Non-violence/harm toward all living things for nuns and monks, avoidance of violence/harm to all living things to the best of one's ability, no violent thoughts for lay Jains.

    2. To be truthful.

    3. No stealing.

    4. Celibacy for nuns and monks, premarital celibacy and marital fidelity for lay Jains.

    5. No possessions for monks and nuns, avoidance of material attachments and possessions for lay Jains.

In addition to these five vows, lay Jains also follow the four Vows of Instruction/Discipline that provide guidance related to spiritual rituals and practices. The Three Subsidiary Vows focus on how to live simply in day-to-day life.[3,5,13]

- The core principle of Jainism relates to non-violence, called *ahisma*.[2,6] This principle is related to the belief that souls reside not only in human beings, but in everything and are created equal. Although an individual may not be able to avoid non-violence to every single thing, the Jain makes a concerted effort to the best of his or her ability. Souls are classified according to the number of senses that they possess:[11,13,14,15]

  - **Level 1** – Possess only one sense – touch: These include the elements of fire, water, earth, air, and microorganisms. It also includes plants. Roots are thought to contain clusters of souls.

  - **Level 2** – Possess two senses – touch and taste: These include worms, snails, leeches, mollusks, including shellfish.

  - **Level 3** – Possess three senses – touch, taste, and smell: Includes certain insects such as ants, moths.

  - **Level 4** – Possess four senses – touch, taste, smell, and sight: These include many insects such as butterflies, flies, and spiders.

  - **Level 5** – Possess five senses and include humans, higher-level animals, birds, reptiles.

- The universe, in Jain cosmology, is shaped like a huge human figure, broad at the top, narrow in the middle, and larger again at the bottom. It is called the *loka puruṣa*. It is here that souls reside at various levels based on karma and where rebirth occurs. There is believed to be nothing outside of the loka. The universe is divided into five levels.[3,13,16]

  - **Uppermost Level** (Siddaloka) or Realm of the Perfected Ones: Reserved for those who have achieved moksha. Rebirth does not occur here. The souls remain there forever in bliss.

  - **The Upper World:** Occupied by those souls who have achieved a positive rebirth, but have not achieved moksha. There are multiple heavens at this level

- **The Middle World:** Occupies the smallest area of the universe, consisting of oceans, continents, the galaxy, and is where humans, other creatures, and plants live. It is the only area from which rebirth occurs.

- **The Lower World:** Consists of seven levels of hell, with each level progressively colder, darker, and more unpleasant. The seventh hell is the worst.

- **The Base:** Some sources indicate that nothing resides at this level. Other sources indicate that only the very lowest levels of life live here.

- Essentially, the world (universe) is composed of two substances: matter (*ajiva*) and souls (*jiva*). Matter is inert, having no life. The body is matter. The soul is life and resides in the body (matter). Therefore, when the soul leaves the body, nothing is left but lifeless matter. However, the soul does not die; it only takes up residence in another body or form. Souls can also be reborn in one of the heavens and hells of the universe. The soul cannot die; thus, the cycle of rebirth continues until moksha is achieved.

- In the universe, there are extremely minute particles of matter that bind themselves to the soul and impact the soul's ability to be liberated from the cycle of rebirth (karma). The karmas are attracted to the soul through an individual's thoughts, passions, deeds, etc. Release from the effects of karma can only be achieved through the Jain's actions in life. Jains recognize at least eight types of karma that impact the soul and, consequently, the individual. Examples of how the effect of the karmas can be reflected are: ignorance, intuition, life span of the body, socioeconomic status, pain/suffering, and ability to do good deeds. As long as karmas are bound to the soul, the cycle of rebirth will continue.[6,7,10,14]

- There is no affirmation of a God as known in the Abrahamic religions as a Creator. There is no Higher Power who determines whether an individual is rewarded or punished for acts committed during life. Because there is no beginning or end to the universe and souls continue to occupy matter of various forms, there is no need to have a God who manages the universe and controls salvation. God is seen as one who no longer carries attached karma and is a completely liberated soul, a Supreme Being in a state of infinite bliss, possessing infinite knowledge, vision, and power. One who reaches this level becomes reverent in the view of Jains. Karma determines whether an individual will be rewarded with ultimate freedom, moksha, escaping from the cycle of rebirth/reincarnation. In other words, one's actions, good or bad, will reap joy or suffering respectively, if not in this life, maybe in another life. For these reasons, it is to the Jain's advantage to strive to live a life of good.[3,5,17]

- There is no God who can forgive bad deeds; the individual is totally responsible for joy or suffering.

Special/Religious Observations[7,10]

- Celebrations/observations are based on the lunar calendar.
- **Mahavira Jayanti:** Birth of Mahavira. Celebrated in early April.
- **Devali:** Commemorates Mahavira's liberation. Celebrated in October/November.
- **Pajjusana:** Celebrates the end of the Jain year. Celebration lasts for eight days and occurs in August or September. Jains fast and perform acts to try to amend any wrong doings and to begin the New Year on a positive note.
- Worship areas with shrines may be found in the home. These areas should not be entered unless given permission.
- Periods of meditation and prayer may be observed daily. Ask about specific times so that care/treatment can be arranged so that the individual is undisturbed during these times, to the extent possible.

Health Beliefs/Practices

- An individual is expected to keep the body and mind as healthy as possible. A healthy body and mind is conducive to good spiritual health, although one can be spiritually healthy while physically weak.[7]
- Provide non-capsulated medications if possible since many capsules are made from meat products. Heparin, pork insulin, and other medications from animal sources should be avoided.
- **Blood Transfusions:** Personal choice of the individual.[18]

Birth/Children

- Self-control, including control of sexual activity, is stressed to prevent unplanned pregnancy, sexually-transmitted diseases, etc. Married couples may use their own discretion related to contraception.[7]
- **Sutak**: A ten-day period of purification is observed by the mother. During this time, there is no participation in the usual religious rituals.[10, 19]
- Because of the belief in no-violence, abortion is not acceptable to most Jains. Among others, abortion may be chosen when it is perceived that abortion will prevent greater harm.[7, 20]

Dietary Considerations

- Jains are strict vegetarians. Among some Jains, the types of vegetables and fruits are also limited because of the potential of life or the likely presence of micro-organisms. Ask specifics about preferred foods and request dietary consults as needed. In addition to meat, fish, eggs, the following dietary restrictions are common.[1, 2, 21, 22] The strictest vegetarians may not want to eat food that has been cooked in a pan that has been used to cook meat.[10]
  - Foods containing animal fat.
  - Honey.
  - Root vegetables such as beets, potatoes, onions, turnips, garlic, carrots.
  - Vegetables where insects often live within the leaves such as cauliflower, cabbage.[22]
  - Certain fruits and vegetables that have lots of seeds such as figs and eggplant.
  - Dairy milk products and foods containing milk (may be accepted by some), soy or rice milk may be substituted.
  - Gelatin and gelatin-containing foods.
  - Spicy foods.

- Foods/drinks containing cochineal/carmine-based dye, often red in color.
- Alcoholic beverages.
- Tap water may be refused. Provide purified, filtered or boiled water instead. Beverages should not be left uncovered.
- Fresh foods are most desirable. Leftover food may be refused.

- Eating after sunset or before sunrise may be refused because of the decreased risk of ingesting a living creature that would be more difficult to see. Eating before sunset is also thought to contribute to better sleep.
- Fasting is common. Explore fasting habits and adapt treatment regimens as much as possible to be respectful of fasting while achieving the goals of treatment.

Death

- Death is accepted as a natural part of the life cycle. The soul leaves the body at the time of death. Karma determines the type of body that the soul will occupy in the next life.[3] A quiet and peaceful state of mind is desired immediately prior to death so that good karma can be bound to the soul to improve conditions in the next life.[6]
- It is important that family members be allowed to stay with the dying patient. The family may perform prayers, chants, and hymns to facilitate a peaceful state of mind for the patient.[18]
- Family members will want to perform ritual washing and dressing of the body following death. Cremation is the preferred method of final disposition.[18]
- **Self-Starvation** (Sallekahanā or santhārā): This practice of fasting until death is very rare and reserved in most cases for monks and nuns. This highly spiritual process is not considered suicide. The act is undertaken with a lucid mind and must be approved by family and the spiritual leader. It is reserved for those who are facing inevitable death because of conditions such as old age, incurable disease/injury, etc. Sallekahanā is the ultimate act of non-violence and detachment from worldly attachments. While meditating and fasting, it is believed that the individual is able to cleanse the soul of negative karma and prevent

the entrance of any additional negative karma. The individual and the family look toward death in a state of peace and anticipation that the individual will be released from the cycle of rebirth.[3,5,23]

- **Autopsies:** Autopsies are allowed based on necessity. However, these should be completed as quickly as possible so that appropriate steps can be taken for final disposition.[24]
- **Organ Donation:** Permissible as long as the donor incurs no harm.
- **Withdrawal of Life Support:** Individual choice. A decision may be delayed until spiritual leaders are consulted.[21]

---

1 Hubbard, B., Hatfield, J. & Santucci, J. (2007). *An educator's classroom guide to America's religious beliefs and practices*. Westport, CT: Libraries Unlimited.

2 Pollock, R. (2002). *The everything world's religion book*. Avon, MA: Adams Media Corporation.

3 Long, J. (2009). *An introduction to Jainism*. New York, NY: I. B. Tauris & Co., Ltd.

4 Religion Facts. (2010). *Jain beliefs*. Retrieved from http://www.religionfacts.com/jainism/beliefs.htm

5 Dundas, P. (2002). *The Jains* (2nd ed.). New York, NY: Routledge.

6 Jain, S. C. (2006). *Introducing Jainism*. Delhi, India: B R Publishing Corporation.

7 Shah, B S. (2002). *An introduction to Jainism*. New York, NY: The Setubandh Publications.

8 Association of Religion Data Archives. (2005). *Most Jainist nations*. Retrieved from http://www.thearda.com/QuickLists/QuickList_45.asp

9 Jainism. (2011). In Encyclopædia Britannica. Retrieved from http://www.britannica.com/EBchecked/topic/299478/Jainism

10 Hopfe, L. M. & Woodward, M. R. (2007). *Religions of the world* (10th ed.). Upper Saddle River, NJ: Pearson Prentice-Hall.

11 Jordan, M. (1998). *Eastern wisdom*. New York, NY: Marlowe & Company.

12 Jainism Global Resource Center. (2011). *The way of salvation*. Retrieved from http://www.jainworld.com/book/jainism/ch12.asp

13 Cort, J. (2001). *Jains in the world: Religious values and ideology in India*. New York, NY: Oxford University Press, Inc.

14 HinduWebsite. (2011). *Jainsim and the concept of karma*. Retrieved from http://www.hinduwebsite.com/jainism/karmainjainism.asp

15 Chapple, C. K. (2001). The living cosmos of Jainism: A traditional science grounded in environmental ethics. *Daedalus, 130*(4). Retrieved from http://www.questia.com/read/5000888462

16 University of Michigan. (n.d.). *Jaina geography: Jain universe*. Retrieved from http://www.umich.edu/~umjains/universe/universe.html

17 JainUniversity.org. ((2011). *Concept of God in Jainism*. Retrieved from http://www.jainuniversity.org/jainism_god.aspx

18 Metropolitan Chicago Healthcare Council (2002). *Guidelines for health care providers interacting with patients of the Jain religion and their families*. Chicago, IL: Author.

[19] Indian Mirror. (2011). *Jain rituals*. Retrieved from http://www.indianmirror.com/culture/cul2.html

[20] Feminist Women's Health Center. (2007). *Summary of sacred choices*. Retrieved from http://www.fwhc.org/abortion/religion.htm

[21] Jain Centre. (2002). *Jainism*. Retrieved from http://www.jaincentre.com/

[22] Jain, M., Jain, L. & Dalal, T. (2005). *Jain food: Compassionate and healthy eating*. Retrieved from http://www.mjain.net/cookbooks/jain_book.pdf

[23] Jainism Global Resource Center. (2011). *Sallekhanā*. Retrieved from http://www.jainworld.com/education/senior15.asp

[24] Dobrin, A. (Ed.). (2004). *Religious ethics*: A sourcebook. Mumbai, India: Hindi Granth Karyalay.

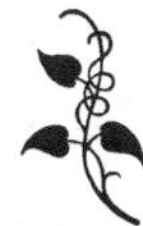

JEHOVAH'S WITNESS

Background

During the 1870s in Alleghany, PA, Charles Taze Russell organized the group formerly known as the *Russelites*, now known as Jehovah's Witnesses.[1] The group's name, Jehovah's Witnesses, refers to their "bearing witness concerning Jehovah, his Godship, and his purposes."[2] There are approximately 7.6 million Witnesses worldwide in two hundred thirty-six lands. Countries with the largest numbers are the United States (1.2 million), Brazil (about 742,400), and Mexico (about 739,900). The world headquarters and home of the Governing Body of Jehovah's Witnesses is located in Brooklyn, NY. The worldwide membership is divided as follows: zones → branches → districts → circuits → congregations (approximately twenty per circuit). The *Watchtower* magazine, a publication distributed by the Jehovah's Witnesses' membership, is published in more than four hundred languages worldwide, including sign languages and braille.[2]

Religious Representatives

- **Elder**: May be used to refer to male representatives.

Religious Beliefs

- **The Holy Bible**: The Old and New Testaments are referred to as the *Hebrew* and the *Christian Scriptures*, respectively.[2]
- There is no recognized Sabbath. Each day is considered holy.
- No national holidays are observed, including Christmas. Do not attempt to involve patients or family in related celebrations.[3]
- Followers believe that when the end of the world comes, 144,000 of those who have followed God's laws will rise from the dead and spend eternity in heaven. Those that do not go to heaven will experience paradise on earth for eternity. Witnesses, most often, abstain from accepting blood and most blood fractions. These beliefs are based on religious passages from the Bible (Acts, Genesis, Leviticus, and Deuteronomy). Those who have violated God's laws by receiving blood into the body (one's soul is associated with blood), celebrating birthdays (placing themselves above God), or worshiping idols (e.g., saluting the American flag, veneration of religious symbols) will spend eternity in a state of nothingness.
- Service in the military, holding public office, voting, and other political activities are prohibited. Witnesses believe that they hold citizenship in Jehovah's organization. Therefore, there is no need to exhibit acts of allegiance to more than one 'kingdom.'[4]

Special/Religious Observations

- An annual service reminiscent of the Last Supper is held, which commemorates the Memorial of Christ's Death. The date of the event is the 14th day of the Jewish lunar month of Nisan and varies between the latter part of March to early April.[2,3]

Health Beliefs/Practices

- The use of tobacco and abuse of drugs are prohibited.[5,6]

- Reading of the scriptures is encouraged during illness to comfort the individual, leading to mental and spiritual healing. Members of the congregation will visit, pray, and read scriptures with the sick.

- Opposed to all blood transfusions involving blood obtained **from a blood bank** through autologous or donated sources.[7] The refusal of blood is based on various Bible passages that are interpreted to view blood as a sacred symbol of life and as a substance that should not be taken into an individual's body.

- Witnesses may be receptive to some types of autologous transfusions and/or volume expanders. A Witness may accept *albumin*, *globulins*, *fibrinogen*, *clotting factors*, and *stem cells* based on personal conscience. Many individuals carry cards indicating types of blood fractions that are acceptable to them and/or have completed an advance directive and/or health care power of attorney documents indicating their preferences. Physicians can make the decision to administer blood to children in life-threatening situations without a court order. However, **every** effort should be made to inform and involve the parents in decision-making.[8, 9] Physicians should familiarize themselves with laws surrounding these care issues and consult facility legal resources as necessary.

- Health care providers must not make assumptions about a Witness' preferences, but should engage in private conversation to identify acceptable treatment options and to facilitate true informed consent.[10] Early identification, communication, and documentation of specific preferences are imperative to optimize care. Informed consents should address specific blood fractions and clearly indicate the patient's wishes on the form.[11]

- Minors deemed 'mature minors' by Jehovah's Witnesses guidelines may make the decision to refuse blood transfusions, even in life-threatening situations. Mature minors are generally adolescents. Though the specific steps and circumstances may differ from state to state, all states have processes in place to seek judicial intervention when blood is deemed medically warranted for minors. A few states recognize the concept of 'mature minor' and support the minor's rights to medical decision-making without adult consent. Medical providers should make every effort to be aware of such laws in their state of medical practice and consult the facility's legal resources, if needed.[8, 9]

- Opposed to eating foods to which blood has been added such as lunch meats and certain types of sausage.

- **Elective Pregnancy Termination**: Unacceptable.
- **Amniocentesis**: Acceptable.
- **Autopsies**: Unacceptable unless required by law. Parts may not be removed from the body since this is viewed as separating man's body from the spirit.[4,5]
- **Birth Control**: Acceptable with the exception of sterilization, which is seen as a form of body mutilation.
- **Circumcision**: Acceptable
- **Organ/Tissue/Bone Marrow/Stem Cell Transplantation**: Individual decision.[9,12]
- **Cremation**: Permitted. The type of burial is the family's choice. Body donation is prohibited.

Other Considerations

- **Pregnancy and Childbirth**[13,14]
  - Explore care issues during early prenatal visits to establish plan of care and to address preferences related to receiving blood/blood products should there be complications surrounding pregnancy and delivery. Document carefully, communicate to appropriate providers, and provide patient with a copy of the written plan of care that can be taken with her when she presents to the Labor and Delivery area. The Neonatal Intensive Care Unit should be notified of mother's admission in case infant requires specialized newborn care.
  - Early identification of conditions such as placenta previa that place the patient at risk for excessive bleeding is critical. Instruct patient to report vaginal bleeding immediately.
  - Reinforce the importance of keeping prenatal appointments that will monitor for early signs of anemia. Stress compliance with taking dietary supplements as ordered and consumption of diet that supports red blood cell production.

- Hospitals should have clear policies and procedures related to care of Jehovah's Witnesses patients. Staff should be familiar with location and content of policies.

- During initial screening/assessment, carefully review medications that the patient takes, including herbal, to identify any drugs having anticoagulant effects. Also, inquire about the presence of any medical conditions related to coagulation deficiencies.[11]

- For patients having planned surgery, medications that stimulate red blood cell production may be ordered several weeks prior to the surgery in an effort to reduce the effects of blood loss. (Medications to stimulate red cell production may be ordered post-operatively also.) Dietary supplements often ordered include iron, multivitamins containing Vitamin C, folic acid, B_{12}. Foods high in Vitamin K may be recommended to help in synthesis of clotting factors. Arrange for nutritional consult, as needed.[11, 15]

- After recovery from surgeries, etc. involving a large blood loss, educate the patient regarding foods high in iron, iron/vitamin supplements, avoidance of foods that interfere with iron absorption such as coffee, tea, milk. Educate regarding symptoms of anemia.[7]

- **Hemodialysis/Heart-Lung Bypass/Surgery**: Determine from the individual or family if these procedures will be permitted. Circuits should be primed with a non-blood solution. Because the person's blood flows in a continuous circuit, some persons view this as an extension of their own circulation and will accept these treatments. Use smallest circuits possible that are compatible with the patient's body size. Implement intra-operative measures to prevent red blood cell loss.[3, 9, 15]

- Collaborate with treatment team on the use of volume expanders other than blood, such as saline, Ringers' lactate, dextran, Haemaccel, Hetastarch, etc.[2]

- Monitor oxygen saturation levels and provide supplemental oxygen as indicated and ordered. Minimize factors and clinical interventions that contribute to increased oxygen needs.

- Implement blood-conservation strategies such as using micro blood samples for labs, collaborate with physicians regarding elimination of non-critical lab tests, etc. Carefully monitor and document blood loss, particularly in children.

- Consult hematologist and/or medical centers specializing in bloodless medicine and surgery management, if needed.[7, 16] Consult local Jehovah's Witnesses resources if unfamiliar with location of such facilities. Jehovah's Witnesses Hospital Liaison Committees are available in many major cities to enhance understanding and communication with the medical community.[12]

- Provide emotional and spiritual support to the family during illness crisis of a family member, respecting their decision to refuse blood products.

Death

- There are no special rituals surrounding death. Inquire about family's desire to notify an Elder who may offer prayers and family support. Provide a quiet, uninterrupted environment.[17]

- Articles of comfort adorned with religious symbols should not be offered to family or placed on the body.[17]

---

1 Mead, F., Hill, S., & Atwood, C. (2010). Handbook of denominations in the United States (13th ed.). Nashville, TN: Abingdon Press.

2 Watch Tower Bible and Tract Society of Pennsylvania. (2012). *Watchtower*. Retrieved from http://www.watchtower.org

3 Thurkauf, G. (1989). Understanding beliefs of Jehovah's Witnesses. *Focus on Critical Care,16*(3), 199-204.

4 Andrews, M. & Boyle, J. (2012). *Transcultural concepts in nursing care* (6th ed.). Philadelphia, PA: Lippincott, Williams & Wilkins.

5 Quintero, C. (1993). Blood administration in pediatric Jehovah's Witnesses. *Pediatric Nursing, 19*(1), 46-48.

6 Watch Tower Bible and Tract Society of Pennsylvania. (2012). *About Jehovah's Witnesses*. Retrieved from http://www.jw-media.org

7 Vernon, S. & Pfeifer, G. (1997). Are you ready for bloodless surgery? *American Journal of Nursing, 97*(9), 40-47.

8 Family care and medical management for Jehovah's Witnesses. (1992). Brooklyn, NY: Watch Tower Bible and Tract Society of New York, Inc.

9 Hughes, D. B., Ullery, B. W. & Barie, P. S. (2008). The contemporary approach to the care of Jehovah's Witnesses. *The Journal of Trauma, Injury, Infections, and Critical Care, 65*(1), 237-247. Doi: TA.0b013e318176cc66

10 Gyamfi, C., Gyamfi, M. & Berkowitz, R. (2003). Ethical and medicolegal considerations in the obstetric care of a Jehovah's Witness. *Obstetrics and Gynecology, 102*(1), 173-180.

[11] Berend, K. & Levi, M. (2009). Management of adult Jehovah's Witness patients with acute bleeding. *The American Journal of Medicine, 122*(12), 1071-1076. doi: 10.1016/j.amjmed.2009.06.028

[12] Doyle, J. (2002). Blood transfusions and the Jehovah's Witness patient. *American Journal of Therapeutics, 9*(5), 417-424.

[13] Braithwaite, P., Chichester, M. & Reid, A. (2010). When the pregnant Jehovah's Witness patient refuses blood. *AWHONN: Nursing for Women's Health, 14*(6), 462-470. Doi: 10.1111/j.1751-486X.2010.01593.x

[14] Mirza, F.G. & Gyamfi, C. (2010). Management of pregnancy in the Jehovah's Witness. *Contemporary OB/GYN, 55*(12), 41-48.

[15] John, T., Rodeman, R., & Colvin, R. (2008). Blood conservation in a congenital cardiac surgery program. *AORN Journal, 87*(6), 1180-1186.

[16] Salipante, D. (1998). Refusal of blood by a critically ill patient: A health care challenge. *Critical Care Nurse, 18*(2), 68-76.

[17] Smith, A. (2010). Care of the older person: A Jehovah's Witness perspective. *Nursing & Residential Care, 12*(4), 195-196.

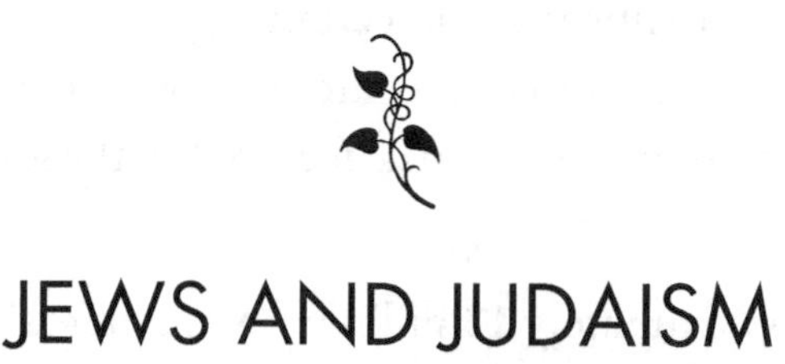

JEWS AND JUDAISM

Background

Jews trace their beginnings to Abraham, who was the first to experience the oneness of God. The Jewish nation grew out of the descendants of Abraham.[1] They developed their own language, Hebrew, and identified Israel as their homeland.[2] Any individual having a Jewish mother or who has formally converted to Judaism according to Jewish law is considered part of the Jewish community. Within the Reform movement, a child born to a Jewish father and a non-Jewish mother is considered Jewish. This remains a controversial issue, with the more traditional divisions of Judaism not recognizing this status. Jews who do not practice Judaism are sometimes called secular Jews. The term *Jewish* reflects both a people and a religion.[1, 3]

Jews may be grouped into four major ethnic groups. The *Ashkenazim* (meaning 'German' in Hebrew) are those who lived in Germany or France prior to migration to Eastern Europe. This group makes up approximately 80 percent of the world's Jews. *Sephardim* are those who lived in Spain or Portugal before expulsion in 1492. The *Oriental Jews* (Mizrahi) are those who lived in Asia or North Africa. Today, Oriental Jews are generally grouped with Sephardic Jews, as their religious rites are very similar. *Yemenite Jews* are Oriental Jews whose social and geographical isolation led to a distinct set of religious rites. There are several much smaller Jewish ethnic groups living in various parts of the world.[3, 4, 5]

Throughout their history, Jews have been the subjects of anti-Semitism. The most horrific acts resulting from this hatred were those of the Holocaust, during which six million Jews were killed over a period of six years in Nazi Germany. The Jewish community has established memorials and other remembrances so that the world will not forget this dark period in history.[1, 6, 7, 8]

Risk factors for Jews of European origin include Tay-Sachs disease, Gaucher's disease, Canavan's disease, familial dysautonomia, Type A Neimann-Pick disease, Group C Fanconi anemia, Mycolipidosis IV, cystic fibrosis, and certain types of breast, ovarian, and colorectal cancer.[9, 10, 11, 12] Because of the continuing exposure to violent acts in and around Israel, post-traumatic stress and depression are health risk factors for those who have been exposed to those events.[13]

Worldwide, there are approximately 13 million Jews. Approximately six million Jews live in the United States, the largest population outside of Israel. Half of the Jewish population in the United States resides in New York City, Los Angeles, and Miami.[8, 14, 15]

Religious Representatives

- Rabbi.
- Each Hasidic group has a spiritual leader known as a *Rebbe* who may also be an ordained rabbi. A Rebbe is thought to have mystic abilities, understand various levels of the soul, and can advise people about their spiritual lives, etc.[16, 17]

Worldview/Religious Beliefs

- Religious texts:
  - Hebrew Bible (the Torah, the Nevi'im, and the Ketuvim)
  - Talmud (the Mishnah and the Gemera)
- In traditional Judaism, one indivisible God exists. By His will, the universe and all that is in it was created.[18] Each man is viewed as an individual created in God's image with a soul that will survive eternally and be returned to God after death.[19]

- Observant Jewish life is centered around living a life that is congruent with written and oral Jewish law or *halakhah*.[3]

- There are a growing number of divisions with Judaism. They differ in their acceptance and practice of Jewish religious traditions. The larger divisions include:

  - **Orthodox**: Members follow strict interpretation of the law. Within the Orthodox group are several groups including the modern Orthodox who have largely integrated into modern society, but practice stricter adherence to Jewish law. Hasidic (Chassidic) Jews live separately from larger society and dress distinctively in dark clothing, full beards, and sidelocks. Most wear black hats, and all extremities are covered.[3,6,20]

  - **Conservative**: Members follow less strict interpretation of the law. Conservatives advocate evolving ideology as long as it does not disrupt Jewish tradition and remains in accord with Jewish law.

  - **Reform**: Members follow a liberal interpretation of the law. Its members continually adapt the traditional practices to modern cultural concerns.

  - **Reconstructionist**: Members stress Jewish culture and humanistic values. Democracy is highly valued among the group. Jewish tradition is valued only to the degree that it contributes to the maintenance and development of Jewish culture.

  Humanistic: A secular group formed in the 1960s. Members have a non-theistic philosophy and focus on human power and responsibility. They celebrate Jewish identity, history, and culture.[21,22]

  Renewal: A recent Jewish movement in the United States. This group is seeking new ways to practice Judaism while staying within the traditions of Judaism.[23]

- Sabbath begins at sundown on Friday and ends at sundown on Saturday. Unless for life-saving reasons, medical and surgical procedures, including labor induction and elective Caesarean Sections, should not be scheduled on the Sabbath or on holy days.

- **Orthodox Jews**:

  - Men must keep the head covered at all times in reverence to God. The small skullcap worn many times by men and boys is known as a *kippah* or *yarmulke*. On the Sabbath, work of any kind is prohibited according to the law of the Torah. This includes looking at television, listening to the radio, driving, writing, using and answering the telephone, pushing elevator buttons, tearing paper, etc. or traveling with food (other than food for a baby). No money or keys will be carried. Operating bed controls and other electrical equipment, including lights, is prohibited. Non-emergency consent forms and other documents may not be signed on the Sabbath and other Holy days. Verbal consent for treatment is acceptable. The only law of the Torah that supersedes Sabbath laws is that one must do everything possible to save a life.[24] Plan assignments and care to accommodate meeting these needs. Pre-determine how the patient/family will notify clinical staff of any needs during Sabbath/Holy days observation.

  - Orthodox Jews will pray three times a day—morning, noon, and evening, before and after meals. Ritual hand washing is done upon awakening and before eating. If the patient is hospitalized and not ambulatory, a pitcher of water, basin, and a towel may be requested to perform this obligation. Provide a quiet, uninterrupted environment during prayer times.

- **Conservative Jews**:
  - Men's heads are covered during worship.
- **Reform Jews**:
  - Men are not obligated to cover heads.
  - May follow kosher dietary laws.

Special/Religious Observations

- Sabbath.
- **Passover** (Pessach): Occurs at or near Easter. Celebrates the Exodus from Egypt.
- **Shavuot** (Festival of Weeks): Celebrates the giving of the Torah at Sinai.
- **Sukkot** (Feast of Tabernacles): Commemorates divine guidance and protection during the wilderness wanderings.

- **Shemini Atzeret**: A special service held the day after the Sukkot ends.

- **Rosh Hoshanah** (Jewish New Year): A solemn festival that introduces a ten-day period of penitence that concludes with the fast of Yom Kippur. Man is to reflect on his destiny and resolve to lead a better life during the coming year.

- **Yom Kippur** (Day of Atonement): A day of pardon and reconciliation with God.

- **Hanukkah** (Festival of Dedication or Lights): Commemorates the rededication of the Temple of Jerusalem.

- **Purim**: Based on the account in the Book of Esther that the Jews in the capital city of Shushan celebrated their deliverance on this day. Individuals may fast the day preceding Purim.

- **Fast of the 9th Av**: Commemoration of the destruction of the Jerusalem temple by the Romans (Orthodox only).

- **Fast of Tammuz**: Celebration of the breaching of the walls of Jerusalem at the time of the destruction of the First and Second Temples (Orthodox only).

- **Fast of Esther**: Based on the account given in the book of Esther (Orthodox only).

- **Asara B'Tevet** (Fast of the 10th of Tevet): Commemorates the siege of Jerusalem by Nebuchadrezzar before the destruction of the First Temple (Orthodox only).

Language

- Hebrew is the official Jewish language and is considered sacred. Hebrew is written and read from right to left.[3,26]

- Hasidic Jews generally speak *Yiddish*, primarily influenced by German, as a first language and English as a second language.

- *Ladino*, sometimes called Judaeo-Spanish, is a hybrid language that resulted when the Jews were expelled from Spain in 1492. It is a combination of Hebrew, Old Spanish, and a few other languages. (A person who speaks Spanish will not be able to speak Ladino).

Ladino is rapidly becoming a lost language. It is spoken in parts of North Africa, Israel, Turkey, the Balkans, and the United States, mainly in New York, Seattle, South Florida, and Los Angeles.[27]

Health Beliefs/Practices

- The body is a gift from God. Hence, the maintenance of the health of the body and the soul is extremely important. Preventive health and wellness measures are stressed. Generally, will quickly seek medical attention for health maintenance and illness.[24]
- The hope of recovery from illness should not be abandoned until death actually comes. Often, second opinions are sought related to health issues, based on the high value of education and knowledge. An 'expert,' including a Rabbi, may be sought to assure that questions are clarified and that the highest level of care is delivered.[27,28,29]
- Do not shave Orthodox Jews. It is believed that God's mercy descends through the beard. Provide emotional and spiritual support to male cancer patients who experience hair loss resulting from treatments.[29]
- **Blood and Blood Products**: Acceptable as part of medical treatment.

Expression of Pain

- Expressive. May tend to expect immediate relief of pain. Family members may verbalize the need for pain relief for the patient.[30]

Male-Female/Kinship/Social Relationships

- **Orthodox**: No casual touching of the opposite sex, including spouse, in public. Handshakes between opposite sexes will be declined or a handkerchief used as a barrier. Health care workers should limit touching to what is required for medical interventions. Provide a third person in the room if two persons of the opposite sex must be in a closed room/space together.[9,29]

- Based on the laws of *niddah*, women are considered impure when blood is emitted from the uterus during menstruation, and for seven days following the menstrual period, a state of nidda exists. Husbands and wives may not sleep in the same bed during this period. Purification takes place through ritual bathing (mikvah).[2,9] Women can also become niddah if the cervix is dilated for procedures as well as during labor and after childbirth. Bleeding resulting from trauma to the uterine outer surfaces and vaginal canal does not generally render the woman in niddah. Whether a state of niddah results from trauma to the inner surfaces of the uterus varies based on the circumstances. When procedures involving the vaginal canal and uterus are necessary, provide detailed information regarding types of instruments that will be used, whether the cervix will be dilated, possibility of bleeding and for how long.[31,32]

- **Orthodox**: Modesty is highly valued. For reasons of modesty, many married Hasidic women shorten the natural hair and wear a wig and/or scarf. **Do not** remove the wig without permission of the family and unless absolutely necessary. If removal is necessary, determine if the woman would like to have a head covering. Provide gowns and cover the knees and elbows. Appropriately shield the woman's body during procedures. Even husbands are not to look directly at the wife's naked body.[17,33]

- **Orthodox**: Male nurses should not be assigned to female clients, if at all possible. Female nurses may attend to male clients. Laws are waived for male physicians, allowing them to attend to female clients. However, same-sex caregivers are most desirable.

- It is Jewish obligation to visit family and friends during hospitalization or illness. Anticipate a generous number of visitors. These visits will be valued and comforting to the patient.

- **Orthodox**: Visitors must live within walking distance to visit on the Sabbath. Spouses will not leave unless within walking distance of residence. Provide a comfortable resting area.[34]

Birth/Children

- Procreation is one of the most important duties of Jews, fulfilling the commandment to be fruitful and multiply. Therefore, children are cherished and viewed as a precious gift.[9,33]

- The average number of children in Hasidic families is five.[17]

- An Orthodox husband may choose not to participate in the delivery. If he does participate, support will only be through verbal means, including reading Biblical passages. The father should not be interrupted during reading/prayer unless for an emergency. There will be no touching of the wife during labor because of laws dictating separation during any type of vaginal bleeding. He will not view the wife's genital area during birth. Any mirrors used should be positioned so that the mother's perineum is not visible to her husband. Consequently, the husband may stay at his wife's head or behind a curtain/screen during the birth and will not participate in cutting the umbilical cord. Allow female support persons to stay during the birth, if requested by the mother and father. An Orthodox father may not be comfortable having the baby handed to him by a female. Clean any blood from the baby's body, place the baby in a crib first, allowing the father to take the baby directly from the crib.[3, 9, 33, 34, 35, 36]

- Breastfeeding is generally the feeding method of choice and has no religious restrictions. Assure that any formula offered meets the kosher requirements. Soy-based formula is allowed. A limited number of formulae are certified as *cholov yisroel* (prepared under Jewish supervision).[33, 34, 37, 38]

- Recommend that couples discuss with their spiritual advisor how engorgement and providing breast milk for an infant who is unable to nurse but needs milk will be handled on the Sabbath and Holy days, since there are restrictions on using breast pumps and saving milk on these days. Generally, for reasons related to the well-being of the mother and baby, exceptions/alternatives will be suggested and approved by the advisor.[38]

- **Orthodox**: On the Sabbath and some Holy days, be attentive to the prohibition of operating electrical equipment such as lights, bed controls, etc. Expect that family members will be very attentive to the mother, especially during the first seven days post-partum. At least six weeks of rest for convalescence is expected following childbirth.[34]

- Completion of birth certificates may be delayed until after the new baby's name has been revealed in conjunction with appropriate religious rites. Provide information to the family about how to complete the birth certificate after the naming ceremony has occurred.[9, 33]

- Women are considered in a state of impurity for seven days after the birth of a son or fourteen days after the birth of a daughter. Ritual bathing must be performed for purification.[2]

- Circumcision is considered a sacred ritual. It is generally performed in the parents' home on the eighth day of life in a celebration called a *berit milah* by a trained person known as a *mohel* (circumcisor). In some cases, the child's father or a pediatrician will perform the circumcision.[39] Physicians performing the circumcision should be Jewish. An ill or premature infant's circumcision is performed when health permits. It is important for the nurse to cover information about circumcision care for full-term infants prior to discharge from the hospital.[35]

- A family member or friend of the family will stay with the hospitalized child at all times.

- **Elective Pregnancy Termination**: Therapeutic abortion is permitted if the mother's health is in danger. Non-therapeutic termination is not supported.

- **Birth Control**:

  - **Orthodox**: Birth control discouraged.

  - **Conservative, Reform, Reconstructionist, Renewal, Humanistic**: Birth control measures at the couple's discretion.

Dietary Considerations

- Family and community members will provide food unless kosher food can be provided through a caterer or through other means. Kosher food should not be warmed using microwave or traditional ovens that have been used for non-kosher food unless double-wrapped. Allow the patient/family to remove wrappings. Provide disposable utensils, etc., since use of utensils used for preparation of non-kosher food is not permissible.[9, 34, 36]

- Individuals may fast for twenty-four hours on Yom Kippur. Fasting occurs on several other Holy days for varying lengths of time. Fasting is not required for sick individuals, those with special dietary requirements such as diabetics, and children under the age of thirteen. Explore any fasting obligations in the initial assessment.

- Determine specific foods that the client considers kosher.

- Soy milk or dairy products that are certified as chalav yisroel are permitted.

- The laws of *kashrut* demand that 'proper' (kosher) foods be eaten. Very careful attention will be paid to the ingredients and preparation of foods. These laws also apply to medicines and nutritional supplements. The degree of observance of dietary laws varies among individuals. Inquire about individual dietary preferences and requirements. Orthodox Jews will strictly follow a kosher diet.[24]

- Kosher meat is from animals that both chew their cud and have cloven hoofs, such as cows, sheep, goats, and deer. They must be slaughtered strictly in accordance with defined procedures. Poultry should be slaughtered in the same manner. Poultry traditionally permitted includes chicken, turkey, geese, ducks, and doves. All traces of blood must be removed. Fish with both scales **and** fins is permissible. Shellfish are forbidden. The eggs, milk, and oil from non-kosher animals are forbidden. Honey is permissible. Dairy products and meat (including poultry) are not consumed together. Dairy products are not consumed immediately before or after consuming meat. Separate utensils and dishes are required for preparing and serving dairy and non-dairy products.

- There are additional food restrictions during Passover. These include bread, cakes, etc. made with baking powder, and foods containing grain products or by-products not specifically designated as permissible. These prohibitions extend to medications.[2,3,4,30,41]

Death

- Someone will stay with a critically ill or dying family member until death. By religious law, someone should stay with the dying individual so that the soul will not feel alone and the dying person maintains a sense of connectedness to family, friends, and the community.[27]

- The dying individual is encouraged to recite the confessional or the affirmation of faith (shema), if possible, before death. If the dying client is unable to do so, family members are encouraged to recite the confessional for the dying family member.

- Contact the nearest synagogue or rabbi if no family or friends are available to provide support for the terminally ill patient.

- A son or the nearest relative may want to close the eyes and mouth of the dead family member. An individual of the opposite sex should not touch the body of an Orthodox Jew.

The body should be laid flat, legs should be extended, arms and hands (opened) should be extended at the sides of the body, incisions covered, and the body, including the face, covered with a sheet. Any dressings with the patient's blood on them must be left in place. The body will be washed and prepared for burial by same-sex individuals. Some Jews may want to have the position of the body oriented so that the feet are toward the door. Amputated limbs must be buried with the body.[18, 24, 42, 43, 44]

- It is believed that the spirit leaves the body at the time of death. Caregivers should leave the body untouched for approximately one-half hour after death to allow the soul to depart. After death, Judaic law requires that the body not be left alone.[18]

- Infants who die after thirty full days of life are ritually prepared, then wrapped in a blanket. Some Jews may want to have a male infant circumcised prior to burial.[9, 28]

- **Traditional Judaism**: Cosmetic restoration and measures to retard decomposition of the body (embalming) by artificial means are discouraged. If the body cannot be buried within three days or there is a legal requirement, embalming is permissible.[28]

- The body is to be buried as soon as possible, preferably within twenty-four hours. If death occurs on the Sabbath, the family may request that the body remain in the morgue (not travel) until the Sabbath is over.[18] Bodies are generally buried, including fetuses of any gestation.[39]

- Sending floral arrangements as an expression of sympathy is inappropriate. Often, donations will be accepted to an organization of the family's choice.[9, 44]

- **Autopsy**:

  - **Orthodox**: Not allowed unless required by law. Autopsy is allowed if the dead person had a heredity disease or another known person is suffering from a deadly disease that information gained from an autopsy may be of value. All organs should be returned to the body for burial.[39]

  - **Conservative, Reform, Reconstructionist**: Acceptable. All organs should be returned to the body.[18]

  - **Organ Donation**: Permitted only if it would lead to saving the life of another.[9, 30]

Other Considerations

- Capsules and insulin made from pork products are not permissible. Consult the pharmacist if needed. Pharmaceutical companies that manufacture capsules will know what products are used to make their capsules. Gelatin and cellulose in medications or foods make them non-kosher.[9]

- If a large population of Sabbath-observant Jews is served, consider programming a designated elevator to automatically stop on each floor. With this option in place, Sabbath-observant Jews will not have to press the elevator buttons during the Sabbath.[9] Research and development of equipment incorporating the use of *grama* (indirect) technology is currently underway that automates equipment such as telephones, electric wheelchairs, and other devices that use electricity, eliminating the violation of Jewish law related to activating an electrical circuit.[36, 45]

- Many Jewish women light candles at the beginning of the Sabbath each week. Consider having electric or battery-powered candles available for illumination during hospitalization. The woman, however, would be excused from this obligation if her medical condition prohibits her doing so.[9]

- Individuals may refuse to be discharged from the hospital during the Sabbath because of the prohibition of riding in vehicles.[9]

- Allow the patient/family to tear open any needed non-sterile packaged items prior to the Sabbath. Do not discard toilet tissue that may be pre-torn in preparation for the Sabbath.[9]

---

1 Keene, M. (1993). *Believers in one God: Judaism, Christianity, Islam.* Great Britain: Cambridge University Press.

2 Havely, H. (1991). *To be a Jew: A guide to Jewish observance in contemporary life.* New York, NY: HarperCollins Publishers.

3 Selekman, J. (2013). *People of Jewish heritage.* In Purnell, L.(4th ed.), pp. 339 - 356. Philadelphia, PA: FA Davis Company.

4 *WordIQ: Dictionary and Encyclopedia Definitions Online.* (2010). Retrieved from http://www.wordiq.com

5 PBS: Public Broadcasting System Online. (2008). The Jewish Americans. Retrieved from http://www.pbs.org/jewishamericans/about/index.html

6 Goring, R. & Whaling, F. (Eds.). (1994). *Larousse dictionary of beliefs and religions.* New York, NY: Larousse Kingfisher Chambers, Inc.

[7] United States Holocaust Memorial Museum. (2012). *Introduction to the Holocaust.* Retrieved from http://www.ushmm.org/wlc/en/article.php?ModuleId=10005143

[8] Schaefer, R. (2012). *Racial and ethnic groups.* (13th ed.). Upper Saddle River, NJ: Pearson Prentice Hall.

[9] Lewis, L. (2003). Jewish perspectives on pregnancy and childbearing. *American Journal of Maternal Child Nursing, 28*(5), 306-312.

[10] Weinstein, L. (2007) Selected genetic disorders affecting Ashkenazi Jewish families. *Family Community Health, 30*(1), 50-62.

[11] Niell, B., Long, J., Rennert, G. & Gruber, S. (2003). Genetic anthropology of the colorectal cancer-susceptibility Allele APC|1307K evidence of genetic drift within the Askhenazim. *American Journal of Human Genetics, 73*(6), 1250-1260.

[12] Einstein Victor Center for the Prevention of Jewish Genetic Diseases. (2012). *Jewish genetic diseases.* Retrieved from http://www.victorcenters.org/faqs/jewish_genetic.cfm

[13] Johnson, R., Palmieri, P., Varley, J., Canetti, D., Galea, S., & Hobfoll, S. (2009). A prospective study of risk and resilience factors associated with posttraumatic stress symptoms and depression symptoms among Jews and Arabs exposed to repeated acts of terrorism in Israel. *Psychological Trauma: Theory, Research, Practice, and Policy, 1*(4), 291-311.

[14] North American Jewish Data Bank. (2010). *World Jewish population, 2010.* Retrieved from http://www.jewishdatabank.org/Reports/World_Jewish_Population_2010.pdf

[15] Wagner, M. (2008, September 26). *World Jewish population grows by 70,000.* Retrieved from http://www.jpost.com/JewishWorld/JewishNews/Article.aspx?id=115679

[16] Gershom, Y. (1999). *Frequently asked questions on Hasidic culture and customs.* Retrieved from http://www.pinenet.com/~rooster/hasid1.html

[17] Harris, L. (1985). *Holy Days: The world of a Hasidic family.* New York, NY: Simon and Schuster.

[18] Charnes, L. & Moore, P. (1992). Meeting patients' spiritual needs: The Jewish perspective. *Holistic Nurse Practitioner, 6*(3), 64-72.

[19] Lutwak, R., Nay, A. & White, J. (1988). Maternity nursing and Jewish law. *Maternal-Child Nursing Journal, 13*(1), 44-47.

[20] Rich, T. (1999). *Judaism 101: Movements of Judaism.* Retrieved from http://www.jewfaq.org/movement.htm

[21] Society for Humanistic Judaism. (2011). *Society for Humanistic Judaism answers 13 tough questions about Humanistic Judaism.* Retrieved from http://www.shj.org/FAQs.html

[22] Cohen, D. (1995). *Focus on issues: Secular humanistic Jews seeks to attract.* Retrieved from http://archive.jta.org/article/1995/11/13/2883397/focus-on-issues-secular-humanistic-jews-seeks-to-attract-unaffiliated

[23] Alliance for Jewish Renewal. (2007). FAQs about Jewish Renewal. Retrieved from https://www.aleph.org/faq.htm

[24] Horowitz, S. (2001, December). Ancient wisdom for modern medicine: Jewish perspectives on health. *Alternative & Complementary Therapies,* 7(6), 355-359.

[25] Sommer, J. (1995). Special considerations for Orthodox Jewish patients in the emergency department. *Journal of Emergency Nursing, 21*(6), 569-570.

[26] The Hebrew Language. (2013). Retrieved from http://judaism.about.com/od/jewishhistory/a/Hebrew-Language-Origins-History.htm

[27] Bonura, D., Fendler, M., Roesler, M. & Pacquiao, D. (2001). Culturally congruent end-of-life care for Jewish patients and their families. *Journal of Transcultural Nursing, 12*(3), 211-220.

[28] Kolatch, A. (1993). *The Jewish mourner's book of why.* New York, NY: Jonathan David Publishers, Inc.

[29] Mark, N. & Roberts, L. (1994). Ethnosensitive techniques in the treatment of the Hasidic patient with cancer. *Cancer Practice, 2*(3), 202-208.

[30] Schwartz, E. (2013). Jewish Americans. In Giger, J.N. *Transcultural nursing: Assessment and intervention* (6th ed.) (pp. 508-530). St. Louis, MO: Mosby.

[31] The Jeanie Schottenstein Center for Advanced Torah Study for Women. (2008). *Becoming niddah.* Retrieved from http://www.yoatzot.org/index.php

[32] The Jeanie Schottenstein Center for Advanced Torah Study for Women. Jewish Women's Health. (2008). *Gynecology.* Retrieved from http://www.jewishwomenshealth.org/topic.php?topicID=56

[33] Semenic, S., Callister, L. & Feldman, P. (2004). Giving birth: The voices of Orthodox Jewish women living in Canada. *JOGNN, 33*(1), 80-87.

[34] Zauderer, C. (2009). Maternity care for Orthodox Jewish couples. *Nursing for Women's Health, 13*(2), 112-120.

[35] Callister, L. (1995). Cultural meanings of childbirth. *JOGGN, 24*(4), 327-331.

[36] Noble, A., Rom, M., Newsome-Wicks, M., Engelhardt, K., & Woloski-Wruble, A. (2009). Jewish laws, customs, and practice in labor, delivery, and postpartum care. *Journal of Transcultural Nursing, 20*(3), 323-333.

[37] Orthodox Union. (n.d.). *Chalav Yisroel.* Retrieved from http://oukosher.org/index.php/common/article/chalav_yisroel/

[38] The Jeanie Schottenstein Center for Advanced Torah Study for Women. Jewish Women's Health. (2008). *Lactation.* http://www.jewishwomenshealth.org/topic.php?topicID=61

[39] Andrews, M. & Boyle, J. (2012). *Transcultural concepts in nursing care* (6th ed.). Philadelphia, PA: Lippincott Williams & Wilkins.

[40] Toropov, B. & Buckles, L. (2011). *The complete idiot's guide to the world's religions* (4th ed.). New York, NY: Alpha Books.

[41] Burke, T. (1996). *The major religions: An introduction with texts.* Cambridge: Blackwell Publishers.

[42] Ponn, A. (1998). Judaism. In C. Johnson and M. McGee (Eds.). *How different religions view death and afterlife* (pp. 154-159). Philadelphia, PA: The Charles Press, Publishers.

[43] Lamm, M. (1969). *The Jewish way in death and mourning.* New York, NY: Jonathan David Publishers.

[44] Collins, A. (2002). Judaism. *Nursing Times, 98*(9), 34-35.

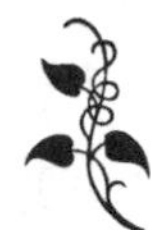

LESBIANS, GAYS, BISEXUALS, AND TRANSGENDERS (LGBTs)

Background

Individuals whose sexual expression and gender expression falls outside of the surrounding society's more accepted heterosexual traditions are referenced by many terms and acronyms. They include, but are not limited to:[1, 2, 3, 4]

- **LGBT** or **GLBT**
- **GLBTQ** (gays, lesbian, bisexual, transgender, and queer): The 'Q' may also refer to those individuals questioning their personal gender identity and/or sexual orientation.
- **GNC**: Gender noncomforming
- **LBTQ2S** (lesbian, bisexual, transgender, queer, two-spirit): The term 'two-spirit' is used among some Native Americans in referencing those who identify as LGBT or individuals who exhibit both the male and female spirit.
- **FF**: Refers to family and friends and may be added to either of the above acronyms.
- **I** (intersex) and **A** (allies): May be added to either of the above acronyms.

One's 'sex' and expected behaviors pertaining to sexuality have traditionally been defined at the time of birth by looking at a newborn's genitalia. The inability to determine an infant's sex at birth or exhibition of behaviors that fall outside those expected of a male or female, tend to cause great distress, and sometimes fear, among persons closest to the individual and to many members of a given society. In many cultures and societies, non-heterosexual intimacy is not readily accepted. Individuals who do not practice heterosexual lifestyles risk negative consequences that can impact all aspects of their lives. In some societies, however, more ambiguity is allowed and not necessarily seen as "abnormal." In fact, certain individuals may be viewed as having spiritual powers.[1,5,6]

Documentation of same-sex and transgender behaviors have been found in literature throughout history. The words *homosexual* and *heterosexual* appeared in medical literature in 1869 and 1892, respectively. Both terms referred to forms of mental illness.[7,8] Early sexologists advanced the idea that heterosexuality was in need of limited further explanation by focusing most of their research on homosexuality. Case studies were conducted, and theories emerged concerning the origins of homosexuality. Disagreements among medical and psychoanalytical authorities continued for many years. In 1973, after much deliberation, the American Psychiatric Association removed homosexuality from the *Diagnostic and Statistical Manual of Mental Disorders (DSM)*.[8] The term *transgender* appeared in the 1980s secondary to the beliefs that other terms did not adequately portray the person who desired to live as another gender.[9]

Although education regarding the care of LGBTs is sorely lacking in health care curricula, health care providers encounter LGBTs in all aspects of life. It is believed that at least one in ten persons is lesbian, gay, bisexual, or transgender. Studies reflect both higher and lower estimates and currently, there is no firm agreement. Estimates of transgenderism vary widely because of the many barriers facing transgender individuals. However, the most recent international prevalence is estimated at one in 11,900 for mail-to-female transsexuals and one in 30,400 for female-to-male transsexuals.[3,7,9,10,11,12,13,14]

Heterosexuals are often heard saying, "I have *gaydar*. I can tell if a person is gay, lesbian, bisexual, or transgender." In truth, many LGBTs go through life with few people knowing their sexual identity. Therefore, health care providers encounter LGBTs every day in the patient/client population from all socioeconomic backgrounds, as co-workers, in churches, at the playground with their children, as visitors in providers' homes, as family members, as friends, and in all cultures and ethnic groups.

While heterosexuals sometimes express strong, negative feelings about LGBTs, including extreme aversion and hate, interacting with LGBTs is unavoidable. Significant research has been conducted, confirming frequent displays of negative feelings by health care providers toward LGBTs. These feelings are brought from home into the workplace and are conveyed to LGBTs in the form of unfriendliness, condescension, fear, ostracism, intimidation, breaches of confidentiality, refusal of care, refusal of service, rough handling, and voyeuristic curiosity. Continued exposure to negative behaviors can contribute to higher stress levels, and consequently, stress-related health conditions. Unfortunately, this has also led to some distrust of the health care system which can consequently, lead to a delay in seeking needed treatment.[2, 3, 15, 16, 17]

While personal feelings, values, and beliefs cannot be checked at the entry door to our health care facilities, LGBTs make up a significant number of persons belonging to a disadvantaged subculture that seeks and needs health care. Health disparities among LGBTs and heterosexuals have been identified in the Healthy People 2020 objectives developed by The Department of Health and Human Services.[18] A critical step for providers is to examine personal feelings towards LGBTs so that respectful health care services can be offered to assist LGBTs in attaining/maintaining optimal health and/or support with facing death.

LGBTs may be hesitant to truthfully answer assessment questions related to their sexual orientation and/or gender identity for fear of negative impacts on their care. To adequately address health needs, risk factors, and education needs, health care providers should routinely–in a very sensitive manner, gain information about an individual's sexual practices during the initial visit, and whenever evidence suggests a change in sexual behaviors. Individuals should receive a careful explanation regarding the need for sexual information to accurately screen and counsel. Health care providers should stress that information will be held in strictest confidence. Consult with the individual about information to be included in the medical record since this information may affect insurance benefits, etc.[11, 19]

Heterosexuality or homosexuality should not be assumed. As a beginning to gathering an accurate sexual assessment, it is helpful if health care providers know and use correct terminology when working with patients/clients.[11] The following are helpful definitions in working with this population:

- **Sexual Orientation**: Refers to an individual's pattern of physical and affectional response toward other persons–who one finds sexually attractive. Sexual orientation is generally categorized as *heterosexual, gay, lesbian,* or *bisexual.* There is some debate about whether *asexual* (persons with no sexual attractions) should be included as a sexual orientation.

Sexual orientation is believed to be the result of genetic, biological, and hormonal influences during fetal growth. Health care providers should remember that sexual orientation (which may be displayed publicly) does not necessarily provide any information about the person's actual **sexual behavior** (which is generally displayed privately). For example, a person who identifies himself or herself publicly as heterosexual by wearing a wedding band, displaying pictures of spouses, etc., may engage in sexual behavior in private that is traditionally thought, by some persons, to be homosexual behavior.[3, 4, 14, 20, 21]

- **Gender Identity**: Refers to an individual's internal sense of self as being male or female–how an individual sees him/herself **socially**. For example, an individual may have a penis, but prefers to relate to others socially as female. Sometimes individuals will relate socially as male and female. **Gender role** refers to an individual's **overt** expression of being male or female. Generally, societies define expected roles and behaviors of males and females. Gender identity and gender role are usually congruent with an individual's anatomical/biological sex assigned at birth. Some individuals' gender identity does not match their anatomic or chromosomal sex. This is sometimes called *gender identity disorder* or *gender dysphoria* in psychiatric settings. The terms should not be used loosely to "label" individuals. It is important to know that many LGBTs do not see this incongruence as a "disorder." LGBTs' sexual orientation will be heterosexual, gay, lesbian, or bisexual.[3, 4, 14, 20, 21]

- **Heterosexual**: A person whose persistent sexual and affective attraction is to persons whose sex is different from his/her own.

- **Heterosexism**: The belief that heterosexuality is superior to homosexuality and is the only normal option for human sexual relationships.[8]

- **Homosexual**: A person who has persistent sexual and affective attraction to persons of one's own sex.[22] The term 'gay' may be used to refer to both men and women. However, in recent years, the term gay is commonly used to describe men, and 'lesbian' is used to refer to women. Also, the term 'queer,' once seen as offensive, has become a popular substitute to refer to both gays and lesbians and is sometimes used to refer to those persons who don't accept being placed in a category based on widely accepted gender roles and sexual expression. The term, *homosexual*, is becoming less acceptable.[2, 3, 7]

- **Bisexual**: A person who is attracted sexually and affectively to persons of both sexes. A lifestyle that is receiving more attention is known as "living on the down low" or "living on the DL." Men who live on the DL secretly have sex with men while maintaining sexual relationships with wives and girlfriends. Unprotected sex is common in DL relationships. Wearing a condom is often seen as "taking away from the thrill of spontaneity." The men will often speak out strongly against homosexuality and, many times hold much respected career positions and positions within their communities. DL lifestyles are a major factor in the rising incidence of HIV/AIDS, particularly among African Americans and Hispanic heterosexual women, when their male partners engage in DL sexual activity.[17,22,23]

- **Transgender**: The term *transgender* is used many times, as an umbrella term that references a variety of gender identities and displays of behavior that are contrary to the expected gender behaviors of the dominant culture. The gender variations may be lived full- or part-time. Some individuals explore transgender lifestyles, but do not consider themselves transgender. Transgenders may refer to themselves simply as "trans." Transgenders face profound isolation not only from mainstream heterosexual society, but also from the gay, lesbian, and bisexual communities. As a result, they are at risk for being victims of violence, mental health illnesses including suicide, and substance abuse.[17,24,25]

- Transgender persons include the following:

  - **Transsexual**: The transsexual person has the belief that s/he belongs to the gender other than that suggested by his or her genitalia and seeks to correct their gender through various avenues including, sometimes, self-mutilation. Transsexual persons often state that they feel as though they were born into the wrong body. Some transsexuals attempt to disguise their birth sex by the use of various types of clothing and other articles. Others have surgical and medical treatments, including hormonal treatments to alter their body appearance to more closely match their psychological sexual identity. The ultimate goal is to live full-time as dictated by their gender identity. Common terms used to refer to transsexual gender identity include *female-to-male* (FTM or transman) and *male-to-female* (MTF or transwoman). FTMs were deemed females at birth, but identify as male; MTFs were deemed males at birth, but identify as female.

    Surgery to alter the body to be more congruent with the individual's gender identity can range from a single surgery to sex reassignment surgery. FTMs may have surgeries that include bilateral mastectomy, hysterectomy, salpingo-oophorectomy, urethroplasty, placement of a testicular prosthesis, and creation of a neophallus. MTF surgeries may include penis and scrotal removal, creation of a neovagina, breast augmentation, reshaping of the nose and Adam's apple, hair transplants, and facial surgery. Gender transition is a lengthy process requiring intense psychological and physical care and support. Transsexuals identify themselves as male or female based on their sexual identity and may be heterosexual, bisexual, gay, or lesbian in their sexual identity.[1, 7, 21, 23, 26, 27]

- **Transvestite (TV)/Cross-dresser (CD)**: A person, usually a heterosexual male, who periodically wears clothing of the opposite gender for enhanced relaxation. Women who cross-dress are often not identified in Western society because of wider acceptance of women dressing in clothing that is sometimes viewed as masculine (i.e., pants, certain styles of shirts, etc.). Men who cross-dress are frequently married, have children, and have traditionally masculine jobs and hobbies. **Fetish cross-dressers** do so for sexual gratification and frequently gain the gratification through wearing a specific type of clothing. These persons usually do not wish to undergo any medical or surgical treatments to permanently change their physical features.[5, 17, 27]

- **Drag Queen/King**: Drag Queen refers to a gay male who dresses as a woman–usually flamboyantly. Often, their destination is to a club or bar when dressed in drag. Drag King refers to a woman who dresses as a male and takes on a traditional male role intermittently.

- **Female Impersonators**: Men, sometimes gay, who work in the entertainment industry.

- **She-Male**: Refers to a man who lives as a woman, but retains his male organs. Sometimes select physical features are changed such as undergoing breast augmentation. She-males are often involved in adult entertainment jobs and may be involved in prostitution.[5]

- **Intersex**: Refers to persons who have mixed sexual physiology. This may be caused by various medical conditions in which an individual's genetic sex (chromosomes) and phenotypic sex (genital appearance) do not match, or are somehow different from the 'standard' male or female. About one in 2,000 babies are born with ambiguous genitalia, while some other intersex conditions are not detected until later in life. The current medical protocol calls for the surgical 'reconstruction' of these different, but healthy bodies to make them "normal." This practice has become increasingly controversial as adults who went through the treatment report being physically, emotionally, and sexually harmed by such procedures.[28, 29]

• **Homophobia**: The irrational fear, distrust, and/or hatred LGBTs because of their sexual orientation.[30] New terms such as "homo-ignorance," "homonegativity," or "homohatred" are replacing this term since it is not a "phobia" in the sense of the word.[10]

Heterosexuality is assumed and sanctioned among most health care providers.[16, 31] This assumption is reflected in policies and procedures, questions used in gathering information for histories/assessments, literature in waiting rooms, etc.[8] Health care providers must be careful to maintain confidentiality in medical records and discuss **explicitly** with non-heterosexuals whether documentation of sexual identity can be placed in the patient chart, since the ramifications can have a lifelong impact on employment, family relationships, insurance coverage, etc. This should be done in private with the patient, unless s/he gives permission for other individuals to be present.

Some health care providers have developed symbols to use in documentation or use phrases that serve as personal reminders so that patient confidentiality is not breached. Although patient records are ideally confidential, the reality is that many persons have access to the record, such as other office staff, other physicians, insurance company representatives, etc. **Remember to support parents and other family members who may be learning for the first time that a loved one is gay, lesbian, or bisexual and for the individual who is disclosing their sexual identity for the first time to family members.** Health care providers may observe emotional displays of shame, denial, anger, blaming of the individual's partner (if present), blaming of the health provider, and/or shock.

Health risk factors for adolescents struggling with sexual identity issues include fear of humiliation, bullying, harassment, physical injury, emotional/social isolation, and pregnancy as a result of trying to hide sexual identity. There may be frequent absences from school leading to lower grades. Homelessness and prostitution, with its associated risks, may be a result of being barred from the familial home, and may be used as a method of financial support and gaining social interactions. Approximately 26 percent of adolescents are forced to leave the family home after identifying themselves as gay, lesbian, or bisexual. Up to one-half of those forced from the family home resort to prostitution to support themselves. LGBT adolescents comprise approximately 40 percent of homeless youth.[10, 32] Self-hatred, shame, depression, substance abuse, suicidal ideation, and suicide are common. LGBT adolescents are two to seven times more likely to attempt suicide than non-LGBT adolescents. Their attempts are more serious and more often lethal. Furthermore, they comprise 30 percent of completed youth suicides each year.[17, 24, 33, 34]

Health risk factors for lesbians include breast, ovarian, and endometrial cancer, which may be related to the higher incidence of not becoming pregnant and decreased preventive gynecological exams.[35, 36] Gay and bisexual men may be at risk for gastrointestinal infections and anal pathology, including anal cancer. Gay and bisexual men are seventeen times more likely to develop anal cancer than those who have sex with women only. In addition, individuals who participate in unprotected oral sex are at risk of pharyngeal gonorrhea, chlamydial infection, and hepatitis A infections. Sexually transmitted diseases continue to be a risk factor for men who have sex with men. Approximately 78 percent of new HIV/AIDS cases occur among men who have sex with men (MSM). Hispanic and African American communities have been severely impacted. Anal human papillomavirus is seen in more than 60 percent of HIV-negative MSMs. Lesbians appear to have lower rates of certain sexually transmitted diseases than heterosexual or bisexual women.[11, 30, 37, 38, 39, 40]

Gay men and lesbian women tend to have fewer preventive screenings such as blood pressure and cholesterol screenings.[41] Because of repeated experiences with rejection, sexual harassment, and violence, mental health problems such as depression, suicide, alcoholism, etc. may be seen.[26, 30] In a 2011 study conducted by the National Center for Transgender Equality, 41 percent of the participants had attempted suicide.[42] LGBTs may present with advanced symptoms of chronic diseases because of lack of insurance coverage, lack of primary care physicians, and fear. Chronic conditions may be poorly controlled because of the same reasons. The use of feminizing or masculinizing hormones place many transgenderists at risk for side effects of such hormones.[11, 13]

Depending upon whether hormone therapy is for feminizing or masculinizing purposes, health risk conditions for transgender persons undergoing hormone therapy include Type 2 Diabetes, cardiovascular disease, venous thrombosis, osteoporosis, elevated liver enzymes, cholelithiasis, breast cancer, ovarian cancer, liver cancer, and prostate cancer. Consider the effects of hormones when evaluating lab values, monitoring drug interactions, and prior to surgery and other treatments. HIV, STDs, and Hepatitis B and C are disproportionately seen in the transgender community.[1, 13, 25]

Special Celebrations

- LGBTs observe the traditional celebrations of the dominant culture, their ethnic group, and/or their religious affiliation. In addition, National Coming Out day is celebrated in the United States by some LGBTs each October 11th, commemorating the 1987 gay and lesbian rights march on Washington, DC. The celebration is actually a visibility campaign to encourage people to tell the truth about their lives and to "come out of the closet."[7]

- Various Gay Pride parades and celebrations are held throughout the world at varying times of the year.

Language

- LGBTs primary language will be that of the dominant culture and/or ethnic group.
- LGBTs may use coded language among themselves, sometimes called 'lavender language.' The color of lavender is used because it is often seen in gay-friendly environments.

Worldview/Religious Beliefs

- Based on culture, ethnic group, and religious affiliation.

Health Beliefs/Practices

- Health care will be sought for all the reasons that other men and women seek health care. However, LGBTs may avoid seeking health care until the disorder or illness is at the advanced stage or crisis stage because of past negative experiences with health care providers.[35, 43]
- There are no known illnesses/problems that are exclusively found among LGBTs.
- Lesbians may prefer to have female providers.[35]
- Among lesbians, smaller vaginal specula, including pediatric specula, may be needed for pelvic exams to decrease discomfort.[35]
- **Intimate partner violence (IPV) screening should be applied to both females and males.** LGBTs may be victims of IPV and hate crimes, but may be hesitant to present for assistance because of fear related to their sexual identity. Screen for abuse, offer support, and make referrals to agencies and counselors with skills in working with this population of people, if available. Gay and bisexual men who are victims of rape should be treated with sensitivity. Protect privacy and confidentiality as a female rape victim would be treated. Men are often afraid to come to hospitals for fear the staff will not believe that they were raped, fear of publicity, and/or fear that it will be thought that the man "asked for it." A male bisexual may be married and fear that his family will find out about his bisexuality. Male rape victims often sustain other injuries when raped.[44, 45, 46]

- Transgenders who are in a state of transition from one gender role to a desired gender role may present to health care facilities exhibiting characteristics of both genders. Two names may be used–the birth name and the chosen name. Be respectful during interactions; maintain confidentiality. Ask preferred name.[13]

- Residual prostate and breast tissue may remain after sex reassignment surgery. Therefore, male-to-female transgender individuals should receive preventive screening for prostate cancer. Female-to-male individuals should receive routine breast examinations and Pap smears. A pediatric vaginal speculum may be needed in the event that testosterone therapy has led to atrophic changes in the vaginal mucosa that cause painful pelvic exams. The individual's biological sex, surgical status, use of hormone therapies, and declared gender should be considered when determining health screening needs. Use extreme sensitivity in explaining the necessity and preparation for screenings that are based on his/her biological sex vs. the individual's chosen gender.[12,13,25]

- Inquire about self-treatment with non-prescribed hormonal substances, including body-enhancing substances such as silicone. These substances may be obtained from friends, underground drug markets, or the Internet. Over-the-counter plant-derived estrogens/androgens may be taken as dietary supplements.[13]

Expression of Pain

- Variable based on culture.

Male-Female/Kinship/Social Relationships

- "Family" includes partners unless otherwise specified by the adult patient. Allow visitation and inclusion in supportive activities such as care issues, visitation in hospitals, including critical care units and participation in office visits, as for other family members. (As of November 2010, hospitals that receive Medicaid and Medicare funding must allow visitation based on the patient's choice and respect the wishes of same-sex partners related to designated persons making medical decisions on the patient's behalf, if needed.)[47]

- Older LGBTs may refer to their partner as "my friend" or "my roommate." Gently explore the meaning and/or relationship of 'friends' or 'roommates.'

- Determine the position of critical referral services in the hospital, such as the clergy, before a crisis arises. Some religious denominations are strongly antigay.[48]

- Refer to the transsexual by his/her desired name and pronoun. If in doubt ask, "What do you prefer to be called?"[12, 26]

- Family members, other than the client's partner, may not be aware of the LGBT's sexual orientation. The individual should have control over when, or if, their sexual orientation is shared with other family members. Family members may need professional referrals to assist them with dealing with their feelings. Support groups such as *Parents, Families & Friends of Lesbians & Gays* (PFLAG) can also be of tremendous support. PFLAG affiliates are located in all 50 states and have international affiliates. Since 1998, PFLAG has included transgenders in the organization's mission.[49]

- Assign transsexuals to private rooms, if possible, when hospitalized.

- Health care facilities should explore designating some restrooms as unisex/family instead of having all restrooms labeled as "Women" or "Men."

Birth/Children

- Discuss methods and options for sperm/fertilized embryos preservation prior to beginning hormone therapy for transsexuals.[1, 50]

- Lesbian, gay, and bisexual couples may have children from previous marriages and/or adoption. Lesbian couples may opt to have artificial insemination or may enter an agreement to have the child fathered through actual sexual intercourse with a male. While adults often wonder what children will call two mommies or two daddies, children usually quite easily come up with names to differentiate the two adults.[7] The correct term for same-sex parents sharing the parenting of a child or children is *co-parenting*.

- Lesbian women often have the fear that they will receive inadequate and/or unsafe care during childbirth if their sexual orientation is known.[8]

- For lesbian couples desiring to have a child by artificial insemination, provide referrals to reputable semen donor banks. Patients may want to select their own donors.

- Provide antenatal, birth, and postpartum education to lesbian couples, as with traditional couples.

- Explore breastfeeding plans during prenatal period. Both partners may want to breastfeed the baby. Refer to the physician and lactation consultant for discussion of methods to stimulate lactation in the non-birth mother.[35]

- Allow partners to participate in the birth process by serving as support partners, etc.

- During pregnancy, discuss topics that are unique to same-sex parents such as parenting concerns, advising to get legal assistance to assure custody for both parents–particularly in the event of the death of one parent.

- In asking questions about the family of children of same-sex couples, consider the following:[43]

  1. Who are ____________'s parents?

  2. Who else is a part of ____________'s family?

- Teach parents and other caregivers to take seriously any signs of depression or suicidal ideation exhibited by children, particularly adolescents. Signs of depression may include running away from home, decline in school performance, truancy, disruption in personal/family relationships, promiscuity, substance abuse, etc.[22]

Death

- Allow the partner and other family members to stay with the dying patient and participate in terminal care as much as possible.

- Provide religious and grief support, being cognizant of any religious affiliation or religious beliefs.

- Refer the partner and other family members to appropriate grief counselors for follow-up assistance in coping with the death of his or her partner.

Patient and Family Teaching/Other Considerations

- Examine personal attitudes and feelings toward LGBTs prior to interaction, if possible, to decrease the possibility of negative interactions. Pay close attention to personal non-verbal behavior such as distancing self from client, tone of voice, etc.[8]

- Assess support systems (family, friends, etc.) available after discharge from the hospital, particularly when working with elderly LGBTs, who often have limited support systems.

- Health care providers should become familiar with community resources for LGBTs so that appropriate referrals can be made to assist with issues of coping, special services, etc. Referrals should be to physicians and other individuals/agencies that are not homophobic and who will provide supportive care for the individual.[30]

- In conducting health assessments/sexual histories, evaluate questions that assume hetero-sexuality, consider the following:

  1. Substitute terms such as "partner," "life partner," "domestic partner," or "significant other" for the terms "husband/wife/boyfriend/girlfriend." Other questions might include: "With whom do you live?" or "Who is important to you?" or "I see that you've indicated that you are not married, but are there any significant loved ones/ friends?"[19, 43]

  2. For demographic forms, add 'Transgender' (male-to-female and female-to-male) as a choice of identities vs. only Male and Female. A choice of 'Decline to State' should also be added as well as 'Other,' allowing the individual to define his/her own identity.[19]

  3. When inquiring if one is sexually active, add "with men, with women, or with both." "Are you in an intimate relationship?" "Do you regularly use protective barriers during sexual encounters? If yes, what kind?"

4. When assessing birth control needs, ask "Do you have a need for birth control?" vs. "What type of birth control are you using?"

5. For eliciting sexual histories from adolescents, questions may include the following:[30]

   "Many girls/boys your age are thinking about dating. What are your thoughts about this?" "Have you started dating anyone yet?" or "Is there any one person that you're pretty serious about?" or "Do you date several different people?"

   If an adolescent acknowledges being gay: "How do you feel about that?", "Are you comfortable with being gay?", "Does it make you or others upset?" or "Have you told persons significant to you, such as your parents, family members, friends, or teachers?"

6. Feldman and Bockting (2003) suggest inclusion of the following questions when taking transgender-specific histories:

   - "Have you undergone sex reassignment surgery or other masculinizing/feminizing procedures? If not, do you plan to pursue surgery in the future?"

   - "Are you currently taking cross-gender hormones (including over-the-counter herbal hormones)?" "Which ones and for how long?"

   - "Have you had any complications or concerns?" "Have you used hormones in the past? If not, do you plan to pursue hormone therapy in the future?"

   - "Are you currently seeing a therapist?" Does s/he specialize in gender and/or sexual health issues?"

   Other than penile-vaginal intercourse, LGBTs use the same sexual methods that are practiced among heterosexual couples to give and receive sexual pleasure. Educate regarding safe sexual practices.[10]

   - Some individuals may not be aware that women can transmit sexually transmitted diseases to other women during sexual contact. The risk may be increased further if there has been previous sexual activity with male or bisexual partners.[51]

   - Avoid sex-play that involves exposure to body fluids when there are breaks in the skin or mucous membranes. Cuticles and nail beds should be protected, even in the absence of breaks in the skin.

- Protect against the exchange of body fluids between multiple partners. Dental dams (a latex barrier between the mouth and genital area/anus) should be used, but may be hard to find and expensive. A condom or glove that has been cut open length-wise, or household plastic wrap may be used if dental dams cannot be found or afforded.[51, 52, 53]

- Sex toys used between multiple partners should be washed/cleaned between partners. Encourage condom use on sex toys.[51]

- Use separate objects for vaginal and anal penetration. If unable to afford two of the same objects, changing condoms between vaginal and anal penetration is recommended.[53]

- Use only water-based lubricants because oil-based lubricants may cause breakdown of the integrity of latex and plastic barriers.[54]

- Spermicides should be used in addition to condoms with multiple male-female or anal sexual encounters.[10, 54]

• Include information in health care curricula that addresses care issues of LGBTs. Provide in-service.[31] Assure that the medical library contains references that provide non-biased research and information related to LGBTs.

• Standards of care for transgender patients have been developed by the World Professional Association for Transgender Health (formerly the Harry Benjamin International Gender Dysphoria Association) and can be accessed at http://www.wpath.org.

• A number of resources are available on the Internet and from health care facilities that specialize in the care of transsexuals and sexual reassignment surgery.

---

1 World Professional Association for Transgender Health. (2012). *Standards of care for the health of transsexual, transgender, and gender nonconforming people* (7th version). Retrieved from http://www.wpath.org/documents/SOC%20V7%2003-17-12.pdf

2 Pettinato, M. (2012). Providing care for GLBTQ patients. *Nursing 2012, 42*(12), 22-27.

3 Eliason, M., Dibble, S., DeJoseph, J., & Chinn, P. (2009). *LGBTQ Cultures: What health care professionals need to know about sexual and gender diversity*. Philadelphia, PA: Lippincott, Williams & Wilkins.

[4] The Joint Commission. (2011). *Advancing effective communication, cultural competence, and patient-and family-centered care for the lesbian, gay, bisexual, and transgender (LGBT) community: A field guide.* Oak Terrace, IL: Author.

[5] Brown, M. & Rounsley, C. (2003). *True Selves: Understanding transsexualism.* San Francisco, CA: Jossey-Bass Publishers.

[6] Tofoya, T. (2003). Native gay and lesbian issues: The two-spirited. In: Garnets, L. & Kimmel, D. (Eds.). *Psychological perspectives on lesbian, gay, and bisexual experiences*, pp. 401-409. New York, NY: Columbia University Press.

[7] Marcus, E. (1993). *Is it a choice: Answers to 300 of the most frequently asked questions about gays and lesbians.* New York, NY: Harper Collins Publishers.

[8] Eliason, M. (1996). Caring for the lesbian, gay, or bisexual patient: Issues for critical care nurses. *Critical Care Nursing Quarterly, 19*(1), 665-72.

[9] Carroll, L., Gilroy, P., and & Ryan, J. (2002). Counseling transgendered, transsexual, and gender-variant clients. *Journal of Gerontological Nursing, 29*(7), 44-49.

[10] Apleby, G. and & Anastas, J. (1998). *Not just a passing phase: Social work with gay, lesbian and bisexual people.* New York, NY: Columbia University Press.

[11] Knight, D. (2004). Health care screening for men who have sex with men. *American Family Physician, 69*(9), 2149-2156.

[12] Berreth, M. (2003). Nursing care of transgendered older adults: Implications from the literature. *Journal of Gerontological Nursing, 29*(7), 44-49.

[13] Feldman, J. and & Bockting, W. (2003). Transgender health. *Minnesota Medicine, 86*(7), 25-32.

[14] Gay and Lesbian Medical Association. (n.d.) *Quality healthcare for lesbian, gay, bisexual & transgender people.* [Webinar series]. Retrieved from http://www.glma.org/_data/n_0001/resources/live/GLMA%20 Cultural%20Competence%20Webinar_Part%201_June%2019%202012.pdf

[15] Kane-Lee, E. & Bayer, C.R. (2012). Meeting the needs of LGBT patients and families. *Nursing Management, 43*(2), 43-46.

[16] Stevens, P. (1992). Lesbian health care research: A review of the literature from 1970 - 1990. *Health Care for Women International, 13*(2), 91-120.

[17] Institute of Medicine. (2011). *The health of lesbian, gay, bisexual, and transgender people: Building a foundation for better understanding.* Washington, DC: The National Academies Press.

[18] US Department of Health and Human Resources. (2012). *Healthy People 2020: Lesbian, gay, bisexual, and transgender health.* Retrieved from http://www.healthypeople.gov/2020/topicsobjectives2020/overview.aspx?topicid=25

[19] Coren, J.S., Coren, C.M., Pagliaro, S.N. & Weiss, L.B. (2011). Assessing your office for care of lesbian, gay, bisexual, and transgender patients. *Health Care Manager, 30*(1), 66-70.

[20] Frankowski, B. (2004). Sexual orientation and adolescents: Clinical report. *Pediatricians, 113*(6), 1827-1832.

[21] Wylie, K. (2004). Gender related disorders. *British Medical Journal, 329*(7466), 615-617.

[22] Kreiss, J. and & Patterson, D. (1997). Psychosocial issues in primary care of lesbian, gay, and bisexual, and transgender youth. *Journal of Pediatric Health Care, 11*(6), 266-274.

[23] King, J. (2004). *On the down low: A journey into the lives of straight black men who sleep with men.* New York, NY: Broadway Books.

[24] Moon, M., O'Briant, A., and & Friedland, M. (2002). Caring for sexual minority youths: A guide for nurses. *The Nursing Clinics of North America, 37*(3), 405-422.

[25] Alegria, C.A. (2011). Transgender identity and health care: Implications for psychosocial and physical evaluation. *Journal of the American Academy of Nurse Practitioners, 23*(2011), 175-182.

[26] Ramsey, G. (1996). *Transsexuals: Candid answers to private questions*. Freedom, CA: The Crossing Press.

[27] Israel, G. & Tarver, D. (1997). *Transgender care: Recommended guidelines, practical information and personal accounts*. Philadelphia, PA: Temple University Press.

[28] Intersex Initiative. (n.d.). *Intersex FAQ*. Retrieved from http://www.intersexinitiative.org

[29] Intersex Society of North America. (2008). *What is intersex?* Retrieved from http://www.isna.org/faq/what_is_intersex

[30] Harrison, A. (1996). Primary care of lesbian and gay patients: Educating ourselves and our students. *Family Medicine, 28*(1), 10-23.

[31] Eliason, M., Dibble, S., & DeJoseph, J. (2010). Nursing's silence on lesbian, gay, bisexual, and transgender issues: The need for emancipatory efforts. Advances in Nursing Science, 33(3), 206-218.

[32] Lowrey, S. & Burke, J.C. (Eds.). (2010). *Kicked out*. Ypsilanti, MI: Homofactus Press, LLC.

[33] Suicide Prevention Resource Center. (2012). *Suicide prevention among LGBT youth: A workshop for professionals who serve youth*. Retrieved from http://www.sprc.org/training-institute/lgbt-youth-workshop

[34] Kosciw, J.G., Bartkiewicz, M., & Greytak, E.A. (2012). Promising strategies for prevention of the bullying of lesbian, gay, bisexual, and transgender youth. *The Prevention Researcher, 19*(3), 10-13.

[35] Dibble, S.L. & Robertson, P.A. (2010). *Lesbian health 101: A clinician's guide*. San Francisco, CA: UCSF Nursing Press.

[36] Zaritsky, E. & Dibble, S.L. (2010). Risk factors for reproductive and breast cancer among older lesbians. *Journal of Women's health, 19*(1), 125-131.

[37] Palefsky, J., Holly, E., Ralston, M., & Jay, N. (1998). Prevalence and risk factors for human papillomavirous infection of the anal canal in human immunodeficiency virus HIV-positive and HIV-negative homosexual men. *Journal of Infectious Diseases, 177*(2), 361-367.

[38] Centers for Disease Control and Prevention. (2010). *HIV in the United States: At a glance*. Retrieved from http://www.cdc.gov/hiv/resources/factsheets/us.htm

[39] Dietz, C.A. & Nyberg, C.R. (2011), Genital, oral, and anal human papillomavirus infection in men who have sex with men. *Journal of the American Osteopath Association, 111*(3), S19-S25.

[40] Patel, P., Hanson, D.L., Sullivan, P.S., Novak, R.M., Moorman, A.C., Tong, T.C.,...Brooks, J.T. (2008). Incidence of types of cancer among HIV-infected persons compared with the general population in the United States, 1992-2003. *Annals of Internal Medicine, 148*(10), 728-736

[41] Denenberg, R. (1995). Report on lesbian health. *Women's Health Issues, 5*(2), 81-91.

[42] Grant, J.M., Mottet, L.A., Tannis, J., Harrison, J., & Keisling, M. (2011). *Injustice at every turn: A report of the National Transgender Discrimination Survey*. Retrieved from http://www.thetaskforce.org/downloads/reports/reports/ntds_summary.pdf

[43] Lynch, M. (1993). When the patient is also a lesbian. *AWHONNS Clinical Issues in Perinatal and Women's Health Nursing, 4*(2), 196-202.

[44] Cruz, M. (2003). "Why doesn't he just leave?": Gay male domestic violence and the reasons victims stay. *The Journal of Men's Studies, 11*(3), 309-314.

[45] Ristock, J. (2003). Exploring dynamics of abusive lesbian relationships: Preliminary analysis of a multisite, qualitative study. *American Journal of Community Psychology, 31*(3-4), 329-341.

[46] Ard, K.L. & Makadon, H.J. (2011). Addressing intimate partner violence in lesbian, gay, bisexual, and transgender patients. *Journal of General Internal Medicine, 26*(8), 930-933.

[47] US Department of Health and Human Services. (2012). *US Department of Health and Human Services recommended actions to improve the health and well-being of lesbian, gay, bisexual, and transgender communities*. Retrieved from http://www.hhs.gov/secretary/about/lgbthealth.html

[48] Eliason, M. (1996). Caring for the lesbian, gay, or bisexual patient: Issues for critical care nurses. *Critical Care Nursing Quarterly, 19*(1), 665-72.

[49] Parents, Families and Friends of Lesbians and Gays. (2012). *About PFLAG*. Retrieved from http://www.pflag.org

[50] Greeman, Y. (2004). The endocrine care of transsexual people. *The Journal of Endocrinology & Metabolism, 89*(2), 1014-1015.

[51] Ripley, V. (2011). Promoting sexual health in women who have sex with women. *Nursing Standard, 25*(51), 41-46.

[52] Stevens, P. (1994). HIV prevention for lesbians and bisexual women: A cultural analysis of a community intervention. *Social Science and Medicine, 39*(11), 1565-1578.

[53] Caster, W. (2003). *The lesbian sex book*. (2nd ed.). Los Angeles, CA: Alyson Books.

[54] Rankow, E. (1995). Breast and cervical cancer among lesbians. *Women's Health Issues, 5*(3), 123-129.

NATIVE AMERICANS

Background

There are several theories regarding the origins of Native Americans, the indigenous peoples of the Americas. The theory put forth by Father Joseph de Acosta in 1570 is the most widely accepted. He suggested that Native Americans migrated to North America during the period of 15,000 BC - 12,000 BC. They came from northeast Asia via the Bering Strait (present day Alaska), which joined Asia and North America during the Ice Age. The people inhabited the uppermost point of North America through the southern tip of South America. Each Native American group also has its own theory of origin. At first contact with Europeans, there were approximately sixty to seventy million Native Americans in the Western Hemisphere who made up more than two thousand cultures and spoke hundreds of languages.[1,2,3]

After years of persecution, oppression, racism, and various atrocities, Native Americans make up only 1.7 percent of the United States population. The 2010 United States census indicated a population of only 2.9 million Native American/Alaska Native people and an additional 2.3 million individuals that identified themselves as Native American plus another race. There are over one million Native Americans (First Nations) in Canada. A number of indigenous groups reside in Mexico, and Central and South America; some in remote areas.

In the United States, the largest Native American groups are found in California, Oklahoma, and Arizona respectively.[1,2,4]

Tremendous diversity exists among Native American groups. Clothing styles, music, language, and spiritual/philosophical beliefs are specific to each group.[4] Health care providers should become familiar with specific practices and beliefs of those groups most often cared for. Traditional practices that promote wellness and holistic healing can be incorporated into mainstream medical settings.[5] Organizations and online sites such as the Indian Health Services (IHS), Tribal Government: USA.gov, National Congress of American Indians, and Management Sciences for Health provide many informational resources related to specific groups' beliefs and practices.[6,7,8,9]

In all of the Americas, 28.4 percent of Native Americans are living in poverty.[4] Poor access to health care continues to be a major problem. Health risk factors for Native Americans include alcohol abuse and its subsequent effects, poor dental health, obesity, diabetes, cardiovascular disease, cancer, respiratory disease, and liver disease.[10,11,12,13] Injuries and violence among Native Americans ages one to nineteen years accounts for 75 percent of all deaths; specifically, motor vehicle accidents, suicide, homicide, drowning, and fires, in respective order of frequency. The homicide victims include a significant number of young children.[14,15] Native American women are twice as likely to be victims of sexual violence as women of other races in the United States. Early parenthood is common for Native American families, and almost half of all Indian mothers are under twenty years of age when their first child is born. The infant mortality rates are 22 percent higher than the general population. The incident of infant death from Sudden Infant Death Syndrome (SIDS) and accidents remains high.[16,17]

Statistically, Native American causes of death may be understated due to racial misclassification on death certificates. Leading causes of death are: cancer, heart disease, accidents, diabetes, and liver disease. Suicide is ranked eighth and homicide is the eleventh most frequent cause of death among Native Americans.[18]

Language

- Many Native Americans speak English or the prominent language of their country of residence. However, some individuals may speak only their tribal language. There are at least two hundred tribal languages spoken today.[19] Persons from parts of Mexico, Central and South America may only speak indigenous languages such as *Quechua, Guarani*, etc. and are not able to converse in English or Spanish.

- There is a strong effort to revitalize the languages of the indigenous people since many languages are on the verge of extinction.

Worldview/Religious Beliefs

- There is a sacred relationship with the universe. All things are connected and should be honored and treated with respect. Individuals receive spiritual energy from their natural surroundings. Balance and harmony with the environment, community, and ancestral spirits is optimal. Certain animals carry spiritual meanings. The survival and well-being of individuals is synonymous with the survival and well-being of the community. Cooperation and sharing is required for harmony and balance.[20]

- Storytelling is an important method of transmitting cultural traditions such as moral behavior, beliefs about creation, religious beliefs, survival skills, ceremonies, healing methods, etc.[20, 21]

- Religious expression varies among tribes. The Native American Church (Peyote Religion) and other Christian church memberships are common. The Peyotists combine Christian practices with rituals and beliefs that represent most North American tribes.[22] The Peyotists derive their name from the Peyote button of the mescal cactus plant—the source of the mood, thought, and perception-altering drug *mescaline*. It is sometimes called simply "the Medicine." Peyote is considered sacred and helps to clear the individual's mind for a closer relationship with God's spirit. Peyote may also be used for healing purposes.[23, 24]

Health Beliefs/Practices

- Total harmony with nature and fellow man reflects health. The road of human life is everlasting and endless. Spiritually, many Native Americans strive to walk the Red Path, consisting of balance in life, establishing a feeling of belonging, a sense of mastery, respect for independence, being unselfish, generous, and living according to the rules of the Creator. The body must be treated with respect just as the earth should be treated with respect. If the earth is harmed, the body is harmed and vice versa.[20, 25]

- The Medicine Wheel (or Sacred Hoop) is an important symbol of Native American spirituality and represents the circle of life. The term 'medicine' in this sense references vital life and spiritual forces. It is the symbol of a balanced life giving orientation to the many aspects of life associated with different directions. The circle encloses a cross forming the four spokes of the wheel pointing East, South, West, and North. The interpretation of the directions and other components of the Medicine Wheel may vary according to tribes. Life will be unbalanced and more difficult if important aspects of life are ignored.[20]

- May believe that illness is a price paid because of something that has or will happen.[26] Other causes include supernatural forces such as soul loss and/or spiritual intrusion, natural forces, and human agency.[25]

- Plan to spend additional time to establish positive rapport and trust. Native Americans may be suspicious and skeptical of mainstream medical treatments, believing that the intent is to harm and not heal. For instance, a diagnosis of cancer may still be viewed as a "White man's disease" because the disease was rare prior to European contact in North America. Patients and families may be hesitant to discuss the disease if it is viewed as punishment, with shame, or risk of rejection. Communicate specific interventions that impact recovery via plan of care so that all providers provide consistency in approaches to care.[27,28]

- Folk healers still exist among tribes. Herbal treatments, especially sage, are commonly used. It is important to allow medicine men and folk healers to visit and counsel with the hospitalized client to facilitate spiritual healing.

- Curing not only pertains to physical cures. Spiritual healing must also occur for an individual to regain a health balance. Origins of illness, preventive healing, and health maintenance practices vary among groups.[29]

- Medicine bags may be worn around the neck or waist for the purpose of protecting the individual from harm. The bags are considered sacred in some cases and are always very personal and private. If there is a risk that the bag will become wet during treatments, application of plastic wrap may be acceptable to the individual to protect the bag from moisture. Health care providers should not open the bag or remove it from the individual's body unless absolutely necessary. If it must be removed, it should be given to a family member for safekeeping. In the case of death, the bag should be left in place so that it can be buried with the individual.[30]

- Prayer and prayer-chants are important in the healing process.

- Eagles are considered sacred and to possess special energies. Eagle feathers may be used in healing ceremonies, or a hospitalized Native American may want to have an eagle feather(s) present in the room.

- A healing method known as *smudging* is popular among Native Americans. It is done for the purpose of cleansing an individual of negative energies. Sage, tobacco, or cedar and sweet grass are burned in a bowl or pot. The smoke is fanned over the person using an eagle feather. Smudging is often combined with other healing modalities such as fasting, praying, etc.[20, 30, 31]

Expression of Pain

- Stoicism will likely be displayed to avoid the guilt and shame of public suffering. The patient may be resistant to disclosing the presence of pain or true pain levels. Offer comfort measures if the patient does not ask.

- Displays of disability may be seen as bringing unwanted attention to self and family. Explain the need for assistive devices such as crutches, wheelchairs, etc.[32]

Male-Female/Kinship/Social Relationships

- Extended family relationships are extremely important, especially during illness and death. 'Family' is a matter of blood and spirit.[22] Decision-making will include family, particularly elders. Elders and children are highly valued. Include respected leaders and elders in health care efforts directed toward the community.

- May avoid direct eye contact with nurses, physicians, and elders as a sign of respect. Direct eye contact and staring is sometimes considered impolite or aggressive.

- Modesty among men and women is valued. Provide appropriate privacy measures. Determine if a same-sex provider is preferred. Explore privacy measures that will make the patient feel more protected.[19]

- Professional demeanor is important. A provider may be evaluated on moral appearance and approach rather than natural appearance or approach.[30] Assertiveness may be offensive. Honesty and keeping one's word are highly valued.

- Silence is considered essential to understanding and respecting another person. A pause by a Native American when questioned indicates that careful consideration is being given. Health care workers should avoid the appearance of being hurried or impatient.

- Avoid taking notes during conversations such as admission assessments, etc. Much information is passed through verbal means among Native Americans. Note-taking is considered insensitive. If note-taking is necessary, provide explanation prior to beginning.[28]

- Native Americans may speak in a low tone of voice. A quiet setting should be used when talking with these clients.

- Vigorous handshaking may be considered aggressive.

Birth/Children

- Childbirth practices vary among Native American groups. Ideally, these practices should be explored with the mother prenatally.

- Mothers may wish to have the placenta returned to them at the time of discharge for ceremonial disposition.[33]

- May seem permissive in child-rearing practices.

- May be considered taboo to cut a child's hair. Parents should always be consulted first if the child's hair must be shaved or trimmed for medical treatment purposes.

Death

- Expressions of grief and practices surrounding death vary among groups.

- Generally, do not believe that autopsies will help to explain the reason of death.

Patient Teaching/Dietary Considerations

- Popular foods include beans and corn.

- Frequently lactose-intolerant.

Other Considerations

- If amputation of a limb is required or other organs/tissues are removed, the individual/family may want to bury the limb or carry out ceremonial disposal rather than utilizing hospital disposal methods. Give special instructions about handling if the tissues have been exposed to formalin or other preservatives.[34]

- If hair must be shaved or cut in preparation for surgery, consult the patient or family before disposing of hair.

---

[1] Oswalt, W. *This land was theirs: A study of North American Indians* (9th ed.).New York, NY: Oxford University Press.

[2] Josephy, A. (1991). *The Indian heritage of America.* Boston, MA: Houghton Mifflin Company.

3 Rights, D. (1991). *The North American Indian in North Carolina* (2nd ed.). Chelsea, MI: BookCrafters.

4 U.S. Census Bureau. (2011, November 1). *Profile America facts for features: American Indian and Alaska Native heritage month: November 2011.* (CB11-FF-22). Retrieved from http://www.census.gov/newsroom/releases/archives/facts_for_features_special_editions/cb11-ff22.html

5 Horowitz, S. (2012). American Indian health: Traditional Native healing practices and western medicine. *Alternative & Complementary Therapies, 18*(1), 24-30.

6 U.S. Department of Health & Human Services (n.d.). *Indian Health Service.* Retrieved from http://www.ihs.gov/

7 Tribal Governments:USA.gov. (2012). Retrieved from http://www.usa.gov/Government/Tribal-Sites/index.shtml

8 National Congress of American Indians. (n.d.). Retrieved from http://www.ncai.org/

9 Management Sciences for Health. (n.d.). *The providers guide to quality & culture: Cultural groups: Native Americans.* Retrieved from http://erc.msh.org/mainpage.cfm?file=5.4.7.htm&module=provider&language=English

10 Mahoney, M. & Michalek, A. (1998). Health status of American Indians/Alaska natives: General patterns of mortality. *Family Medicine, 30*(3), 190-195.

11 Centers for Disease Control and Prevention. (2011, October 24). *Faststats A to Z.* Retrieved from http://www.cdc.gov/nchs/fastats/default.htm

12 Centers for Disease Control and Prevention: Office of Minority Health & Health Disparities. (2010, November 30). *American Indians & Alaska Native (AI/AN) populations.* Retrieved from http://www.cdc.gov/omhd/Populations/AIAN/AIAN.htm

13 National Center for Health Statistics. (2011,February). *Health, United States, 2010: With special feature on death and dying.* Retrieved from http://www.cdc.gov/nchs/data/hus/hus10.pdf#026

14 Green, J. (1999). *Cultural awareness in the human services: A multi-ethnic approach* (3rd ed.). Boston, MA: Allyn and Bacon.

15 Story, M., Stevens, J., Himes, J., Stone, E., Rock, B., Ethelbah, B. & Davis, S. (2003). Obesity in American-Indian children: Prevalence, consequences and prevention. *Preventive Medicine,* 37, S3-S12.

16 McWhirter, P., Robbins, R., Vaughn, K., Youngbull, N., Burks, D., Willmon-Haque, S., & Nael, A. (2010). Honoring the ways of American Indian Women: A group therapy intervention. *The Journal for Specialists in Group Work, 35*(2), 134-142.

17 Centers for Disease Control and Prevention: Office of Minority Health & Health Disparities. (2007, June). *Highlights in minority health & health disparities: October 2006.* Retrieved from http://www.cdc.gov/omhd/Highlights/2006/HOct06SIDSIF.htm

18 National Vital Statistics Reports. (2012, June 6). *Deaths: Leading causes for 2008.* Retrieved from http://www.cdc.gov/nchs/data/nvsr/nvsr60/nvsr60_06.pdf

19 Blount, M. (1996). Social work practice with Native Americans. In D. Harrison, B. Thyer, & J. Wodarski, *Cultural diversity and social work practice* (2nd ed.) (pp. 157-298). Springfield, IL: Charles C. Thomas Publisher, Ltd.

20 Rybak, C. and Decker-Fitts, A. (2009). Theory and practice: Understanding Native American healing practices. *Counseling Psychology Quarterly, 22*(3), 333-342.

21 Lewis, R. (1990). Death and dying among the American Indians. In J. Parry, *Social work practice with the terminally ill* (pp. 23-32). Springfield, IL: Charles C. Thomas, Publisher.

22 Garrett, J. & Garrett, M. (1996). *Medicine of the Cherokee: The way of right relationship.* Rochester, VT: Bear & Company Inc.

[23] Hodge, F., Pasqua, A., Marquez, C. & Geishirt-Cantrell, B. (2002). Utilizing traditional storytelling to promote wellness in American Indian communities. *Journal of Transcultural Nursing, 13*(1), 6-11.
[24] Henderson, G. & Spigner-Littles, D. (2006). *A practitioner's guide to understanding indigenous and foreign cultures* (3rd ed.). Springfield, IL: Charles C. Thomas Publishing.
[25] Amen, K. (1992). *Navajo drypainting as medicine*. Unpublished master's thesis, Wake Forest University, Winston-Salem, North Carolina.
[26] Smith, H. & Snake R. (1996). *One nation under God: The triumph of the Native American Church*. Santa Fe, NM: Clear Light Publishers.
[27] Loftin, J. (1983). The harmony ethic of the conservative Eastern Cherokees: A religious interpretation. *Journal of Cherokee Studies, 8*(1), 40-43.
[28] Ramer, L. (1992). *Culturally sensitive caregiving and childbearing families*. New York, NY: March of Dimes Birth Defects Foundation.
[29] York, C. & Stichler, J. (1985). Cultural grief expressions following infant death. *Dimensions of Critical Care Nursing 4*(2), 120-127.
[30] Null, G. (1998). *Secrets of the white buffalo: Native American healing remedies, rites, and rituals*. Upper Saddle River, NJ: Prentice Hall.
[31] Frank-Stromborg, M. & Olsen, S. (2001). *Cancer prevention in diverse populations*. Pittsburgh, PA: Oncology Nursing Society.
[32] Haozous, E., Knobf, M.T. & Brant, J. (2010). Understanding the cancer pain experience in American Indians of the Northern Plains. *Psycho-Oncology*, 20, 404-410. doi: 10.1006/pon.1741.
[33] Whiteman, W. (1992). *Sacred sage: How it heals*. Ashland, VA: Whiteman.
[34] Birdson, W. (1998). The placenta and cultural values. *Western Journal of Medicine, 168*(3), 190-192.

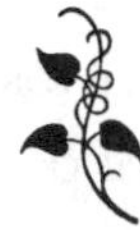

PACIFIC ISLANDERS

Background

The islands of the Pacific Ocean comprise more than one-half of the total islands of the world.[1] Some are uninhabited and extremely isolated. The people of the inhabited islands comprise a group of the most heterogeneous cultures in the world.[2]

The islands and people are broadly categorized as *Melanesian*, *Micronesian*, and *Polynesian*. The total population is approximately 13.6 million people. Melanesia is so named because many of the native people are dark-skinned. The prefix *mela* means "dark." A number of the islands of Melanesia are large with dense populations. Micronesia's islands are much smaller and more separated. Polynesia encompasses thousands of islands. Hence, the word *Polynesia* means "many islands." Most Pacific Islanders who have migrated to the United States are from Polynesia. The indigenous people of New Zealand are the *Maori*.[3,4,5]

There have been cultural and political struggles over the years since Europeans first discovered the islands in the early 1500s.[2,6] Hawaii especially suffered severe cultural damage as a result of exploitation and depopulation. This was strongly related to diseases introduced by foreigners, to which the natives had no immunity. Today, there are less than eight thousand Hawaiians of pure lineage (piha kanaka maoli).[7]

Popular islands located in Melanesia include Papua New Guinea, the Solomon Islands, Fiji, and New Caledonia. Melanesia is the largest of the regions in population. The islands of Micronesia are the least populated and have fewer natural resources. Islands within Micronesia include the Marshall Islands and Guam. Polynesia is the largest of the regions. Included in Polynesia are Hawaii, Tahiti, Tonga, Western Samoa, American Samoa, French Polynesia, and New Zealand. Hawaii and New Zealand were originally populated by Polynesians. However, today the populations are predominately non-Polynesian.[8, 9]

Approximately 85 percent of Pacific Islanders in the United States are Polynesians primarily from Hawaii, Tonga, and the Samoan Islands. Most of the persons from Micronesia and Melanesia are from Guam (Chamorros - the native people of Guam and the Marianas Island) and Fiji, respectively.[10, 11] The ten states with the largest populations of Pacific Islanders are Hawaii, California, Washington, Texas, New York, Florida, Utah, Nevada, Oregon, and Arizona.[12]

The Compact of Free Association agreement creates a special relationship between the United States and the Marshallese people and others from the Freely Associated States (FAS) group. As a result of the agreement, the United States allows the people of the FAS to enter or leave the United States without the normal immigration requirements. The Marshallese, FAS group, or Palau are also eligible for benefits and services offered in the United States in exchange for military use of their islands by the United States government.[13]

Common values among Pacific Islanders include a sense of group affiliation with family, respect for nature, modesty, humility, generosity, sharing with family, respect for status and hierarchy within the social network, and positive interpersonal relationships. As Western influences have been adopted by Pacific Islanders, more health problems have resulted. Health risk factors include obesity, cardiovascular disease, and cancer. Stomach, lung, and uterine cancers are common. Breast cancer is the most common cancer site among Somoan and Chamorro women.[14, 15, 16, 17] Infectious diseases include tuberculosis, drug-resistant mycobacterium marinum, and leptospirosis. Rheumatic fever resulting in rheumatic heart disease when prophylaxis treatment is not received remains a risk.[8] Gout and hyperuricemia are common throughout the Pacific Islander populations resulting from a hereditary decrease in renal fractional excretion of uric acid.[8]

The prevalence of diabetes has increased dramatically among urban Pacific Islanders resulting in markedly higher morbidity rates than Whites.[18, 19] Daily cultural conflicts and struggles regarding the practice of traditional values versus pressure to adopt Western values and practices contribute to risks of substance abuse, depression, and suicide–particularly among young males.[7, 20]

Language

- The people of the Pacific Islands speak approximately 1,200 languages. However, many native islanders speak either English or French.[9, 21] In the Island of Micronesia, at least eleven languages are spoken, which are not mutually intelligible across cultures. Polynesian languages are closely related and can often be understood by diverse groups and speakers.[13]

- Pacific Islanders who live in the United States speak English at varying levels of proficiency. Native languages may be spoken in the home. Use interpreters who are fluent in the language and in communicating medical information. It may be difficult to find interpreters for some of the languages such as *Marshallese*. The larger private and military hospitals in Honolulu may be helpful with finding interpreters if the usual efforts have been exhausted. Most Hawaiians do not speak their native language with proficiency.[7, 10]

- Pacific Islanders may be conservative in communicating with unfamiliar persons, particularly those in authority. The limited communication with those in authority is out of respect. Respect for authority is exhibited by listening and limiting conversation.[10]

- Health providers should ask questions about household, transportation, availability of resources and wait patiently for answers. Offer alternatives, encourage choices, and express care and concern in interactions.[22]

Worldview/Religious Beliefs

- Strong sense of connection to homeland.

- Family gods, spirits, and supernatural beliefs may play important roles in individuals' lives and beliefs about the origin of illnesses.

- Christianity has been introduced to the people of most islands, primarily Protestantism and Catholicism.[3] Religious beliefs may be a blend of Christian and native religious beliefs. Religion is an important part of everyday life. Adjust treatment regimens and provide privacy to accommodate daily prayers.

Health Beliefs/Practices

- Herbal and massage treatments are common. Prayer is thought to aid the healing process. If native healers are nearby, treatment may be sought from them before seeking mainstream treatments. The love and power of the spirit world and of God is expressed through the healer. Only spiritual healers have the power to cure spiritual illnesses. Therefore, it is advantageous to combine mainstream medical approaches with traditional folk medicine when possible.[23]

- Among native Hawaiians, health is reflected by a balanced relationship between God, the environment, and human beings. Illness is a result of imbalance or disturbance of harmony.[24]

- *Ho'oponopono*, "making things right," involves prayer, forgiveness, and discussion. It is utilized among some native Hawaiians to restore harmony and balance to family relationships. It is usually led by a Hawaiian elder or healer.[19, 24]

- Samoans and Chamorros may believe that behavioral illnesses have spiritual origins called 'ghost illnesses' (ma'i aitu). For Samoans, the incorporation of 'spirit priests,' if available, may be useful. Christian ministers may be acceptable also.[25]

Expression of Pain

- May approach pain with stoicism. Be observant of nonverbal signs of pain. Offer pain medication, even if the patient does not ask.

Male-Female/Kinship/Social Relationships

- Individuals have strong, shared identity and interdependence with family. *Family* consists of immediate and extended family. There are clearly defined roles in families. Several generations of families may live together.[26]

- Interactions within families may be based on status such as age, gender, etc. Traditional Samoan culture is changing so that the previous power of matais has been weakened.

In traditional Samoan culture, *chiefs* (matais) have status over untitled persons, elders over younger persons, and men over women.[9, 26] A Samoan matai has responsibility for the leadership and care of all members of families under his control. Obedience is required at all levels. The matai may have to be consulted for health care decisions. Health care providers should respect such roles and status levels when interacting with individuals and families for problem-solving, decision-making, etc.[7, 27]

- Approach patients/families with an attitude of equality, not superiority; genuineness, not pretense. Establish positive rapport with clients by informal conversation prior to addressing more serious and/or personal issues.[7]
- Family members often travel long distances to participate in the care of an ill relative. Allow liberal visitation and involvement of family members in care, whether in the home or in a health care facility. Placing the ill person in a private room may be helpful if the family is a large one.[28, 29]

Birth/Children

- Couples may stay with parents or siblings until they have several children.
- Among native Hawaiians, children are expected to respect elders, and complete assigned duties and responsibilities. Corporal punishment may be a method of discipline.[25]
- Among Samoans, children are loved and cherished, but are at the bottom of the social hierarchy. They are expected to provide service and to be obedient to their parents, other titled persons, and to older persons.

Death

- Death may be seen as both a transition and a translocation to a higher level of being.[28]
- Outward expressions of grief may be minimal as death is seen as a natural life occurrence and God's will.[28] Among native Hawaiians, death is seen as a reunion with one's deceased elders in the spiritual world.[7]

- Ask family members if they would like to be involved in postmortem care.
- Allow liberal time for family to be with the person who is dying and after death.

Patient Teaching/Dietary Consideration

- May be conservative about asking questions. Confirm understanding of teaching with return demonstrations, etc. Individuals may say they understand out of respect for the professional.[16]
- May believe that eating larger portions of food is associated with good health status, which may be detrimental if food consumed is not nutritious.[16]
- Pacific Islanders culturally value larger body size and may not have the desire to lose weight for better health.[30]
- Ethnic and traditional foods may have special meaning and influence food preferences of Pacific Islanders. Therefore, meaningful dietary teaching for patients with Type 2 Diabetes should include these foods or versions of their healthier alternatives.[31]
- Compliance with taking medications and follow up care must be explained to patients and family members in very practical terms. Preventive care is not a common concept within the culture and, once relief is obtained, individuals may not see a need to prolong treatment.[8, 13]
- Because many Pacific Islanders lack experience with recovery from a serious illness such as a heart attack or stroke, there is the belief that their condition is fatal. Efforts at rehabilitation to restore mobility and self-care following a serious illness might be resisted, and the family is much more likely to lovingly care for an elder providing their last days with comfort.[8]

---

1 Center for Pacific Island Studies (2005). *Oceania.* Retrieved from http://www.hawaii.edu/cpis/oceania_1.html

2 Campbell, I. (1996). *A history of the Pacific Islands.* Berkeley, CA: University of California Press.

[3] Management Sciences for Health. (n.d.). *The providers guide to quality & culture: Cultural groups: Pacific Islanders.* Retrieved from http://erc.msh.org/mainpage.cfm?file=5.4.8a.htm&module=provider&language=English

[4] GEOHIVE. (2013). Global Statistics. Retrieved from, http://www.geohive.com

[5] Spickard, P., Roondilla, J. & Wright, D. (Eds.) (2002). *Pacific diaspora: Island peoples in the United States and across the Pacific.* Honolulu, HI: University of Hawaii Press.

[6] Williams, B., Lye, K. & Porter, M. (1994). *The Kingfisher reference atlas.* (Rev. ed). New York, NY: Kingfisher Books.

[7] Blaisdell, K. & Mokuau, N. (1991). Kanaka Maoli: Indigenous Hawaiians. In N. Mokuau (Ed.), *Handbook of Social services for Asian and Pacific Islanders* (pp. 131-154). Westport, CT: Greenwood Press.

[8] Wergowski, G. & Blanchette, P.L. (2001.). *Health and health care of elders from Native Hawaiian and other Pacific Islander backgrounds.* Retrieved from http://www.stanford.edu/group/ethnoger/

[9] Strathern, A., Stewart, P., Carucci, L., Poyer, L., Feinberg, R. & Macpherson, C. (2002). *Oceania: An introduction to the cultures and identities of Pacific Islanders.* Durham, NC: Carolina Academic Press.

[10] Barringer, H., Gardner, R. & Levin, M. (1993). *Asians and Pacific Islanders in the United States.* New York, NY: Russell Sage Foundation.

[11] Untalan, F. (1991). Chamorros. In N. Mokuau (Ed.), *Handbook of social services for Asian and Pacific Islanders.* (pp. 172-182). Westport, CT: Greenwood Press.

[12] U.S. Census Bureau. (2010, March 21). *Profile America facts for features: Asian/Pacific American Heritage Month: May 2012.* Retrieved from http://www.census.gov/newsroom/releases/pdf/cb12ff-09_asian.pdf

[13] Kroeker, J.W. (n.d.) *Question submitted by Hana Like staff of Parents and Children Together (PACT): Responses by Julie Walsh Kroeker, Small Island Networks.* Retrieved from http://www.hawaii.edu/cpis/mi_workshop/files/hana_questions.htm

[14] Fong, R. & Mokuau, N. (1994). Not simply "Asian Americans": Periodical literature review on Asians and Pacific Islanders. *Social Work, 39*(3), 298-305.

[15] Tanjasiri, S., Wallace, S., & Shibata, K. (1995). Picture imperfect: Hidden problems among Asian Pacific Islander elderly. *Gerontologist, 35*(6), 753-760.

[16] Queensland Health Information Network. (2011). *Community health profiles: Samoa and Tonga.* Retrieved from http://www.health.qld.gov.au/multicultural/health_workers/cultdiver_guide.asp

[17] Tanjasiri, S., LeHauli, P., Finau, S., Fehoko, I. & Skeen, N. (2002). Tongan-American women's breast cancer knowledge, attitudes, and screening behaviors. *Ethnicity & Disease, 12*(2), 784-790.

[18] Foliaki, S. (2003). Prevention and control of diabetes in Pacific people. *British Medical Journal, 327*(7412), 437-439.

[19] Colagiuri, S., Colagiuri, R., Na'ati, S., Muimuiheata, S., Hussain, Z. & Palu, T., (2002). The prevalence of diabetes in the Kingdom or Tonga. *Diabetes Care, 25*(8), 1378-1383.

[20] Mokuau, N. (2002). Culturally based interventions for substance use and child abuse among Native Hawaiians. *Public Health Reports, 117*(Supplement 1), 582-587.

[21] Center for Pacific Island Studies. (2005). Retrieved from http://www.hawaii.edu/cpis/resources_1.html

[22] Kroeker, J.W., & Aaron, W. (2004, January 15). *A micro-orientation to Micronesian attitudes and beliefs about health care.* Retrieved from http://www.hawaii.edu/cpis/mi_workshop/files/strategies.htm

[23] Toafa, V., Moata'ane, L. & Guthrie, B. (2001). Traditional Tongan medicine and the role of traditional Tongan healers in New Zealand. *Pacific Health Dialog, 8*(1), 78-82.

[24] Kinney, G. (1996). Native Hawaiian health. *Reflections, 22*(4), 21.

[25] Mokuau, N., & Chang, N. (1991). Samoans. In N. Mokuau (Ed.), *Handbook of social services for Asian and Pacific Islanders* (pp. 155-169). Westport, CT: Greenwood Press.
[26] Ewalt, P. & Mokuau, N. (1994). Self-determination from a Pacific perspective. *Social Work, 39*(3), 168-175.
[27] Furuto, S. (1991). Family violence among Pacific Islanders. In N. Mokuau (Ed.), *Handbook of social services for Asian and Pacific Islanders* (pp. 201-215). Westport, CT: Greenwood Press.
[28] King, A. (1990). A Samoan perspective: Funeral practices, death and dying. In J. K. Parry (Ed.), *Social work practice with the terminally ill: A transcultural perspective* (175-189). Springfield, IL: Charles C. Thomas Publishing.
[29] Finau, S., Wainiqolo, I. & Cuboni, G. (2002). Health transition among Pacificans: Unpacking imperialism. *Pacific Health Dialog, 9*(2), 254-262.
[30] Siaki, L.A., & Loesches, L.J. (2011). Pacific Islanders perceived risk of cardiovascular disease and diabetes. *Journal of Transcultural Nursing, 22*(2), 191-200.
[31] Hsu, W.C., Boyko, E.J., Fujimoto, W.Y., Kanaya, A., Karmally, W., Karter, A., … Arakaki, R. (2012). Pathophysiologic difference among Asian, Native Hawaiians, and other Pacific Islanders and treatment implications. *Diabetes Care, 35*, 1189-1198.

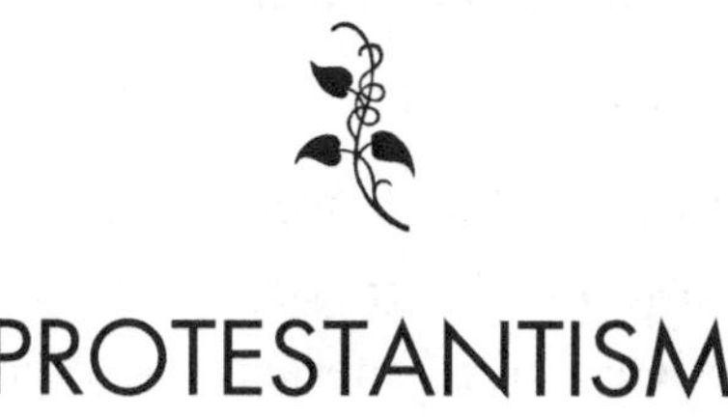

PROTESTANTISM

Background

Protestantism is one of three major branches of Christianity and the most diverse. The original Christian church began approximately 2,000 years ago in Palestine. Early Christians believed that, even though Christ had left the earth (after His crucifixion), He was continuing His mission through a new physical body, the church, of which He remained the head. The Holy Spirit was the soul of the church.[1,2]

The message of Christianity was carried to places such as Greece and Rome. With the Roman Conquest of the Greek East, a firm Graeco-Roman civilization was formed. The Roman Empire was eventually divided and essentially had two capitals–one located in Greece (the East) and one located in Rome (the West). However, the church essentially remained one body until 1054, when it split into the Orthodox Church in the East and the Roman Catholic Church in the West. The reasons for the split are complex, but include geography, culture, language, politics, and religious issues.[1]

During the fifteenth century, the Renaissance marked a critical period in history, leading to more emphasis on individualism and the position that people could take a much more active role in changing their own circumstances and the world's. As people took a scholarly approach to the exploration and study of various classical literary works, the contents of the Latin translation of the Bible came under scrutiny. Subsequently, as people were able to read the scriptures in languages other than Latin and compare their content with earlier Hebrew and Greek translations, they began to look more toward the Bible as the authority of their faith, and not to the interpretation of the Roman Catholic papacy.[4, 5, 6, 7, 8]

As the integrity of the papacy continued its decline during the sixteenth century, conditions became conducive for a religious revolution. In 1517, Martin Luther challenged the Church leadership to debate through posting his *95 Theses* on the church door in Wittenberg Cathedral in Germany and touched off the period in history known as *The Reformation*.

The news of the challenge to the Church spread throughout Europe, and many people supported his cause. Persons who supported this evangelical movement of protest against the Catholic Church became collectively and generically known as *Protestants*. The word Protestant comes from the word *protestari*, meaning not only to protest, but also to acknowledge openly or confess.

There are approximately 801 million Protestants and Independents worldwide, comprised of an extensive number of denominations and movements. Almost 160 million Protestants live in the United States. Terminology often used to describe various Protestant movements include: liberal, conservative, evangelical, holiness, fundamentalist, Pentecostal, charismatic, neo-evangelical, and many others. To trace the evolution of all Protestant groups is beyond the scope of this text. However, some of the major Protestant denominations and their evolution are indicated in the table below. Likewise, religious structure, practices, and doctrines of Protestant groups vary significantly. Obtain information from the patient or family about specific practices that may impact care.[5, 6, 7, 8, 9, 10, 11, 12]

The Development of Some of the Major Protestant Denominations in the United States[9]

(Table does not include all denominations. Many denominations splintered and separated into additional groups.)

Catholic Church	Anabaptist Churches			
	European National Groups ↓	**Mennonite** ↓	**Brethren** ↓	
	North American Baptist (German) Baptist General Conference (Swedish) Advent Christian Seventh-Day Adventist	Amish Conservative Mennonites General Conference Mennonite Old Mennonite Church	Brethren in Christ Hutterite Brethren Independent Brethren Mennonite Brethren	
	Lutheran Churches			
	Scandinavian ↓	**Danish/ General Synod** ↓	**German** ↓	**Moravian** ↓
	Lutheran Brethren Evangelical Covenant Evangelical Free	Evangelical Lutheran Church in America	Missouri Synod Lutheran Wisconsin Synod Lutheran	Moravian Church

<table>
<tr><td rowspan="4">Catholic Church</td><td colspan="6">Reformed Churches</td></tr>
<tr><td colspan="2">Presbyterian (Scottish)
↓
Presbyterian Church in USA
Presbyterian Church in America
Orthodox Presbyterian
Reformed Presbyterian</td><td>Dutch
↓
Reformed Church in America
Christian Reformed</td><td colspan="2">Irish
↓
Churches of Christ
Disciples of Christ
Christian Churches</td><td></td></tr>
<tr><td colspan="6">Angelican Churches</td></tr>
<tr><td>Puritans
↓
United Church of Christ (Congregational)</td><td>Separatists
↓
Baptists
↓
Free Will Baptist
Conservative Baptist
Progressive National Baptist
American Baptist</td><td>Episcopal</td><td>Plymouth Brethren
↓
Independent Bible Churches</td><td>Friends
↓
Friends United
Friends General Conference</td><td>Methodists
↓
United Methodist
African Methodist Episcopal
Nazarene Wesleyan
Free Methodist Assemblies of God
Pentecostal Church of God</td></tr>
</table>

From: Collins, M. and Price, M. (1999). *The story of Christianity: 2000 years of faith*. Great Britain: Dorling Kindersley Limited.

Religious Representatives

- Religious leaders are addressed by various titles including, but not limited to: Reverend, Pastor, Elder, Deacon, Bishop, Brother, and Sister.
- Representatives may be male or female, based upon the doctrines of their Protestant affiliation.

Religious Beliefs

Although there are variations within various Protestant groups, the **original** tenets of Protestantism stressed the following:[2, 6, 7, 8, 12, 13, 14, 15, 16, 17, 18, 19]

- **Sola Scriptura**: The acceptance of the Bible alone, as the sole source of authority for believers. The authority of the Pope was rejected.
- Christians are justified in their relationship to God by faith alone. His grace is extended directly to individuals and was demonstrated by Christ's death on the cross to pay the price for mankind's sins. To believe and/or renew one's commitment to Jesus Christ as one's personal Savior is often referred to as being "born again."
- The priesthood of all believers (i.e., every Christian can communicate directly with God without the need to go through a priest or other intermediary).
- God chooses whom to save and when the person will be saved. He, alone, judges one's moral weaknesses. Good works, alone, cannot guarantee God's salvation. Good works flow as a result of an individual's forgiven heart. Luther labeled this the *doctrine of predestination.*
- A strong embracement of the New Testament, especially the letters and writings of Paul.
- Preaching of the Word.
- A decrease in the ritualism traditionally a part of Catholic worship. All sacraments that had not been instituted by Christ were rejected. The two formal sacraments that are recognized most universally by Protestants are *Baptism* and *Holy Communion* (the Eucharist). There is variation related to other sacraments.

- The Holy Bible. However, interpretations of the Bible vary widely. This has contributed to the formation of the many denominations and movements within Protestantism.

Protestant Diversification

- **Baptists**: Baptists are the largest United States Protestant group. There are over 100 million worldwide and numerous denominations. Doctrines and practices may vary widely among Baptist groups and span a spectrum of very conservative to liberal. Some Baptist groups include:
  - Free Will
  - Southern Baptist
  - American Baptist
  - General Baptist
  - Bible Baptist Fellowship
  - Baptist Missionary
  - National Baptist
  - Primitive Baptist, and
  - Many more
    - In addition to the central tenets of Protestantism, beliefs include baptism of believers by immersion, and autonomy of churches.
    - Sunday is generally recognized as the Sabbath.
    - Supportive acts for those who are sick or shut-in commonly include regular visits by ministers and church members, bringing Communion to the sick, scripture reading, prayer, prayer cloths, anointings.
    - Ministers may be involved with counseling members related to health care decisions.
    - Most health care decisions are based on individual choice.

- **Methodists**: The term *Methodist* arose as a result of the methodical habits of John and Charles Wesley and their *Holy Club*. Members adhered to a strict schedule of duties such as visiting the sick, prayer, teaching, etc. There are over 70 million members worldwide. Some Methodists groups include:
  - Wesleyan
  - African Methodists Episcopal (AME)
  - African Methodists Episcopal Zion (AMEZ)
  - Free Methodist
  - United Methodist
  - Southern Methodist, and
  - Several others
    - Historical ties to the Angelical Church. Some of the Angelican Church liturgy has been retained in more conservative Methodist churches.
    - A Methodist lives by the 'method' specified in the Bible.
    - Emphasis on the importance of the Holy Spirit.
    - Doctrine of the Trinity.
    - Salvation is for all individuals who develop a cooperative relationship with God and His grace.
    - Sacraments include Baptism (infants and adults–often by sprinkling) and Holy Communion.
    - Health care decisions are based on individual choice.
- **Presbyterians**: So named because the church is governed by *presbyters* (representatives/ elders). There are approximately 75 million worldwide. Some Presbyterian groups include:
  - Presbyterian Church USA
  - Cumberland Presbyterian

- Orthodox Presbyterian
- Reformed Presbyterian Church of North America, and
- Several others
  - The Church is a universal community of persons, with their children, who have professed faith in Jesus Christ as Lord and Savior. Christ is the head. All members are equal under Christ.
  - Baptism and Holy Communion are recognized sacraments. Baptism is a symbol and seal of incorporation into Christ.
  - Doctrine of the Trinity.
  - Health care decisions are based on individual choice.

- **Quakers/Society of Friends (of Jesus)**: The term *Quaker* was a nickname given to the group who was said to have trembled or 'quaked' with religious zeal. There are over 350,000 worldwide. Some Quaker groups include:
  - Hicksites
  - Orthodox
  - Gurneyites
  - Wilburites
  - Evangelicals
  - In the United States, Quakers are most commonly found in Indiana, Oregon, Texas, Pennsylvania, North Carolina, and California.
    - Religious gatherings are called *meetings*. However, worship can occur anywhere between individuals seeking God's presence. Provide a quiet, undisturbed environment when an individual is hospitalized. There are no clergy.
    - An 'Inner Light' (God's Spirit) is present in each individual. Therefore, each individual has direct access to God through which she or he can discover spiritual

truth. The truth can be found in the Bible, but it may not be viewed with finality as it relates to conduct and doctrine.

- Individual spiritual searching is stressed to come to a closeness with God.
- Strong emphasis on equality and the worth of all individuals.
- No formal rituals. All of life is sacramental. Baptism in the Holy Spirit occurs from within. Although *meetings* may occur on Sunday, all days of the week are considered holy.
- Simplicity, honesty, integrity, humility, and moral purity are valued.
- The taking of an oath is refused since an individual is to be honest at all times.
- Christian religious celebrations such as Easter and Christmas may not be celebrated since the true meaning of these events should be celebrated on a daily basis.
- Diverse beliefs in life after death. No formal rituals at the time of death.

Special Religious Observations

- Sundays observed as holy days among the majority of Protestant groups. However, a few recognize other days, such as Saturday, as the Sabbath.
- The traditional Christian celebrations and holidays are observed among the majority of Protestants.

Birth/Children

- **Birth Control**: Individual choice.
- **Elective Pregnancy Termination**: Individual choice.

Health Beliefs/Practices

- Generally culturally based.

Death

- There are few rituals surrounding death, unless culturally based. Ask the family about any special end-of-life rituals or practices.
- Presence of clergy or church members will be comforting to many Protestants during terminal illness and to support the family after the death of a loved one.
- **Organ/Tissue Donation**: Individual choice.

---

[1] Smith, H. (1991). *The world's religions: Our great wisdom traditions.* New York, NY: HarperCollins Publishers.

[2] Pollock, R. (2002). *The everything world's religion book.* Avon, MA: Adams Media Corporation.

[3] Smart, N. (1989). *The world's religions: Old traditions and modern transformations.* London, England: Cambridge University Press.

[4] Edwards, L. (2001). *A brief guide to belief: Ideas, theologies, mysteries, and movements.* Louisville, KY: Westminster John Knox Press.

[5] Dowley, T. (Ed). (2002). *Introduction to the history of Christianity.* Minneapolis, MA: Fortress Press.

[6] Bell, J. & Sumner, T. (2002). *The complete idiot's guide to The Reformation & Protestantism.* Indianapolis, IN: Alpha Books.

[7] Goring, R. (Ed.). (1994). *Larousse dictionary of beliefs and religions.* Great Britain: Clays, Ltd.

[8] The Pew Forum on Religion & Public Life. (2011, December). *Global Christianity.* Retrieved from http://www.pewforum.org/christian/global-christianity-protestant.aspx

[9] Collins, M. & Price, M. (1999). *The store of Christianity: 2000 years of faith.* Great Britain: Dorling Kindersley Limited.

[10] Farrington, K. (2002). *Historical atlas of religions.* New York, NY: Checkmark Books.

[11] Toropov, B. & Buckles, L. (2011). *The complete idiot's guide to world religions.* (4th ed.). New York, NY: Penguin Group.

[12] Balmer, R. & Winner, L. (2002). *Protestantism in America.* New York, NY: Columbia University Press.

[13] Smart, N. (1989). *The world's religions.* Melbourne, Australia: University of Cambridge.

[14] Ontario Consultants on Religious Tolerance. (2012). *Christianity.* Retrieved from http://www.religioustolerance.org

[15] Friends World Committee for Consultation. (2012). *About Quakers.* Retrieved from http://www.fwccworld.org/quakers

[16] Rosten, L. (1975). *Religions in America*. New York, NY: Simon & Schuster.
[17] McClain, W. (1984). *Black people in the Methodist church*. Nashville, TN: Abingdon Press.
[18] Presbyterian Church (USA). (2011-2013). *The book of order: The constitution of the Presbyterian Church (USA), Part II*. Louisville, KY: The Office of the General Assembly.
[19] Earlham School of Religion. (2012). *18th century quietism & 19th century schisms*. Retrieved from http://esr.earlham.edu/support/comprehensive-case/the-vine/18th-century-quietism-19th-century-schisms

RASTAFARIANS

Background

Rastafarianism began in the early 1930s in Jamaica as one of the outgrowths of resistance against European dominance. The religion is linked to the African Myal religion, the Revivalist Zion churches, and runaway slave societies.[1] Another influence to its development was the teachings of Marcus Garvey, who attempted to improve the conditions of Jamaicans, as well as the conditions of Blacks throughout the world.[2] When Garvey left Jamaica to come to the United States in the early 1900s, it is said that he told his followers, "Look to Africa where a Black King shall be crowned; he shall be your redeemer."[3]

The original makeup of the group included Jamaican peasants, those who were underpaid in a changing economy, and the dispossessed citizenry.[4] On November 2, 1930, Ras Tafari Makonnen was named Emperor of Ethiopia. He took the throne name of *Haile Selassie I* (Power of Trinity). He remained Emperor until his death in 1975.

Remembering Garvey's prophetic statement, it was believed that God (*Jah* – a short form of Jehovah) had returned in the form of Haile Selassie; God and the Christian doctrine no longer belonged only to Whites.[5] Because Selassie was Black, it allowed the development of a new feeling of empowerment because 'God' was now seen as Black instead of White. To be Black had traditionally meant that there was some imperfection or debility. The group rejected the notion of God being a White man and looked to Haile Selassie I to lead the descendents of Africa out of 'Babylon' (Western society) back to Africa (Ethiopia).[6] The religion takes its name from the word 'Ras,' meaning *prince* and *'Tafari,'* the Emperor's given name.[5,7]

The established 'colors' of Rastafarianism are black, red, green, and yellow. Black represents the color of Africans; red symbolizes the blood shed by Jamaican martyrs; green represents the beauty and vegetation of Ethiopia, and yellow represents the wealth of the African continent, the Rastas' homeland.[8] These colors are often seen in Rastafarians' clothing, hats, crafts, etc. Currently, there are over 800,000 Rastafarians worldwide. However, there are more than two million if one includes those persons who follow the Rasta lifestyle, but not the faith.[9] There are a number of groups within the Rastafarian faith. The largest include *The Twelve Tribes of Israel* (headquarters in Brooklyn, NY) and the *Bobo* (primarily in Jamaica).[10] Others include the *Ethiopian Orthodox Church* (headquarters in Jamaica and New York City), and the *Coptic Zion Church* (headquarters in Florida).[2]

Persons under the religious guise of Rastafarians have been involved in serious crimes in some United States cities. True Rastafarians are known to be peace lovers and refrain from violence.[4]

Language

Rastafarian speech may be a combination of English, Jamaican Creole, and African languages. Rastafarians believe that word sound is power and many times speak in what has come to be known as *dread talk*. Through the use of correct and positive word sounds, an individual can acquire the full power of Rastafarianism. A unique pattern of speaking is by substituting the letter 'I,' reflecting Jah or self, for a syllable(s) of words or by substituting one word in front of another. The word 'I' may be singular or plural, reflected in the phrase "I and I" which may have a singular or plural meaning.

This is symbolic of placing Jah and the Spirit ahead of everything and of making a word more positive. For example, the word *continually* may be changed to *i-tinually,* or the word *unity* may become *i-nity*. 'Irie' is used as a frequent form of greeting. Certain English words such as 'dead' and 'hate' carry particularly negative connotations among Rastas.

Therefore, words that carry forms of words perceived to be negative will have more positive syllables substituted. For example, the word **ded**icate and **dead**line may be changed to **liv**icate and **life**line, respectively; appreci(h)**ate** may be changed to be appreci**love. During conversations, clarify word meanings**. *Livity* refers to the Rastafarian way of life.[7,11,12]

Religious Representatives

- Titles vary among groups. An elder is a highly respected member of a group.

Religious Beliefs

- **Religious Books**: Sections of the Holy Bible (with a strong emphasis on the book of Revelations) and the Kebra Negast, the Bible of Ancient Ethiopians.

- One God exists who is called *Jah*. Jah is believed to have been revealed through Haile Selassie. Rastafarians are highly concerned about positive or negative vibrations (energy) that are encountered or that they personally emanate in all interactions. Jah represents the ultimate positive vibration. Establishing a closer channel of communication with the positive vibrations of Jah is a spiritual goal. Rastafarians strive to *know* Jah and the truth of Rastafarianism. To only *believe* implies doubt.[1,7]

- Living in harmony with nature and the Earth is central to Rastafariansim. To live an *I-tal* way of life reflects the Rastafarian's goal of organic purity, and the rejection of lifestyles that are associated with the Western way of life which is viewed as having many 'artificial' practices. The I-tal way of life is reflected in the Rastafarian's diet, dress, hair care, etc. Positive or negative vibrations (i-brations) may be encountered through the environment, interactions with other people, foods, etc. These positive or negative vibrations influence the Rastafarians' choices in vocabulary, foods, behaviors, and all other aspects of life.[11,13]

- Ethiopia is the symbolic kingdom of Heaven.[14]

- Among some Rastafarian groups, *ganja* (weed, holy herb, callie, wisdomweed, lambsbread, sensi) is used as part of religious rituals. Generally, ganja is not used recreationally. Ganja is better known by non-Rastafarians as *marijuana*. The ganja plant is a specially cultivated type of Indian hemp and is derived from the female plants. The variety differs from Mexican marijuana and is said to be as much as four times stronger. Its spiritual use is based on several Biblical texts that refer to the 'green herb.'[15] It is used both in private and as an aid to meditation and religious worship. The smoking of ganja as a religious sacrament is said to do the following:[2,11]

- Increase the positive state of an individual's vibrations (energy or I-brations), allowing closer communication with Jah.
- Produce psycho-spiritual effects.
- Produce visions.
- Heighten unity and communal feelings.
- Dispel gloom and fear.
- Reduce stress.
- Bring tranquility and peacefulness to the mind.

- Among some Rastafarians, the hair is not cut, nor do they shave. This is based on the Biblical scripture Leviticus 21:5. The Rasta's hair also symbolizes his or her roots, in contrast to the straight hair that is valued in Western mainstream society. The dreads are believed to be very powerful and holy, providing a means of 'telepathic communication with Jah.' The hair on the head is referenced by names such as African or Nubian locks, locks, or dreadlocks.[7, 90, 91] The hair of the beard may also be allowed to tangle and form locks. The locks form naturally as the hair tangles when it is not combed. Long locks take years to grow. Some persons cover locks with knitted hats referred to as *crowns*.[14] **It is a myth that hair worn in locks is dirty and unkempt. Not all Rastafarians wear locks, and all persons who wear locks are not Rastafarians.**

- Health care personnel should ask family members if they have herbal solutions that they would like to bring into an inpatient setting for washing the hair. **Do not attempt to untangle the locks; it cannot be done.** The locks are seen as a strong symbol of naturalism and spiritual power. All measures should be taken to prevent cutting the hair or shaving the body hair among Rastafarians who observe this religious symbolism.[11]

Special/Religious Observations

- **Reasoning Sessions**: Comparable to Communion ceremony among Christians. Small groups gather, share discussions of faith, ceremonially smoke ganja, and pray. The reasoning sessions may last all night.[7, 10]

- **Nyabinghi** or **Binghi**: Celebrations of special events such as Haile Selassie's coronation (November 2nd), his ceremonial birthday (January 6th), his visit to Jamaica (April 21st), his personal birthday (July 23rd), the emancipation from slavery (August 1st), and the birthday of Marcus Garvey (August 17th). The celebration may last for several days. It consists of reasoning sessions during the day and singing, drumming, and dancing at night.[17]
- **January 7th**: Christmas (Ethiopian).
- **September 11th**: The beginning of the Ethiopian New Year.

Health Beliefs

- Orthodox Rastafarians are likely to present late in illness, or not at all, to health care facilities because of rejection of mainstream health care approaches.
- Illness may result from accumulated negative vibrations. Special anointing, prayer, and other purification rituals may be performed to bring the individual back to a healthy state. Fasting and use of purgatives may be methods used to cleanse the interior of the body.[4, 11]
- Rastafarians strive to return to the most natural state of living possible. Therefore, commercial drugs may be rejected. Generally, herbs and other natural substances are utilized for treating illnesses. Ganja teas, tonics, baths, and ganja in food preparation may be used for health maintenance and for illness, as it is believed to be healing. It is used among all age groups. There is liberal use of folk medicine. Often, there are individuals within Rastafarian communities who specialize in the use of plants for treating illness and/or health maintenance.[1, 7, 8, 11]
- During, and for variable periods following menstruation and childbirth, women are considered unclean. During this period of time, they may not cook or prepare food and are generally secluded from social contact until they are considered purified.[17]
- Shaving, trimming, cutting, and tattooing the flesh are considered taboo by some Rastafarians. It is seen as desecration of the body.[2]
- Smoking of tobacco is prohibited in some groups.

Male-Female/Family/Social Relationships

- Women must receive divine knowledge through their spouse and are incapable of receiving it directly.[1]
- Strong sense of self-sufficiency.
- Generally, very family-oriented. May seem to value male children more than females.
- Men may be referred to as 'king-man' by the spouse. Women may be referred to as *daughter*, *Daara*, or *sistren*, regardless of age.[1]
- Women may show deference to males. Generally, hair is covered, make-up is not worn, and ankle-length clothing is worn in public.[17] Same-sex caregivers should be provided, if at all possible. Women may be uncomfortable with men other than their spouses and male family members. Leave hair coverings in place or provide coverings for hair as needed.

Dietary Considerations

- Rastafarians generally consume a low fat, low cholesterol, low sodium diet; many are vegetarians. Some may consume certain types of fish. The foods eaten are referred to as *ital*, meaning 'natural.'[1] Ital foods are free of chemicals and preservatives, condiments, not canned, cooked in metal pans, or processed. Food may be cooked, but is eaten as close to raw form as possible.[8] Natural spices and herbs may be used to season foods. Natural coconut oil may be used for cooking foods.[2, 92] Family members will likely bring food prepared at home.
- There are several foods that are prohibited among Rastafarians, which include: animal flesh, salt and other artificial additives, alcoholic beverages, coffee, soft drinks, shellfish, milk ('white blood'), some fruits with large seeds, and food of unknown sources. Fish without scales or longer than 12" is also prohibited. Fish longer than 12" symbolizes Westerners who feed off of each other.

Death

- Rastafarians celebrate life. Therefore, some Rastafarians may be unwilling to associate themselves in any way with death, including the death of a family member. This may be related to fear of contamination by the dead. The cause of death is irrelevant.
- It is believed that one never dies as long as one remains faithful to Haile Selassie.
- Death may be explained by saying that the deceased departed from the chosen path of the Rastafari or violated some divine doctrine of Jah.
- May refuse to attend funerals.[1]

Political/Legal

- Rastafarians are often stereotyped as violent or drug-addicted individuals because of their alternative appearance and lifestyle. There is a strong movement among Rastafarians to counter these negative stereotypes. The result has been a growing number of 'converts' of all ethnic and socioeconomic levels to Rastafarianism. Be aware of personal biases when interacting with Rastas.[7]
- May be resistant to activities such as voting, joining the military, or working for tax-paying businesses. May favor independent occupations.[4]
- Rastafarians continue to seek approval for legal use of ganja as part of religious services.

Other Considerations

- Use of commercial soap and toothpaste may be rejected by some Rastafarians. Ask the patient about choices for personal hygiene, or ask family members to bring preferred herbal preparations for hygienic purposes.[2]
- Birth control is generally forbidden related to the idea of 'natural' sex (ital) and self-control. Natural childbirth is preferred. Herbal preparations such as raspberry and ganja

teas/tonics may be ingested during pregnancy to control nausea, relieve fatigue, as a sleep aid, and after childbirth.[19]

- Abortion is prohibited.
- **Blood Transfusions:** Generally not acceptable because of fear of body contamination.
- Some groups of Rastafarians may not use combs because combs and brushes are viewed as 'modern' tools and are not mentioned in the Bible.

---

1 Chevannes, B. (1994). *Rastafari: Roots and ideology*. Syracuse, NY: Syracuse University Press.

2 Barrett, L. (1997). *The Rastafarians*. Boston, MA: Beacon Press.

3 Barrett, L. (1996). *Rastafarianism*. Vol. 19, Colliers Encyclopedia.

4 Lewis, W. (1993). *Soul Rebels: The Rastafari*. Prospect Heights, IL: Waveland Press, Inc.

5 *Who is Ras Tafari Haile Selassie I and who are the Rastafarians*. Retrieved from http://web.syr.edu/~affellem/rasta.html

6 Miller, T. (1995). *America's alternative religions*. Albany, NY: State University of New York Press.

7 Glazier, S. (2001). *Encyclopedia of African and African-American religions*. New York, NY: Routledge.

8 *Rastafarian*. Retrieved from http://www.cwrl.utexas.edu/~e..rley/history/rastafar/symbols.html

9 Lieblich, J. (1998, August 15). *Beyond dreads, to roots of Rastafari*. Star Tribune, p. 07B.

10 Dow, J. & Kemper, R. (1995). *Encyclopedia of world cultures*, Volume III. Boston, MA: G. K. Hall & Co.

11 Van De Berg, W. (1998). Rastafari perceptions of self and symbolism. In P. Clarke. *New trends and developments in African religions*. (pp. 159-174). Westport, CT: Greenwood Press.

12 Pollard, V. (2000). *Dread talk*. Montreal, Canada: Mc-Gill-Queens University Press.

13 *The beloved Prophet Gad*. Retrieved from http://web.syr.edu/~affellem/Gad.html

14 Jones, L. (1996, August 11). The Rasta Way. *The Dallas Morning News*, p. 1F.

15 Redington, N. (1995). *A sketch of Rastafari history*. Retrieved from http://www.nomadfx.com/old/rasta1.html

16 Bailey, R. (1997, February 26). More black people wear natural locks to evoke pride, battle prejudice. *The Gannett News Service*, pp. arc.

17 BBC Religions. *(2012). Rastafari*. Retrieved from http://www.bbc.co.uk/religion/religions/rastafari/

18 Edwards, L. (2001). *A brief guide to beliefs: Ideas, theologies, mysteries, and movements*. London, England: Westminster John Knox Press.

19 Dreher, M., Nugent, K. & Hudgins, R. (1994). Prenatal exposure and neonatal outcomes in Jamaica: An ethnographic study. *Pediatrics, 93*(2), 254-260.

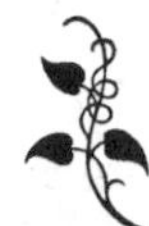

RUSSIANS (NON-JEWISH)

Background

Russia lies in both Europe and Northern Asia. In land area, it is the largest country in the world, almost twice the size of the United States, and spans nine time zones. Russia's population is approximately 139 million. Ethnic Russians comprise about 80 percent of the population. The remaining 20 percent is made up of as many as 175 other ethnic groups, the largest being Tatars, Ukrainians, Bashkirs and Chuvash.[1,2,3]

The people of Russia have a rich cultural history. However, their history has not been without struggles. Russia's history has been dominated by monarchies, war, and religious persecution.[4] These and other factors have left a lasting effect on individuals of Russian heritage.

The first people to occupy parts of Russian territory were nomadic. Archeologists have found evidence suggesting the existence of diverse communities in southern Russia 35,000-10,000 BCE.[5] For centuries, various groups fought for control and expansion of the land. Around the sixth century AD, the Eastern Slavs expanded into Russia and left lasting influences on Russian heritage. Three major languages developed: Great Russian, which is often just referred to as 'Russian,' Ukrainian, and White Russian (Belarussian). The Eastern Slavs also established the first united Russian state, Kievan Rus, during the ninth century and controlled many surrounding areas.[5,6] Vladimir, one of the rulers of the Kievan Rus region, adopted Christianity (Eastern Orthodoxy) for himself and also for the Kievan Rus state during the tenth century. Since that time, Eastern Orthodoxy has been a powerful influence on Russian culture and religious thought.

Through centuries of war and dictator rule, the Russian people suffered. Most Russians were peasants and relied on communal living and family for survival. There was very little opportunity for individuality in decision–making. The experiences of serfdom and communal life carried a lasting imprint on Russian culture.[3] Industrialization expanded greatly during the 19th century, followed by a depression at the beginning of the 20th century. The early 20th century also marked increasing unrest among the poor, resulting in several revolutions in an effort to improve their living conditions, expand civil rights, and citizen involvement. One major result was the increase in opportunities for education, although a high percentage of Russians remained illiterate. However, the expansion in education provided the opportunity for changes in Russian thought and culture. Throughout the upheavals, the Orthodox Church remained influential in Russian life.[5]

In 1917, a series of riots, uprisings, and revolutions resulted in major changes in the ruling powers of Russia. Vladimir Lenin took power, followed by Joseph Stalin. It was in 1922, under Lenin's reign, that the Union of Soviet Socialist Republics (USSR) was established. It consisted of fifteen culturally-diverse surrounding republics, with Moscow serving as the capital.[7] The hope of the people to gain better lives through new leadership was squelched by the dictatorship, brutality, and the continued spread of Communism under Stalin's reign. Civil rights were non-existent, poverty and religious persecution were widespread, and hardships were a way of life. Any opposition could result in imprisonment and even death.[8] Stalin died in 1953.

In the years following Stalin's death, changes in leaders' ideology have evolved and reforms have occurred. Major ones include attempts to change policies related to economic management (*perestroika*), underlining the need for social justice and human rights, governmental transparency, and increased liberty in public expression among the people (*glasnost*). In 1991, the USSR and Communist rule of the Soviet Union collapsed and were abolished.[5] Today, the country is known officially as both Russia and the Russian Federation.

Relocation from Russia has been extensive during its history for various reasons. Unlike most other Europeans who entered North America from the east coast, the first Russians reaching North America came as explorers seeking trading opportunities on the west coast, specifically, the Pacific Rim. The first settlement was established in what is now known as Sitka, Alaska. As trading expanded and Orthodox missionaries attempted to convert Natives already occupying the Pacific Rim, additional settlements were established through Canada and along the coast into southern California. Subsequent waves of Russians resettled in other countries primarily for reasons such as religious persecution, poverty, ethnic discrimination, political and social injustices.[4, 7] Russia is experiencing another wave of citizens relocating to other countries. This, and other factors, are contributing to what is being referred to as a 'demographic crisis.'[9, 10] Many of those leaving the country are highly educated individuals looking for more lucrative work. Almost 100 percent of Russians fifteen years of age and over can read and write.[1]

Today, Russians reside in many countries around the world. The United States is home to one of the largest Russian populations. It is estimated that up to 5.5 million people of Russian heritage live in the United States. Although Russians can be found in many states in the United States, the largest populations reside in the New York area, California, Illinois, Pennsylvania, Massachusetts, Florida, and the District of Columbia/Maryland area.[11]

Health Risks

Despite the major changes that have occurred in Russia, many health risks persist and are important factors to consider when caring for members of this cultural group. If resettlement occurs, the resulting health sequelae will likely be present. Poverty continues to be a major concern in Russia. Associated factors such as homelessness, malnutrition, violence, prostitution, substance abuse, and suicide are disturbing health concerns.[5] As of 2009, approximately 13 percent of the population lived in poverty, an improvement over 40 percent in 1999.

Alcoholism, smoking, and subsequent sequelae are other major health issues in Russia. Russia has the fifth highest death rate in the world.[1] Sixty percent of males and 22 percent of females use tobacco. Cardiovascular disease, stroke, injuries, lung cancer, poisonings primarily related to alcohol consumption, HIV/AIDs, liver disease, stomach cancer, colo-rectal cancer, and suicide are the ten leading causes of death in Russia.[12] Additional rising major health and social concerns are tuberculosis, human trafficking, birth defects, and child abandonment.[13] Seasonal Affective Disorder is a risk for persons living in Russia during winter months.[3] Additionally, persons exposed to radiation as a result of the1986 Chernobyl power plant explosion may be at risk for physical effects such as thyroid cancer, leukemia, etc. The overall life expectancy is 66.29 years. Life expectancy for women is 73.17 and for men, 59.8years.[1, 14]

Many of the deficits in positive health outcomes and mortality rates among Russians, particularly men of working age, are related to alcohol ingestion. For many Russians, alcohol consumption is a part of daily life and is frequently served around the dinner table with meals, business gatherings, etc. Vodka is a common drink. The equivalent of 15.7 liters of pure alcohol per capita/year is consumed. A home-brewed form of alcohol, *Samogon*, is also commonly ingested. In the absence of available distilled alcohol, toxic products containing alcohol not meant for ingestion may be consumed. Beer is also common and was only recently classified as an alcoholic beverage instead of a food item as part of efforts to decrease levels of alcohol consumption. The alcoholism rate is higher among men than women; although, alcohol consumption among women contributes to the high incidence of fetal alcohol syndrome and birth defects among Russian children, particularly those in orphanages.[3, 15, 16] There are approximately 2.5 million registered alcoholics in Russia; 80 percent of them are men. Ten million children 10-14 years of age already consume alcohol.[13, 17] Men between the ages of 15-60 years have a 48 percent probability of death primarily related to alcohol-related causes.[9]

In 2007, the ethnic Russian population in the United States was estimated at three to four million, with a median age of approximately 43 years. Over one-third are 55 years of age and older. Ninety-six percent of the Russian population in the United States holds at least a high school education or equivalent, and almost one-third hold graduate or professional degrees. Approximately 55 percent are employed in fields such as science, health care, education, the arts, and management. Russians, as a group, have some of the highest earnings in the United States. The largest populations are found in California, Massachusetts, New York and Pennsylvania.[11, 18]

Language

- Standard Russian is the official language of Russia. Most Russians are bilingual. Major Russian dialects are broadly divided regionally into Northern Russian and Southern Russian. More than one hundred languages are spoken in Russia.[19, 20]

- In the United States, many younger Russians understand and speak English well. Newly immigrated Russians may not be proficient in English. Older Russians may not understand or speak English well. Overall, approximately 99 percent of Russians in the United States speak some English.[18, 21] Keep in mind that persons who speak English reasonably well may have difficulty doing so when under stress due to illness, hospitalization, or pain.[22] Ethnic Russians born and raised outside of Russia may not speak the language fluently.

- When using interpreters, allow additional time. Because of the difference in structure of Russian versus English language, it may take 10-15 percent longer to express the same message in Russian. Some English words do not exist in the Russian language.[4] Patient assignments should be made with consideration of the longer time required to communicate effectively.

- Conversational distance may be as close as twelve inches or less. Until trust is established, responses may be reserved and without smiles. Trust may be difficult to establish because of past experiences in Russia. Once trust is established, responses may be lengthy, even to simple questions. A person's word is extremely important. Do not make promises that cannot be kept. Honesty and sincerity is valued. Humor, light-hearted approaches are not appreciated when discussing serious/potentially serious issues of health. Physical touching is common among family members and among non-family members once trust has been established. Hands, gestures, and facial expressions may accompany speech.[4,23,24]

- Non-verbal behaviors of healthcare providers are closely observed, and respectful behavior is expected. On the other hand, patients may expect health providers to recognize their needs based on their non-verbal behaviors. The patient may be hesitant to ask questions, particularly older Russians and more recent immigrants. Feet that are placed on furniture are considered impolite as well as sitting with soles of shoes showing toward an individual. Other actions include standing with hands in pockets, widespread legs when sitting or verbalizing the need to go to the rest room.[3]

- Patients and families may express themselves by using negative phrases. For instance, when asked about pain levels, the response may be "not much" instead of specific pain severity. Seek further clarification if responses are vague.[4]

- For centuries, Russians have received information through oral rather than written methods. Importance may not be placed on written documents.[4,25] Assess learning style. Written educational information may not be as effective as oral or visual methods. Other health/medical information sent by mail may also not be effective. May be hesitant to sign documents.

- The metric system is the standard unit of measurement versus system of measurement commonly used in the United States.

- The order of dates is generally written as day, month, and year. Assure that the patient understands the order commonly used in the United States (e.g., month, day, and year). Patients/families may be accustomed to weeks beginning with Monday instead of Sunday.[26]

Time Orientation

- A relaxed view of time is common. Attention to social time frames may not be valued, although health appointment times are usually met.

Worldview/Religious Beliefs

- The most common religious affiliations among ethnic Russians are:
  - Russian Orthodox (see *Eastern Orthodoxy*).
  - As a result of revisions to some of The Orthodox Church's rituals, dogma, and literature during the 17th century, several religious sects formed after disagreeing with some of those revisions. Some of the most well-known sects are:
    - **Old Believers** (Starovery): Members believe in the original Church dogma, rituals, and literature. This group is further divided into the Popovtsy (priest-possessing) and Bezpopovtsy (priestless). Among the Popovtsy, ordained priests are Church leaders and Church hierarchy is maintained. The Church hierarchy is not supported among the Bezpopovtsy, and the requirement for ordained priests is not supported.[4]
    - **Doukhobor** (spirit wrestlers): Doukhobors believe that God's spirit is present in each individual person's conscience, and the individual's goal in life is to reflect His unconditional love. Each person interacts with that Spirit on an individual basis. Therefore, the Church hierarchy, rituals, and symbols such as the Christian cross, scriptures, baptism, etc. are rejected. There is a belief in the spiritual intent of the writings of the Bible, but there is also the belief that other religious books are just as spiritually credible. Their core beliefs in toil and peace are symbolized by bread, water, and salt and these items will be present in all services. Doukhobors are

usually vegetarians based on the belief in not harming living creatures. However, a few may eat fish, fowl, or other meat occasionally. The use of alcohol and tobacco is discouraged.

- Major celebrations include The Burning of Arms (Peace Day or Peter's Day), commemorating the destruction of the group's weapons in 1895 and refusal to participate in Russian activities that involved killing others. The celebration occurs on or around June 28th. Christmas and Easter are also observed. Most Doukhobors in North America live in Canada.[4, 27, 28]

  ▪ **Molokans**: The name is from the Russian word meaning "milk." The group was originally given this name in the 1760s because of their refusal to abstain from consuming dairy products, including milk, during the Russian Orthodox fasting days, particularly during Lent. The group split from the Doukhobors and refer to themselves as the True Spiritual Christians. They reject the Orthodox hierarchy, rituals, and sacraments but accept the teachings of the Bible (with Apocrypha).

- Molokans are further divided into Pryguny (Jumpers) named because of dancing and jumping as a part of worship services, Postoiannye (Constant/Steadfast/Unchanged), and Maksimisty who have some beliefs in mysticism. The Book of Spirit and Life is a companion book to the Bible among Jumpers. Most Molokans in North America live in Canada, Mexico, and in western states such as California, Oregon, and Arizona.[4, 29]

  – Protestant (Baptist, Pentecostal).

  – Non-practicing believers and non-believers.

- Superstitions are common. Common ones include not shaking hands, greeting someone, or saying goodbye over a door threshold as it is thought to bring bad luck. Even numbers may be looked upon as unlucky, including the number of flowers in a vase. Some persons can cast an evil eye resulting in harm to babies by looking at either the baby or its mother.[3,25,26]

- Astrology, numerology, and dream interpretations can play an important role in decision-making.

- Because of the influence of past history, Russians may appear pessimistic and fatalistic.[26]

- Free health care is available to Russian citizens. Private insurance is also available. Newer immigrants may be unfamiliar with some United States health care system components such as having access only to certain doctors, insurance policies, etc.
- Religion and spirituality can be seen as important to overall health. For non-believers, explore ways to support spiritually, if desired.

Health Beliefs

- Harmony in mind, body, and spirit defines health.[22]
- Health promotion activities, preventive care, and disease screening may be viewed as "looking for trouble" and not valued. In Russia, many individuals only visit a physician if home treatments have not worked and they are feeling very ill. Illnesses may be attributed to non-pathological reasons such as stress, not eating the right foods, etc. Explore patient's perception of illness origin.[30, 31, 32]
- Health maintenance and illness treatments/actions include frequent use of herbal preparations, cupping, enemas, minerals, aromatherapy, and massage therapy. Certain crystal and gem stones are also thought to have healing properties and should be left in place if worn by the patient.[22, 33]
- Russian massage (also known as Russian Clinical Massage, Russian Curative Massage, and Russian Therapeutic Massage) is a frequently used form of healing therapy for many health conditions and may be prescribed by physicians in Russia. It involves more than forty massage movements and four major techniques: vibration, rubbing, stroking, and kneading. Raw honey is sometimes used on the skin as part of the massage.
- Illnesses such as colds and headache can originate from becoming chilled. If this is the case, provide warm blankets and warm fluids. Protect from overhead drafts.
- Ask direct questions during health assessments and visits. In Russia, physicians take the lead role when interacting with patients for assessing, diagnosing, and treatment. Russians may not see the necessity of the patient having to provide information to determine a diagnosis and treatment. The health care provider may be expected to know what is wrong. Be definitive and thorough with treatment directions and care.[24]

- Prescribed medications may be considered too strong and herbal treatments substituted instead. Inquire about herbal use and purpose. Stress the importance of taking prescribed medications as ordered and why.[26,32]

- Pain thresholds tend to be high, and patients may not ask for pain medications based on the belief that the medications may be harmful. Provide careful explanations concerning the effects of pain medications, and invite questions. Assess for non-verbal signs of discomfort and pain. Offer medication even if patient does not ask.[31]

- Mental health services are limited in Russia. Distrust and suspicion of sharing information related to mental health status may be displayed because of past experiences as a whole, with mental health treatment approaches in Russia. Mental health problems carry a negative stigma and may be seen as a lack of self-control on the part of the ill individual. It can also be seen as an illness of the soul (*dusha*). Mental illnesses are often expressed in terms of resulting physical illnesses such as loss of appetite, headache, etc. Be especially vigilant when working with the elderly who may feel a loss of their traditional family roles. The individual may not be comfortable sharing any familial history of mental illness.[30,34]

- Personal cleanliness and hand washing are valued.[3] For non-ambulatory patients, provide means to wash/sanitize hands prior to eating and after toileting.

- Many Russians do not wear street shoes in the home. Inquire about need to remove shoes when entering a Russian home.[26]

- As a result of the Chernobyl power plant explosion, Russians who lived in the affected areas may carry lingering fears of radiation exposure. Explain the need for any tests/procedures involving radiation exposure, including any types of x-rays.

Male-Female/Family/Social Relationships

- Err on the side of formality in the use of titles during initial greetings. Professional titles are valued. Russian full names often include the given name, patronymic (first name of person's father), and family name. However, individuals sometimes introduce themselves using only the first name and patronymic. Clarify preferred name.[24,25]

- Handshakes are acceptable between opposite genders if the female extends the hand first. The female's hand may be kissed by a male instead of shaken, which is a gesture of respect. Embraces and kisses are common among Russians of the same gender.[3]

- Respect for the elderly is valued and expected from others. Elderly parents are usually cared for in the home, and placement in nursing homes may be resisted by family. It is not uncommon for homes to be multi-generational. Always acknowledge elders when entering the patient's room or home.[31,32]

- Men and women are seen as equal in terms of pursuing education and employment. However, even if working outside of the home, females tend to take care of household duties and children. Men may be the spokesperson for the family, but they involve family in decision-making. Family is important and will want to stay with the patient and participate in care.

- Modesty among middle-aged and older Russians is valued. Questions/directions related to toileting, health issues of a sexual/intimate nature should be discussed in private.[3]

- May offer gifts to health care providers as tokens of gratitude for service in taking care of patient.

- A Russian proverb is, "If he beats you, he loves you." Intimate partner violence is not uncommon in Russia. It is seen as a private matter, and not much assistance is available to the victim legally. Victims may not be trusting of police, social workers, etc. and unfamiliar with services that may be available to victims in other countries. Conduct careful screening, realizing that victims may be unwilling or fearful of revealing abuse to strangers.[35,36]

- **Women's Day**: March 8th - Similar to Valentine's Day in the United States and is a special day for women.

Birth/Children

- Russian women desire to stay healthy during pregnancy and will keep prenatal appointments. During the post-partum period, the mother and infant may be seen as being in a state of 'weakness,' needing to rest and recover from the delivery. This may occasionally contribute to limiting breastfeeding time and supplementing breastfeeding. However, breastfeeding is viewed positively. Herbal supplements may be taken and breast massage done in an effort to increase breast milk supply. Baby massage is popular following childbirth.[37,38]

- Fathers, although proud of the pregnancy and birth, may choose not to be very active in prenatal visits and the birth. A female relative, often the maternal grandmother, may be the support person since pregnancy and childbirth may be seen as women's business.

- Mothers may not share knowledge of pregnancy with outsiders until they are 'showing.' They may also refrain from making preparations (including baby showers) for a new baby until very late in pregnancy for fear of bringing harm to the unborn child. Congratulatory statements should only be given after the baby is born and deemed healthy. Announcements may not be shared about the baby's birth for the same reason. Maternal activity is restricted for forty days following delivery. Mother and baby stay home, and visitors are discouraged in the home for one to two months following delivery to allow time for the mother and baby to rest and to help in the prevention of infections that may be brought in by visitors.[26,37]

- A pin may be placed in the baby's bed or on the baby's stroller as a protective measure against the evil eye.[37]

- Until recent years, abortion was the primary method of birth control. Contributing factors include no charge for abortions in Russia, limited access to birth control methods, high costs of birth control, lack of education about reliable birth control methods, fear of using hormonal and barrier methods, etc. Assess knowledge of contraceptives and attitudes toward use. Assess for complications of multiple abortions, including infertility.[39,40]

- Almost 60,000 children have been adopted from Russia by families in the United States within the last twenty years. Until recent changes in Russian adoption laws, Russia was a popular source for United States adoptions. The children tended to be older than one year of age. Some had resided in orphanages leaving long-term effects. Screen and follow for possible developmental delays and fetal alcohol spectrum disorders.[41]

- Children may live at home with parents until marriage.

Patient Teaching/Dietary Considerations

- Diet is often high in salt, starches, and fat. Three meals a day are common, with lunch being the largest meal.
- Black or rye bread is popular and is a main staple in diet including small, thin pancakes (*bliny*) served with toppings. Meat is generally eaten with all meals. Popular foods include soups (particularly cabbage, beetroot), whole grain porridges, chicken, fish, mushrooms, cucumbers (sometimes salted), fresh vegetables with herbs, and fresh fruit, especially berries, jam, and honey. *Kvas* is a favorite beverage made from grain or fermented dark, natural grain breads. It is considered non-alcoholic with an alcohol content of around one percent. It can be flavored and is sometimes given to children also.
- Alcoholic beverages are often consumed as a part of celebrations, regular meals, etc. Often, vodka is the drink of choice. Assess level and frequency of alcohol consumption, even among young teens, with a non-judgmental approach. Consumption levels may vary from none to heavy. If the individual consumes large amounts of alcohol, inquire about any consumption of alcohol-containing substances not meant for ingestion such as aftershave, cologne, etc.[42]
- Black tea is a favorite beverage. Offer warm beverages, soups, especially when ill. Mineral water is also a popular beverage and is believed to be therapeutic.
- For Russian Orthodox, inquire about diet restrictions related to fasting practices.

Terminal Ilnesss/Death

- Families may be resistant to sharing information with the patient concerning a terminal diagnosis. Often, Russian physicians do not share such information with the patient because it is feared that hope is destroyed.[32, 43]

- Traditionally, Russians are of the belief that family does everything possible to care for a loved one until death occurs. 'Do Not Resuscitate' discussions, advanced directives, and living wills may be foreign and seen as unacceptable.[24]

- Among religious believers, consent for organ donation and autopsy will be influenced by religious affiliation.

- Hospice services are relatively new in Russia. Approach discussion with sensitivity and careful explanation.

- Provide religious support based on patient's religious affiliation.

---

[1] Central Intelligence Agency. (2011). *The world factbook: Russia.* Retrieved from https://www.cia.gov/library/publications/the-world-factbook/geos/rs.html

[2] Insight Guides. (2009). *Russia, Belarus & Ukraine.* Long Island City, NY: Langenscheidt Publishers, Inc.

[3] Richmond, Y. (2009). *From nyet to da: Understanding the new Russia* (4th ed.). Boston, MA: Nicholas Brealey Publishing.

[4] Hardwick, S. W. (1993). *Russian refuge: Religion, migration, and settlement on the North American Pacific Rim.* Chicago, IL: The University of Chicago Press.

[5] Riasanovsky, N.V. & Steinberg, M.D. (2011). *A history of Russia* (8th ed.). New York, NY: Oxford University Press.

[6] United States Department of State. (2011). *Background note: Russia.* Retrieved from http://www.state.gov/r/pa/ei/bgn/3183.htm

[7] Behnke, A. (2006). *Russians in America.* Minneapolis, MN: Lerner Publications Company.

[8] Conquest, R. (2011). *Soviet Union: The Stalin era.* Retrieved from http://www.history.com/topics/soviet-union/page4

[9] Berlin Institute for Population and Development. (2008, November). *Russia's demographic crisis.* Retrieved from http://www.berlin-institut.org/online-handbookdemography/russia.html

[10] Loiko, S. (2011, November 14). *Russians are leaving the country in droves.* Retrieved from http://articles.latimes.com/2011/nov/14/world/la-fg-russia-emigration-20111115

[11] Russian-Americans residence areas. (2012, January 2). Retrieved from http://www.rususa.com/immigration/russian-american-residence.asp

[12] World Life Expectancy. (2012). *USA vs. Russia: Top 10 causes of death.* Retrieved from http://www.worldlifeexpectancy.com/news/russia-vs-united-states-top-10-causes-of-death

[13] USAID. (2010). *Health in Russia.* Retrieved from http://www.usaid.gov/locations/europe_eurasia/health/countries/docs/country_profile_russia.pdf

[14] United Nations Scientific Committee on the Effects of Atomic Radiation (UNSCEAR). (2012). *The Chernobyl accident: UNSCEAR's assessments of the radiation effects.* Retrieved from http://www.unscear.org/unscear/en/chernobyl.html

[15] BBC News Europe. (2011, July 21). *Russia classifies beer as alcoholic.* Retrieved from http://www.bbc.co.uk/news/world-europe-14232970

[16] World Health Organization. (2011). *Management of substance abuse: The Russian Federation.* Retrieved from http://www.who.int/substance_abuse/publications/global_alcohol_report/profiles/rus.pdf

[17] Weitz, R. (2011, February 15). *Global insights: Russia's demographic timebomb.* World Politics Review. Retrieved from http://www.worldpoliticsreview.com/articles/7888/global-insights-russias-demographic-timebombjjdaajj

[18] U.S. Census Bureau. (2011). *Data profile.* Retrieved from http://factfinder.census.gov

[19] Aliprandini, M. (2009). *Russia. Our world.* Russia, 1-6.

[20] Russian language facts. (2012). Retrieved from http://www.languagehelpers.com/languagefacts/russian.html

[21] U.S. English Foundation, Inc. (2009). *Becoming an American: The Russians.* Washington, DC: Author. Retrieved from http://www.usefoundation.org/userdata/file/Becoming%20an%20American_Russians.pdf

[22] Giger, J. N. (2013). *Transcultural nursing: Assessment and intervention* (6th ed.). St. Louis, MO: Mosby Elsevier.

[23] Krakovsky, M. (2009). National poker face: Happy or not, Russians rarely smile in public. *Psychology Today, 42*(1), 20.

[24] Aroian, K.J., Khatutsky, G. & Dashevskaya, A. (2013). People of Russian heritage. In Purnell, L. *Transcultural health care: A culturally competent approach* (4th ed., p. 426-440). Philadelphia, PA: F. A. Davis Company.

[25] Pavlovskaya, A. (2007). *Cultureshock! A survival guide to customs and etiquette: Russia.* Tarrytown, NY: Marshall Cavendish Corporation.

[26] Gerhart, G. ((2001). *The Russian's world: Life and language* (3rd ed.). Bloomington, IN: Slavica Publishers.

[27] Advameg, Inc. (2012). *Countries and their cultures: Doukhobors–religion and expressive culture.* Retrieved from http://www.everyculture.com/North-America/Doukhobors-Religion-and-Expressive-Culture.html

[28] Union of Spiritual Communities of Christ. (2011). *Doukhobors.* Retrieved from http://www.usccdoukhobors.org/about.htm

[29] Molokans and Jumpers around the world: Short description and history. (2011). Retrieved from http://molokane.org/molokan/

[30] Barko, R., Corbett, C. F., Allen, C.B., & Shultz, J. A. (2011). Perceptions of diabetes symptoms and self-management strategies: A cross-cultural comparison. *Journal of Transcultural Nursing, 22*(3). 274-281. Doi:10.1177/1043659611404428

[31] Hobbs, R. (2002). *Knowledge of immigrant nationalities of Santa Clara County: Russia.* Retrieved from http://immigrantinfo.org/kin/russia.htm

[32] Resick, L. K. (2008). The meaning of health among midlife Russian-speaking women. *Journal of Nursing Scholarship, 40*(3), 248-253.

[33] Adams, O.D. (2005). *The art of Russian massage.* Kurtistown, HI: Hoala Productions.

[34] Polyakova, S. A. & Pacquiao, D. F. (2006). Psychological and mental illness among elder immigrants from the former Soviet Union. *Journal of Transcultural Nursing, 17*(1), 40-49).

[35] Balmforth, T. (2010). *Battery in private.* Retrieved from http://russiaprofile.org/special_report/a1293034376/print_edition/

[36] Misner-Pollard, C. (2009). Domestic violence in Russia: Is current law meeting the needs of victims and the obligations of human rights instruments? *Columbia Journal of East European Law, 3*(1), 145-209.
[37] Callister, L.C., Getmanenko, N., Garvrish, N., Eugenevna, M. O., Vladimirova, Z. N., Lassetter, J., & Turkina, N. (2007). Giving birth: The voices of Russian women. MCN, *American Journal of Maternal Child Nursing, 32*(1), 18-24.
[38] Gabriel, C. (2003). The effects of perceiving "weak health" in Russia: The case of breastfeeding. *Anthropology of East Europe Review, 17*(1), 91-104.
[39] Perlman, F. & McKee, M. (2009). Trends in family planning in Russia, 1994-2003. *Perspectives on Sexual and Reproductive Health, 41*(1), 40-50. Doi.10.1363/4104009
[40] Sawyer, L. (2011, July 16). *Russia president signs law regulating abortions. The Jurist.* Retrieved from http://jurist.org/paperchase/2011/07/russia-president-signs-law-reguating-abortion.php
[41] Pickert, K. (2010, June 28). Russian kids in America: When the adopted can't adapt. *Time, 175*(25), 34-39.
[42] Leon, D.A., Sckoinikov, V. M., & McKee, M. (2009). Alcohol and Russian mortality: A continuing crisis. *Addiction, 104*, 1630-1636. Doi: 10.1111/j.1360-0443.2009.02655.x
[43] Calloway, S. (2009). The effect of culture on beliefs related to autonomy and informed consent. *Journal of Cultural Diversity, 16*(2), 68-70.

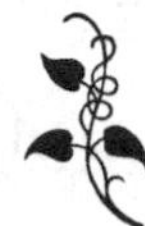

SEVENTH-DAY ADVENTISTS

Background

The Adventist movement in the United States stemmed from the preachings of William Miller (1782–1849), who had prophesied that Christ would return to earth between 1843 and 1844. His followers were called *Millerites* or *Adventists*. After Miller's prophecy did not occur, some of his followers left the group. After continuing to study the Scriptures, searching for an explanation, they concluded that a spiritual event had, in fact, taken place in heaven in 1844.

Leading this group was Ellen White. The Seventh-Day Adventist Church was officially founded in 1863, observing the Sabbath based on the fourth commandment: "Six days thou shalt labor…the seventh day is the Sabbath of the Lord thy God." Hence, the name Seventh-Day Adventists.[1, 2, 3] There are over fifteen million Seventh-Day Adventists worldwide.[4]

Religious Representatives

- Pastor
- Elder

Religious Beliefs

- The Holy Bible.
- Seventh-Day Adventists follow most of the beliefs of conservative Christianity. Some of the exceptions are:[3,5]
  - The written works of Ellen White were inspired by God and can be a source of instruction and guidance. However, the Bible is the standard utilized for all teaching.[4,6]
  - There is no innate immortality of the soul.[7]
  - The second coming of Christ is imminent. It will bring a final catastrophic end to the present evil age and bring with it a one thousand year period of peace, righteousness, and Christian goodness.[1,6]
  - Human suffering is attributed to Satan, never God. God alleviates suffering.[8]
  - Strict dietary laws based on the Old Testament.
  - Non-participation in combatant roles during war. Seventh-Day Adventists do serve in roles as medics and other health providers.[3]

Special/Religious Observations

- Sabbath is recognized as dusk on Friday to dusk on Saturday.[5]

Health Beliefs/Practices

- The body is considered the temple of God and should be meticulously cared for to keep it healthy for the service and glory of God. Care and discipline of the body is vital to true spirituality.[1,7]
- Tobacco, alcohol, caffeine, over-the-counter drugs, and certain foods are avoided.

- Generally, the Church encourages a vegetarian diet. However, some members choose to be non-vegetarians. If non-vegetarians consume meat, it must be derived from an animal that both chews his cud and has a cloven hoof, such as cows, sheep, goats, etc. Chicken, turkey, and fish with fins and scales are acceptable foods.[9]

- Some individuals may practice fasting unless it has adverse effects.

- May refuse medical treatments, procedures, and/or surgery during Sabbath. Schedule non-emergency medical interventions on other days of the week.

- Prayer and anointing of the sick may be seen as therapeutic during illness.

- **Elective Pregnancy Termination**: Elective pregnancy termination is not permitted. Therapeutic pregnancy termination is acceptable only in extreme circumstances such as rape or incest, endangerment of the mother's life with continued pregnancy, or severe congenital anomalies.[4]

- **Amniocentesis**: Acceptable.

- **Autopsy**: Acceptable.

- **Birth Control**: No restrictions.

- **Blood and blood products**: Acceptable.

- **Circumcision**: Acceptable; no special rituals.

- **Organ Donation**: Acceptable.

Death

- The dead wait for the resurrection and are in an unconscious state. There is no progression to heaven or hell immediately after death. The whole person will be resurrected on the last day, with immortality for the righteous.[1, 10]

- Relatives may request that the family member be anointed with oil at the time of death. An elder or pastor of the Church will do the anointing. There are no formal sacraments required at the time of death.[7]

- **Burial**: Individual choice.

---

1 Mead, F. & Hill, C., & Atwood, C.D. (2010). *Handbook of denominations in the United States* (13th ed.). Nashville, TN: Abingdon Press.

2 Goring, R. & Whaling, F. (Eds.). (1994). *Larousse dictionary of beliefs and religions.* New York, NY: Larousse Kingfisher Chambers, Inc.

3 Bergman, J. (1995). The Adventists and Jehovah's Witness branch of Protestantism. In T. Miller, (Ed), *America's alternative religions* (pp. 33-46). Albany, NY: State University of New York Press.

4 General Conference of Seventh-day Adventists. *(2012). Adventists beliefs.* Retrieved from http://www.adventist.org/

5 Ontario Consultants on Religious Tolerance. (2009). *The Seventh-day Adventist church: Its beliefs and practices.* Retrieved from http://www.religioustolerence.org/sda2.htm

6 Edwards, L. (2001). *Beliefs: A brief guide to ideas, theologies, mysteries, and movements.* Louisville, KY: Westminster John Knox Press.

7 Johnston, R. (1998). Seventh-Day Adventist Church. In C. Johnston and McGee, (Eds), *How different religions view death and afterlife* (2nd ed.). Philadelphia, PA: The Charles Press.

8 Taylor, E. & Carr, M. (2009). Nursing ethics in the Seventh-Day Adventist religious tradition. Nursing Ethics,17(6), 707-718.

9 Murphy, F., Gwebu, E., Braithewaite, R., Green-Goodman, D. & Brown, L. (1997). Health values and practices among Seventh-Day Adventists. *American Journal of Health Behavior, 21*(2), 43-50.

10 Maxwell, A. (1975). What is a Seventh-Day Adventist? In L. Rosten, (Ed.), *Religions of America* (pp. 69-81). New York, NY: Simon & Schuster.

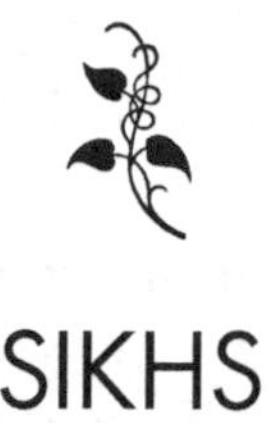

SIKHS

Background

Sikhism was established in northern India approximately five hundred years ago by Guru Nanak.[1] During a period of time when there were conflicts between Muslims and Hindus, Nanak had a divine experience. He reported that he had been in communion with God, the Ultimate Reality or Divine One.[2] God, according to Nanak, had called him to be a guru, a 'spiritual preceptor.'[3] For the remainder of his lifetime, Guru Nanak traveled to countries such as India, Iraq, and Arabia preaching a message of "equality between all religions, love between all men, faith in the one eternal, infinite God who has no rival, is not limited by time and can go anywhere."[4] There were nine other gurus that followed Guru Nanak. The last, Guru Gobind Singh, ended the line of personal gurus and passed the succession of the voice of God to the Sikh holy book.[2]

There are several sects within Sikhism with some practices differing from those of 'orthodox' Sikhs. Sikhs who have undergone the sacred ceremony called *amrit* (a baptism ceremony) are called *Khalsa*. Today, Sikhism is the fifth largest religion with approximately twenty-four million members worldwide. There is a growing population in the United Kingdom, United States, and other areas of North America. The word 'Sikh' means disciple or follower.[5] The most important religious center for Sikhs is the Golden Temple (Harmandir Sahib), located at Amritsar in Punjab.[6]

Religious Representatives

- There is no formal priesthood in Sikhism.
- Each Sikh has a sacred duty to impart knowledge of the religion to others.[7]
- Members of the family and community are expected to visit a Sikh who is hospitalized.

Religious Beliefs

- **Religious book**: Guru Granth Sahib (sometimes called the Adi Granth).
- **Gutka:** A small book containing a collection of Sikh hymns and scriptures (*gutka*) is often carried. The book should be handled with respect and not touched without washing the hands first.[8]
- **Religious place of worship**: *Gurdwara* (or Gurudwara), which means 'door to enlightenment.' A Gurdwara may be a large temple-like building, a smaller more informal building, or a single room in a private home.[2]
- There is one God who is above all things and can be known through meditation. God should be worshipped daily. Tailor care to accommodate prayer times. Be careful not to discard items that may be used during prayer such as prayer beads (*mala*) and holy water (a mixture of sugar and water known as *Amrit)*.[8, 9]
- A person can be released from the cycle of birth, life, death and rebirth (reincarnation) and live forever united with God by living his or her life in a manner that is God-like.[10]
- All persons have equal status in God's eyes.
- The word, *Khalsa* means 'pure ones.' Sikhs who have undergone the Khalsa baptism ceremony adhere to the Khalsa Code of Conduct, which defines social practices, ethical rules of conduct, acceptance of the teachings of the Gurus, and wearing of five physical articles of faith (or five Ks) as follows:
  - **Kes** (also referred to as Kesh, Kais, Kesa): Uncut hair, including body and facial hair. Hair on the head is worn in a topknot.[11] All Sikhs, particularly in Western countries, do not adhere to this practice.[3, 12, 13]

- **Kangha**: A comb carried as a symbol of hygiene, to keep the hair neat, and to hold the topknot in place. Bald Sikhs also wear a kangha.[3]
- **Kara**: A steel or iron bangle worn on the right wrist as a sign of loyalty to the Guru, as a reminder to the wearer to restrain his or her actions, and to remember God at all times.[3,14]
- **Kirpan**: A sword, often a short one, approximately four inches in length or a smaller steel replica. The kirpan is typically worn underneath the clothing and symbolizes defense for all that is just.[3]
- **Kachha**: Knee-length pants tied with a drawstring, generally worn as an undergarment, symbolizing sexual restraint.[3]

- Men who are members of the Khalsa must wear a turban. However, the turban is not one of the five Ks. Women are not required to wear a turban, but may do so if desired. A scarf instead of a turban is acceptable for women.[7] The turban is a method of keeping the hair neat and tidy. It consists of a lengthy piece of cloth and is generally tied as an inverted V over the forehead. The color, shape of the turban, and the manner in which it is tied, can indicate a Sikh's age, geographical origin and/or political preference. A *keski*, or small under-turban about one-fourth the size of the outer turban, may be worn only when not in public.[3]

Special Celebrations/Religious Observations

- There is no fixed day of worship for Sikhs. Persons may gather at any time for worship.[15,16]
- Sikhs celebrate a number of festivals, which follow the lunar calendar. *Gurpurbs* are celebrations of important events in Sikh history. Three gurpurbs celebrated by Sikhs everywhere, are the commemoration of the birth of Guru Nanak (November), the birth of Guru Gobind Singh (December/January), and the martyrdom of Guru Arjan (May/June).[7]
- **Baisakhi**: Celebrates the formation of the first Khalsa. Generally falls during April.[15]
- **Divali**: Also called the Festival of Light. Generally falls in October or November. This festival symbolizes peace and joy.

- **Naming Ceremony**: Religious ceremony performed in the Gurdwara, during which a newborn receives his or her name. The ceremony is one of thanksgiving for the birth of the child.[17]

- Sikhs who have been initiated into the Khalsa take the name *Singh* for men (meaning 'lion') or *Kaur* for women (meaning 'princess').[15]

Health Beliefs

- All humans suffer. Suffering stems from two sources: failure to appreciate God's creation, and failure to control the mind.[10]

- Alcoholic beverages, narcotics, tobacco are avoided by most.

- Cleanliness contributes to good health. Showers may be preferred to baths. To sit in bath water is considered unsanitary.[8, 18]

- The five Ks are worn at all times, even during hospitalization, illness at home, or when washing, bathing, or showering. When there is a need to change the kachha, leave one leg in the unclean pair while placing the other leg in the clean pair. Consult the patient/ family before removing any of these items.[13, 19]

- Women may consider themselves unclean during menstruation.

Kinship/Social Factors

- Sikhs may have a large extended family, which includes all members of the Sikh community. Oftentimes, many people will visit when a person is ill or hospitalized. Elders are valued and cared for by the family.

- Men and women have equal status. However, women are expected to cover their legs.[20] Women may wear loose trousers called *salvars* and a shirt that reaches to the knees.[2]

- Provide same-sex caregivers, including physicians, particularly for women. Protect modesty, leaving the body covered as much as possible.

- Eye contact may be avoided between children and adults, men and women.
- Family members are likely to stay with a relative who is hospitalized. Allow participation in care as much as possible.

Birth/Children

- Children are considered a gift from God. The father will wish to whisper the *Mul Mantra* (Guru Nanak's first poetical statement) into the newborn's ear as soon as possible following birth.[10, 11]
- The mother may be secluded for a period of thirteen to forty days following delivery. This is considered a period of impurity.[3, 19]
- **Birth Control**: Acceptable.
- **Artificial Insemination**: Permitted if sperm is from husband.
- **Elective Pregnancy Termination**: Generally unacceptable.
- Children's hair will be left uncut. Boys may undergo a ceremony of turban-tying in the Gurdwara at ten to twelve years of age. From this point forward, the turban should be treated with the same care and symbolism as with adults. Teenage boys who adhere to traditional Sikh practices will not shave.[2]

Dietary Considerations

- Many Sikhs are vegetarians. In this case, no meat of any kind will be accepted. Alcohol is prohibited. Medications containing alcohol may be refused. Make the patient/family aware of the presence of alcohol in the medication prior to attempting administration. If refused, seek alternative medications.
- Animal-based medications, thickeners, and foods may be refused by Sikhs. This will include medications that are in capsule form and foods that contain gelatin. Consult with the patient/family concerning dietary choices.

- During hospitalization, family members may bring *karah parshad* (a special food that has been blessed) to the ill relative. If at all possible, the hospitalized person should be allowed to have a small piece of the food, even if on a restricted diet.[19] Patients may also request that family members be allowed to bring in food to assure that vegetarian preparation is adhered to during preparation.

Death

- Scriptures will be read and hymns chanted during the last hours of a Sikh's life.
- Hope, rather than sadness, should characterize the death of a Sikh.[10] Expressions of grief for one who has lived a happy and long life are limited or not seen at all. It is believed that crying, etc. will interfere with a peaceful departure of the dying person. Expressions of grief may be more liberal with a person who dies early in life or from some unnatural cause.[2,15]
- The family will likely wish to prepare the relative's body following death. This involves washing and dressing the deceased by wrapping in a white shroud, leaving the five Ks in place. The head will be wrapped in a turban.[19] If no family is available, the head of the deceased should be kept covered. All hair should be left untrimmed. The face should be cleaned and the eyes and mouth closed. Limbs should be straightened and the body covered with a *solid* white sheet. The five Ks and the turban should be left in place.[21]
- Sikhs are generally cremated within twenty-four hours of death, if possible. Stillborns, fetuses from miscarriages, and neonates may be buried.[20]
- **Autopsy**: Acceptable, but generally not desirable unless required by law. Every effort should be made to complete the autopsy promptly so that cremation is not delayed, if possible.[21,22]
- **Organ Transplant/Donation**: Acceptable.[21]

Other Considerations

- Baths are taken daily at dawn, followed by meditation and prayer. Additional prayers are offered in the evening and before going to sleep. Plan care to incorporate these practices. Provide privacy.[23]

- Cutting/shaving of hair should be avoided. Consult the patient/family, except under extreme emergencies, explaining medical reasons, etc.

- If the kachha must be removed for medical examinations or childbirth, discuss keeping them around one leg instead of removing them.[19]

- If the turban must be removed, the majority of Sikh men will want their head and hair covered with a cloth. The turban should be handled with care and held using two hands. Leave the turban near the patient, if possible. It should not be placed in a bag with other clothing or allowed to touch the floor.[19]

- If there is space in the home, a copy of the *Adi Granth* will be placed in a separate room. The holy text will be opened during the morning and put to rest after sunset each day.[23]

- **Blood Transfusions**: Acceptable.[21]

---

1 Fenton, J., Hein, N., Reynolds, F., Miller, A., Neilsen, N., Burford, G. & Forman, K. (1993). *Religions of Asia* (3rd ed.). New York, NY: St. Martin's Press.
2 Singh, N. (1993). *Sikhism: World religions.* New York, NY: Facts on File, Inc.
3 McLeod, H. (1997). *Sikhism.* New York, NY: Penguin Books.
4 Comte, F. (1992). *Sacred writings of world religions.* New York, NY: W&R Chambers, Ltd.
5 Real Sikhism. (2010). *Exploring the Sikh religion.* Retrieved from http://www.realsikhism.com/index.php
6 *Sikhism in Brief.* Retrieved from http://www.sikhs.org/summary.htm
7 Cole, W. (1994). *Teach yourself Sikhism.* Chicago, IL: NTC Publishing Group.
8 Gatrad, R., Notta, H., Panesar, S., Brown, E. & Sheikh, A. (2007). Palliative care for Sikhs. In R. Gatrad, E. Brown, & A. Sheikh (Eds.), *Palliative care for South Asians: Muslims, Hindus, and Sikhs* (pp. 89-93). United Kingdom: Quay Books.
9 SikhiWiki. (2009). *Gutka* Retrieved from http://www.sikhiwiki.org/index.php/Gutka
10 Keene, M. (1993). *Seekers after truth: Hinduism, Buddhism, Sikhism.* Great Britain: Cambridge University Press.
11 Cole, W. & Sambhi, P. (1997). *A popular dictionary of Sikhism.* Chicago, IL: NTC Publishing Group.
12 Lakshmi, R. (2009, May 7). *Younger Sikhs giving up long hair, turbans. The Record.* Retrieved from http://www.highbeam.com
13 Black, P. (2009). Cultural and religious beliefs in stoma care nursing. *British Journal of Nursing, 18*(13), 790-793.
14 Smart, N. (1989). *The world's religions: Old traditions and modern transformations.* Great Britain: Cambridge University Press.
15 Meredith, S. and Hickman, C. (2001). *The Usborne internet-linked encyclopedia of world religions.* London, England: Usborne Publishing, Ltd.

[16] Warrier, S. & Walshe, J. (2001). *Dates and meanings of religious and other multi-ethnic festivals 2002-2005.* New York, NY: Foulsham Educational.
[17] Zaehner, R. (1997). *Encyclopedia of the world's religions.* New York, NY: Helicon Publishing Ltd.
[18] Reimer-Kirkham, S. (2009) Lived religion: Implications for nursing ethics. *Nursing Ethics, 16*(4), 406-417.
[19] Henley, A. & Clayton, J. (1982). The five signs of Sikhism. *Health and Social Service Journal, 92*(August 5), 943-945.
[20] McDonald, R. (1985). Cultural exchange. *Nursing Mirror, 160*(7), 32-35.
[21] Green, J. (1989). Death with dignity. Sikhism. *Nursing Times, 85*(7), 56-57.
[22] Pattison, N. (2008). Care of patients who have died. *Nursing Standard, 22*(28), 42-48.
[23] Doniger, W. (1999). *Merriam-Webster's encyclopedia of world religions.* Springfield, MA: Merriam-Webster, Incorporated.

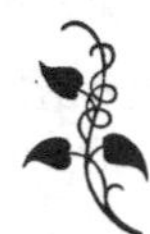

SOUTHEAST ASIANS, CHINESE, KOREANS

Background

Following the Vietnam War, more than one million Southeast Asians arrived in the United States from 1975-1994, primarily as refugees. The persons were primarily from Vietnam, Cambodia, and Laos. The land surface of Southeast Asia is slightly larger than approximately one-half of the continental United States. Southeast Asia is home to almost 600 million people. It is bordered to the north by China, India to the West, and the Pacific Ocean to the East.[1, 2, 3] Countries located in Southeast Asia include Vietnam, Laos, Malaysia, Singapore, Brunei, Myanmar (Burma), the Philippines, Cambodia, Indonesia, Thailand, and Timor-Lest (East Timor). China and Korea are located in eastern Asia. China is approximately the same size in area as the United States, but is home to over one billion people. Chinese are the largest group of Asian immigrants to the United States.[4, 5, 6]

After World War II, Korea split into North and South Korea, forming two separate governments. Today, the relationship between the governments of North and South Korea is antagonistic. North Korea is slightly smaller than the state of Mississippi, and has a population of approximately 24.5 million people. South Korea has a population of almost 49 million people and is slightly larger than the state of Indiana.[7] According to the 2010 United States Census, Chinese, Filipinos, Vietnamese, and Koreans are the largest populations of eastern and southeastern origin in the United States.[8] There is great diversity between and within groups of Southeast Asians, Chinese, and Koreans and care must always be individualized.

Common health risk factors include smoking, depression, post-traumatic stress disorder, anxiety, Hepatitis B, cardiovascular disease, including a high incidence of hypertension among Filipinos, diabetes, and various cancers. New immigrants may also be at risk for internal parasites and tuberculosis. Sudden Unexplained Nocturnal Death Syndrome (SUNDS) is a risk among young, healthy Southeast Asian males, usually refugees. Poverty is a continuing factor that contributes to major health risks among a large portion of Southeast Asians, Chinese, and Koreans. Persons leaving their countries as refugees may suffer long-term emotional scars from their experiences.[6, 9, 10, 11, 12, 13]

Language

- There are many dialects spoken by the people of Southeast Asia, China, North and South Korea. However, major languages include, but are not limited to:[7]
    - **Cambodia:** Khmer, French, English
    - **Vietnam:** Vietnamese, English, French, Chinese
    - **Laos:** Lao, English, French
    - **Maylasia:** Bahasa Malaysia, English, Chinese
    - **Singapore:** Mandarin, English, Malay
    - **Brunei:** Malay, Chinese
    - **Myanmar:** Burmese
    - **Philippines:** Tagalog, Cebuano, Ilocano
    - **Indonesia:** Bahasa Indonesia, English, Dutch
    - **Thailand:** Thai, Chinese
    - **Timor-Lest:** Tetum, Portuguese, Indonesian

- **China**: Mandarin Chinese (pu tong hua) and numerous Chinese dialects that are spoken. The spoken languages are not mutually understandable. However, since the written language uses the same characters, persons may be able to communicate through writing. When seeking interpreters for a Chinese person, the health care worker must find out the specific dialect that the client speaks. Avoid compound sentences using 'and' and 'but' since such sentences may be confusing to the Chinese. Avoid asking questions in the negative tense such as "You've had a bath today, haven't you?" Provide instructions in the order that the task should occur and careful explanation when touching is necessary. Observe for non-verbal cues.[4,6,7]

- **Chinese**: Chinese Names - Use the family name when addressing individuals. The family name is written and stated first, then the given name. Therefore, if one's name is Lin Ying, *Ying* is the given name; *Lin* is the family name. If in doubt, ask how the individual would prefer to be addressed. Women may retain their family name after marriage. Children take the father's family name. Some Chinese adopt English names and reverse their name to traditional Western style if in frequent contact with Westerners who find their Chinese name difficult to pronounce.[4,6]

• The official language of North and South Korea is Korean.[7] Many Koreans speak Chinese and Japanese. Interpreters knowledgeable of these languages may be used in many cases if a Korean interpreter is not available.

- **Korean Names**: The family name comes first, followed by one or two given names, one of which may be a generational name (the second name is not considered a middle name). Individuals may choose to hyphenate the two names. Women in Korea may keep their family names. Korean women living in Western cultures may choose to adopt their husband's name or change the Korean name order. Children are given the father's surname. Ask how the individual prefers to be addressed.[6,14]

• Hmongs are the youngest ethnic group in the United States. Mature interpreters may be difficult to find since the median age of Hmongs living in the United States is twenty years. About 43 percent of the United States Hmong population is less than eighteen years of age.[15]

• Since Hmongs are primarily an oral cultural group, they may not have learned to read Hmong or other languages. The two languages most frequently spoken are *Hmoob Dawb* (White Hmong) and *Hmoob Ntsuab* (Blue or Green Hmong). Because they are primarily an oral culture, written educational materials, treatment plans, etc. may not be effective strategies.[4]

- Be aware that some commonly used words used in Western medicine to explain physical and mental illnesses, treatments, etc. have no comparable words in the languages of Southeast Asians, Koreans, and Chinese.

- Patients/families may not give direct eye contact out of respect to the health care provider. Likewise, patients may not voice a lack of understanding or ask questions.[11]

Worldview/Religious Beliefs

- Balance in life is attained through harmony, interdependence, and loyalty. Psychological, spiritual, and physiological functions are interrelated.[4, 16, 17]

- The group is more important than the individual. The individual's behavior is a reflection of the entire family.[6, 18]

- Roles are defined according to social/family status, age. Conflict should be avoided. Self-control and maintenance of individual and family integrity is valued.[16, 19]

- There are strong worldview influences of Buddhism, Taoism, Confucianism, Falungong, animism, ancestor, and spirit worship.[20, 21] Other religious beliefs include Christianity and Islam.

Health Beliefs/Practices

- Health practices are generally based on a balance of hot and cold, yin and yang principles, and/or harmony with the universe.

- Illnesses may result from a number of causes including weather conditions, wind, contaminated foods or water, strong emotions, punishment by ancestors' spirits, soul loss, etc. Individuals may have little or no concept of bacteria/viruses, etc. as a basis of illness.

- Use visuals to assist with explanation of illnesses. Persons who have had little exposure to Western medicine may have no concept of anatomy and physiology and related disorders that can lead to illness.[22]

- A common belief is that if one is feeling well, there is little need to seek health care services or see a doctor. As a group, cancer screening rates are very low among Asian Americans. Among women, additional reasons contributing to low levels of screening for gynecological cancer screening include: fear that the exam will destroy virginity, lack of knowledge concerning personal risk of cancer, modesty, and finances. Women over 40 years of age are less likely to participate in screening.[13, 23, 24, 25]

- Certain numbers and colors may be seen as positive or negative influences on health and well-being.[4]

- Illness prevention and treatments include herbal preparations, certain foods, massage, acupuncture, acupressure, consulting with folk healers, and persons believed to hold supernatural healing powers.[16] Thoroughly assess types of herbal preparations and question where they are obtained. Herbal preparations obtained from countries not requiring quality controls may contain toxic substances such as mercury, lead, and arsenic.

- Coining, burning/moxibustion, skin scraping, and cupping are practiced as methods of healing for ailments such as headaches, colds, sore throats, coughs, diarrhea, and fever.

- Chanting is often done in conjunction with healing methods. These practices may leave reddened or bruised areas on the skin. The skin discolorations are sometimes mistaken for physical abuse, particularly when seen on children. Ask specifically about the origin of the areas on the skin.[17, 26, 27, 28]

- Individuals, including infants, often wear gold/silver bracelets/necklaces, strings or amulets around the wrist, neck, ankle, waist, or attached to clothes. These have protective and religious significance and should not be removed unless absolutely necessary for medical purposes. Provide a thorough explanation to the family/individual and give the object(s) to family members for safekeeping.[22, 27, 29]

- Individuals may expect to have almost immediate results from prescribed medications. The concept of controlling a chronic disease vs. curing the disease may be unfamiliar. Therefore, medications may be discontinued if speedy relief does not occur. Provide careful explanation regarding the expected effects of the medication. Set short-term goals and follow-up.[22]

- One's head is considered private and personal, being the seat of the soul and of life. It is the most sacred part of the body and considered untouchable except by very close relatives.[27,29,30] Avoid touching the head without permission from the patient or parent, especially among persons of Southeast Asian background. Scalp vein IV sites in ill newborns and infants should be avoided. If these sites must be used, the family should receive thorough explanations and rationales. The infant's fontanel is considered an easy exit site for the soul.[27]

- Drawing blood for lab tests may cause high levels of anxiety or the individual may refuse to have blood drawn. The same reaction may occur if blood transfusions are needed. It is believed that losing blood depletes the body's strength and provides a route for the soul to leave the body (surgery may be perceived in the same way). Blood transfusions give the opportunity for the donor's spirits to enter the client's body. These thoughts are especially strong related to children.[31,32]

- A common belief among Southeast Asians is that a "pool of blood" is located in the chest and is vital for life. Loss of this "pool" is thought to lead to death. Be aware that families may react intensely to CPR, nasogastric tubes, etc. that may be perceived as disturbing this life force and possibly leading to death. It is optimal to have a liaison who can be with the family during such an event to attempt to reassure the family.[22]

- Some Southeast Asians believe that when an individual is unconscious, their souls are at large. Illness and death may result. Because of this belief, anesthesia may be seen as harmful.[31]

- Confucianism teaches that the whole body must be returned at death to ensure a proper afterlife. Therefore, individuals may refuse surgery or other invasive procedures fearing that their body may not be whole at the time of death.[26]

- Mental illness carries a stigma, as does the word "crazy." It may be difficult to impossible to convince one to take psychotherapy or to talk about personal issues or private life. Emotional distress may manifest itself through physical complaints that are seen as more acceptable.[11,16,19,33]

- *Hwa-byung* is a psychosomatic illness found among Koreans resulting from suppression and/or repression of accumulated emotional responses to stress factors over a long period of time. These stress factors cause a disruption in the harmony and balance of vital body energies. Factors that may contribute to the development of hwa-byung include marital, family, and financial problems, poverty/hardship, etc. Symptoms include panic, fear, gastrointestinal symptoms such as indigestion, anorexia, etc. Palpitations, a feeling of a mass in the epigastric area, generalized aches and pains, fatigue, depression, and insomnia may also occur. Current treatment approaches include assisting with identifying causes, social support, and lifestyle changes within the person's cultural boundaries.[6,34,35]

- Incorporate folk healers/practitioners into care. Spiritual healing must also occur for balance to be restored. Folk healing may involve the sacrifice of animals.

Expression of Pain

- Stoicism is often seen, particularly among men, reflecting a common belief of suffering as being a part of life. A fear of loss of self-control may also contribute to stoicism. May not request or accept pain medication. Offering pain medication to the patient acknowledges the likelihood of pain and concern about the patient's comfort level vs. waiting for the patient to ask for pain medication.[4]

Male-Female/Kinship/Social Relationships

- Respect for authority, elders, etc. is highly valued. Individuals may avoid direct eye contact with nurses and physicians as a sign of respect and/or until trust has been established. Likewise, health care providers should acknowledge elder family members when entering the room. Direct eye contact is sometimes considered impolite or aggressive.[20,36]

- True feelings may not be expressed because of cultural beliefs based on avoiding conflict and expressions of anger or other emotions. These emotions may be exhibited by the individual becoming silent. Individuals may also respond with a smile even though she or he is in disagreement with the health care provider.

- Side-by-side or right angle seating arrangements may facilitate more positive interactions.[3] Keep feet flat on the floor since sitting toward a patient/family with the soles of the feet showing is considered impolite.

- Modesty is highly valued. The area between the waist and the knees is viewed as particularly private. It is important to explain in advance the need to touch the patient's body, especially the area between the waist and the knees. Generally, males other than husbands do not touch this part of the woman's body. Provide female practitioners if pelvic exams, urinary cauterizations, etc. must be done. The need to perform such procedures should be carefully evaluated since extreme anxiety is likely to result. Allowing the husband to stay in the room may be comforting. It is also important to explain in advance why there is a need to ask personal questions.

- Most Asian cultures are hierarchical. Males are authority figures and generally act as the spokesperson for decisions. Determine from the patient who the primary decision-maker in the family will be and who will need to have information presented to them for decision-making. There may be a delay in signing consents and other documents until reviewed by such person(s). It may be culturally inappropriate for females to make health care decisions, even about issues related to personal health.

- Families may be resistant to sharing information related to serious or terminal illness with the patient.

- Many Asians live in extended family households and value the family of orientation. Even after marriage, sons often continue to live with parents until the parents die. Family members will likely want to stay continuously with the hospitalized person, providing all personal care. Hospitalizations can be frightening to individuals who are often fearful of spirits and ghosts, particularly at night. It is important that health care providers honor the family's wishes to stay with the patient for reassurance to the patient and the family. The family may equate leaving their loved one to abandonment, causing great distress. Respect and obligation demand that children provide care for parents. Chinese sons may be more involved in the parent's care than the daughter since the daughter's primary responsibility will be to the husband's parents after marriage.[22]

- Health care workers with loud voices or who are very talkative may be perceived negatively since persons from these cultural groups tend to be reserved, quiet, and many times practice nonverbal more than verbal communication. Health care workers must be particularly attuned to nonverbal behavior.

- Affirmative answers (yes) are many times misinterpreted by American health care workers as meaning agreement. However, agreement is often used as an indication of respect or that the person is listening carefully to what is being said. This misinterpretation is often the source of noncompliance among these clients.[4]

Birth

- Children are highly valued. Individuals often marry as teenagers and may have several children.
- May seek prenatal care late during pregnancy or not at all because of fear, cost, and/or lack of need. (Hmong are least likely to seek prenatal care).[30]
- Among Vietnamese and Cambodian women, a large amount of salt in the diet is believed to be beneficial during pregnancy.[37,38]
- Possible cultural taboos and practices among Chinese related to childbirth include:[39,40,41]
  - Ingestion of special soups such as bird's nest soup (made from the nest of the Southeast Asian swiftlet bird that is similar in size to the sparrow) and chicken/chicken broth. The small nest is made from sticky starch-like strands of the bird's saliva produced from large salivary glands under the bird's tongue. It is thought to promote the generation and growth of human cells, rejuvenate human skin, and boost the immune system.
  - Lamb is not eaten during pregnancy with the belief that it may cause the baby to have epilepsy. The pronunciation of the word 'lamb' is similar to the word for 'epilepsy' in Chinese. Eating pineapple is believed to cause miscarriage.
  - Newborn babies are not dressed in used clothing as the baby may take on the characteristics of those that wore the clothes previously. Therefore, the family may bring new clothing for the baby instead of dressing the baby in hospital shirts, etc. Disposable shirts may be acceptable.
  - Talking about how beautiful a baby is may cause the gods to take the baby away.
- Korean and Filipino women may avoid certain foods because they are thought to cause the baby to have similar physical characteristics. These include some types of fish, crab, chicken, etc.[6]

- Vitamins during pregnancy may be refused by Filipino women who believe that congenital anomalies may result.[6]

- Women may not express discomfort during labor. To do so is believed to bring shame to the women. Pain and discomfort must be experienced as a part of childbirth.

- Ideally, the laboring woman's mother or mother-in-law attends during labor rather than the husband. This practice varies among cultures.

- May prefer to assume squatting position during birth.[42]

- Parents may not exhibit *usual* positive bonding behaviors such as cuddling a newborn infant, talking to the infant or stroking the infant's head. Asians from some rural areas believe in spirits who might steal the infant by causing its death. Therefore, the mother does not want to attract the spirits to the infant.

- Breastfeeding is generally supported. However, mothers may be resistant to early breastfeeding, believing that colostrum is "bad milk." For this reason, the mother may insist on bottle-feeding the infant until her *real milk* comes in. Mothers should be provided with privacy while breastfeeding.

- Women often follow the practice of having a "lying-in" period (several weeks) following birth. Because the postpartum period may be considered a 'cold' state, bathing, shampooing the hair, cold liquids, cold air/drafts, and exercise may be avoided. Sponge baths can be substituted for hygiene purposes. Ice packs to the perineum will likely be refused. The woman will want to rest and stay warm. If the baby must stay in the hospital after the mother's discharge, it is possible that she may not accompany the father to the hospital to visit the baby because of this lying-in period. Grandmothers, particularly the husband's mother, are often very involved with the new infant and the new mother's recovery. Their authoritative positions should be acknowledged when caring for the mother and during teaching sessions.[43]

- Mongolian spots are commonly found on infants.

- Bilirubin levels may be higher among Chinese infants.[6]

- During the post-partum period, 'cold' foods such as green vegetables, fruits, fruit juice, meats (excluding chicken), and fish are often avoided. Offer warm liquids. Hmong women frequently eat only steamed rice and boiled chicken for thirty days following delivery. Special herbs specified for the postpartum period are added. Koreans may eat foods especially prepared for mothers following birth such as *miyuk-kuk*, a seaweed soup. During the postpartum period, Chinese may eat certain foods such as pigs feet, ginger and other herbs to assist in removal of any placental remnants, to bring the body back into balance, and to stimulate milk production. Beef may be avoided as it is thought to slow the healing process after birth.[31, 40, 41, 44, 45]

- Hmong and some other Southeast Asian mothers may wish to have the placenta returned to them at the time of discharge for ceremonial disposition. Western medical facilities and personnel may be forced to change laws, rules, and thinking related to handling placentas as medical waste. Patients may be afraid to ask for the placenta, even though they wish to take it. Health care providers can facilitate meeting this need by asking if taking the placenta is part of the individual's tradition related to childbirth. There are several reasons that may lead to a family's desire to take the placenta home.[31, 46, 47]
    - The placenta is considered the baby's first 'clothing.' At the time of death, an individual's soul must be able to retrieve this 'garment' to have safe passage into the spirit world to be united with ancestors. If the soul cannot be united with this first garment, the soul may spend eternity wandering.
    - The dried placenta of first-born sons may be used for medicinal purposes.
    - Tying a knot in the cord of the girl's placenta will lead to the next child being a son.
    - Burying the placenta in a level position will prevent the baby from spitting up.
    - The placenta provides a sense of control over the future health and welfare of the baby, mother, and community.
- Male children may receive preferential treatment, especially the firstborn male because of the expectation to support the family and carry on the family name.[2]
- Vietnamese parents are generally very permissive with children relating to the feeding practices, toileting and sex play. Mothers may masturbate male children during the first five years of life to assure optimal sexual performance during adult years. Female infants' genitals may be fondled as a way of comforting a fussy infant.

- Expose children as little as possible during physical exams. Nudity is believed to make the child vulnerable to "bad winds," which can result in illness.
- Parents may be self-sacrificing to provide a better life for their children.
- Overweight children may be perceived as being healthy.

Death

- Among Filipinos, suicide is viewed as shameful to the individual and to the family.
- When faced with a terminal illness and death, individuals may tend to be stoic and fatalistic.
- Most Southeast Asians prefer to die at home. A common belief is that if an individual dies away from home, his or her spirit will be unhappy and cause disturbances to the survivors.[27]
- A common belief among Hmong is that the body has three souls: one that stays with the body after death, one that returns to live with ancestors, and one that returns to the spirit world to be reincarnated and return to earth in some form. Many Hmong believe that the souls of individuals who die from reasons other than natural causes will not be able to get to their afterlife. The person's soul is then believed to stay around and cause difficulties for the living.[26, 48]
- Among Southeast Asians (Vietnamese, Hmong, Laotians, Kampucheans, Lao-Theung), the family will generally want to prepare the body of the deceased. A coin may be placed in the deceased person's mouth to help the spirit at various stages of its journey.
- **Autopsy**: Likely to be refused believing that if the body is cut, organs or body parts are lost, the person will be incomplete during the reincarnation.[31, 49]

Patient Teaching/Dietary Considerations

- Family members may want to bring food for the patient's meals.

- Offer warm or hot beverages vs. only cold beverages based on the belief in keeping balance in the body.

- Individuals may prefer cooked to raw vegetables. Rice or noodles are popular foods among these cultural groups and may be eaten with each meal or several times a day. Traditional diets vary among individuals from different geographical regions of the same country.[4, 6]

- Frequently lactose-intolerant.

- Usual diet is generally high in sodium, low in fat.

- A lack of understanding or embarrassment may be expressed by nervous laughter or agreement. Dignity and self-esteem are extremely important for most Asians. To admit not understanding information results in a loss of self-esteem. Have the individual demonstrate understanding.

- The progress of male and elder patients with self-care activities may be impeded by the expectation that female family members and children carry out activities for them. Self-care and independence from family are not valued.

- May be uncomfortable in group teaching or therapy sessions.

Other Considerations

- In Vietnam, birthdays are not celebrated as in Western culture. Persons are considered a year older at the beginning of each year (Tet). The Vietnamese client should be asked the 'year' of birth. If unable to give a month and day of birth on arrival to the United States, January 1 is generally the official date assigned by the United States government.[4]

- Some studies have indicated that Chinese, as well as some other Asian groups, may be more sensitive to the effects of alcohol, beta-blockers, atropine, antidepressants, and neuroleptics. Gastrointestinal side effects may also be more heightened among Chinese individuals.[6]

1 One World Nations Online. (2013). *Countries of Asia: Southeast Asia.* Retrieved from http://www.nationsonline.org/oneworld/asia.htm

2 Pho, T. & Mulvey, A. (2003). Southeast Asian women in Lowell. *Frontiers, 24*(1), 101-129.

3 U.S. Census Bureau. (2012). *The Asian population: 2010.* Retrieved from http://www.census.gov/prod/cen2010/briefs/c2010br-11.pdf

4 Giger, J.N. (2013). *Transcultural nursing: Assessment and intervention.* (6th ed.). St. Louis: Mosby.

5 Schaeffer, R. T. (2012). *Racial and ethnic groups.* (13th ed.). Boston, MA: Pearson.

6 Purnell, L. D. (2013). *Transcultural health care: A culturally competent approach.* (4th ed.). Philadelphia, PA: F. A. Davis Company.

7 Central Intelligence Agency. (2013). *CIA world factbook: East and Southeast Asia.* Retrieved from http://www.cia.gov

8 U.S. Census Bureau. (March, 2010). *Profile America facts for features: Asian/Pacific American Heritage Month: May 2012.* Retrieved from http://www.census.gov/newsroom/releases/pdf/cb12ff-09_asian.pdf

9 Dhopper, S. (2003). Health care needs of foreign-born Asian Americans. National Association of Social Workers, 28(1), 63-73.

10 Cheng, J., Makielski, J.C., Yuan, P., Nianqinq, S., Zhou, F., Ye, B., & Lu, C. (2011). Sudden unexplained nocturnal death syndrome in southern China: Epidemiologic survey and SCN5A gene screening. *American Journal of Forensic Medical Pathology, 32*(4), 359-363.

11 Sonethavilay, H., Miyabayashi, I., Komori, A., Onimaru, M., & Washio, M. (2011). Mental health needs and cultural barriers that lead to misdiagnosis of Southeast Asian refugees: A review. *International Medical Journal, 18*(3), 169-171.

12 Battle, R.S., Lee, J.P., & Antin, T.M.J. (2010). Knowledge of tobacco control policies among US Southeast Asians. *Journal of Immigrant Minority Health, 12*, 215-220. doi: 10.1007/s10903-009-9265-4

13 Ho, I.K. & Dinh, K.T. (2011). Cervical cancer among Southeast Asian American women. *Journal of Immigrant Minority Health, 13*, 49-60. Doi: 10.1007/s10903-010-9358-0

14 California State Polytechnic University. (2005). *Cal Poly Pomona Asian Name Pronunciation Guide.* Retrieved from http://www.csupomona.edu/~pronunciation/korean.html

15 Hmong Cultural Center. (2012). *Hmong 101.* Retrieved from http://www.hmongcc.org

16 Kuo, C. & Kavanagh, K. (1994). Chinese perspectives on culture and mental health. *Issues in Mental Health Nursing, 15*(6), 551-567.

17 Davis, R. (2000). Cultural health care or child abuse? The Southeast Asian practice of cao gio. *Journal of the American Academy of Nurse Practitioners, 12*(3), 89-95.

18 Li, J. & Wang, J. (2012). Individuals are inadequate: Recognizing the family-centeredness of Chinese bioethics and Chinese health system. *Journal of Medicine and Philosophy, 37*, 568-582. doi: 10.1093/jmp/jhs046

19 Kim, M., Cho, H., Cheon-Klessig, Y., Gerace, L, & Camilleri, D. (2002). Primary health care for Korean immigrants: Sustaining a culturally sensitive model. *Public Health Nursing, 19*(3), 191-200.

20 Leininger, M. & McFarland, M. (2002). *Transcultural nursing: Concepts, theories, research, and practices.* (3rd ed.). New York: McGraw-Hill.

21 Gale, D. (2003). Falungong: Recent developments in Chinese notions of healing. *Journal of Cultural Diversity, 10*(4), 124-127.

22 Johnson, S. (2002). Hmong health beliefs and experiences in the Western health care system. *Journal of Transcultural Nursing, 13*(2), 126-132.

[23] Jin, X., Slomka, J., & Blixen, C. (2002), Cultural and clinical issues in the care of Asian patients. *Cleveland Clinic Journal of Medicine. 69*(1), 50-60.

[24] Appel, H., Huang, B. Ai, A. & Lin, C. (2011). Physical, behavioral, and mental health issues in Asian American women: Results for the national Latino Asian American study. *Journal of Women's Health. 20*(11), 1703-1711.

[25] Ma, G., Shive, S., Wang, M. & Tan, Y. (2009). Cancer screening behaviors and barriers in Asian Americans. American *Journal Health Behavior. 33*(6), 650-660.

[26] O'Hara, E. & Zhan, L. (1994). Cultural and pharmacologic considerations when caring for Chinese elders. *Journal of Gerontological Nursing, 20*(10), 11-16.

[27] Muecke, M. (1983). Caring for Southeast Asian refugee patients in the USA. *American Journal of Public Health, 73*(4), 431-438.

[28] Yarnell, E. & Abascal, K. (2004). Herbal medicine in Korea: "Alternative" is mainstream. *Alternative & Complimentary Therapies, 6*,161-166.

[29] Miller, J. (1995). Caring for Cambodian refugees in the emergency department. *Journal of Emergency Medicine, 21*(6), 498-502.

[30] Rairdan, B. & Higgs, Z. (1992, March/April). When your patient is a Hmong refugee. *American Journal of Nursing*, 52-55.

[31] Fadiman, A. (2012). *The spirit catches you and you fall down: A Hmong child, her American doctors, and the collision of two cultures.* (1st ed.). New York, NY: Farrar, Straus and Giroux.

[32] D'Avanzo, C. (1992). Bridging the cultural gap with Southeast Asians. *Maternal-Child Nursing, 17*(4), 204-208.

[33] Donnelly, P. (2001). Korean American family experiences of caregiving for their mentally ill adult children: An interpretive inquiry. *Journal of Transcultural Nursing, 12*(4), 292-301.

[34] Park, Y., Kim, H., Kang, H., & Kim, J. (2001). A survey of hwa-byung in middle-age Korean women. *Journal of Transcultural Nursing, 12*(2), 115-122.

[35] Choi, M. & Yeom, H. (2011). Identifying and treating the culture-bound syndrome of Hwa-Byung among older Korean immigrant women: Recommendations for practitioners. *Journal of the American Academy of Nurse Practitioners. 23*, 226-232.

[36] Roberson, C. (2003). ASNA independent study activity—cultural assessment of Koreans. *Alabama Nurse, 3*(3), 13-16.

[37] Frye, B. (1991). Cultural themes in health care decision making among Cambodian refugee women. *Journal of Community Health Nursing, 8*(1), 33-44.

[38] Ramer, L. (1992). *Culturally sensitive care giving and childbearing families.* New York, NY: March of Dimes Birth Defects Foundation.

[39] Sullivan, D. H. (2012). Culturally sensitive insight into Chinese immigrants childbearing traditions. *International Journal of Childbirth Education, 27*(1), 23-27.

[40] Braithwaite, A. & Williams, C. (2004). Childbirth experiences of professional Chinese Canadian women. *JOGNN, 33*(6), 748-755.

[41] Hawaii Community College. (2007). *Childbirth.* Retrieved from http://www.hawcc.hawaii.edu/ucwh/library.html#mags

[42] Morrow, K. (1986). Transcultural midwifery: Adapting to Hmong birthing customs in California. *Journal of Nurse Midwifery, 31*(6), 285-288.

[43] Schneiderman, J. (1996). Pospartum nursing for Korean mothers. *Maternal-Child Nursing, 21*(3), 155-158.

[44] Koltyk, J. (1998). *New pioneers in the heartland: Hmong life in Wisconsin*. Boston, MA: Allyn and Bacon.
[45] Kim-Godwyn, Y. (2003). Postpartum beliefs and practices among non-Western cultures. *MCN, 28*(2), 74-78.
[46] Birdsong, W. (1998). The placenta and cultural values. *Western Journal of Medicine, 168*(3), 190-192.
[47] Helsel, D. G., & Mochel, M. (2002). Afterbirths in the afterlife: Cultural meaning of placental disposal in a Hmong American community. *Journal of Transcultural Nursing, 13*(4), 282-6.
[48] Vawter, D. & Babbitt, B. (1997). Hospice care for terminally ill Hmong patients: A good cultural fit? *Minnesota Medicine, 80*(11), 42-44.
[49] Nuttal, P. & Flores, F. (1997). Hmong healing practices used for common childhood illnesses. *Pediatric Nursing, 23*(3), 247-251.

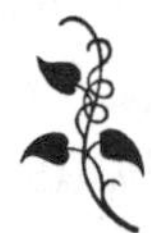

TRADITIONAL FEMALE GENITAL SURGERY (TFGS)

Traditional female genital surgery (TFGS) is often referred to as *"female circumcision"* and more recently *"female genital cutting."* The procedure is not analogous to male circumcision. The anatomical structures affected in females are much more extensive than in male circumcision. Those persons who are working toward abolishment of the procedure more commonly refer to it as *"female genital mutilation"*, implying removal or destruction without medical necessity.[1, 2]

Background

Traditional or ritualistic female genital surgery is more commonly known as female circumcision or female genital mutilation and dates back to the fifth century BC.[3] The procedure may have originated in Egypt as a means of controlling the fertility of slaves.[4, 5] The most severe form of the procedure is most prevalent in countries such as Sudan, Somalia, Eritrea, Dijibouti, Kenya, Ethiopia, Egypt, and some areas of West Africa.[2, 6, 7] Other countries where the procedure can be found to a lesser extent include Oman, Bahrain, Southern Yemen, the United Arab Emirates, Indonesia, India, Pakistan, Malaysia, Java, Sumatra, Eastern Mexico, Peru, and Western Brazil.[3, 8, 9]

No health benefits have been associated with this surgical procedure. The practice crosses socioeconomic classes, ethnic groups, and religions and is seen among Christians, Muslims, Jews, and indigenous African religions.[10] Some people believe that the practice is supported and/or mandated among religious groups, particularly Muslims. However, there is no evidence that any religions mandate the procedure, and the majority of Muslim communities do not practice TFGS.[11] TFGS has very deep cultural meanings that cannot be separated from any other aspect of the practice.

Generally, the procedure is performed on girls between the ages of four and ten years of age. However, in some communities, it is performed on newborns, just before marriage, or after the birth of the first child.[10, 12] Typically, the procedure is performed by village women, midwives, and others. Most have no formal training in human anatomy and learn the skill through apprenticeship.[13] Instruments are often non-sterile and may be used on multiple girls. Razors are the most commonly used instruments, but glass, scissors, sharpened stones, knives, and hot coals may be used. The procedures are performed without anesthesia.[14] Increasingly, families who have the financial resources send their daughters to medical facilities to have the procedure done under sterile conditions and with anesthesia. Currently, approximately 18 percent of the procedures are done under these conditions.[8] The cultural significance of the procedure carries different meanings among different groups.[15] Ongoing efforts to eradicate TFGS are leading to alternative practices such as clitoral flattening and symbolic cutting of pubic hair.[12]

Worldwide, more than 140 million women have undergone traditional female genital surgeries. Up to five million procedures are performed annually.[8] The largest numbers of African immigrant populations (who also have the largest number of women and children who have undergone TFGS or are at risk for TFGS) are located in California, New York, New Jersey, Virginia, Maryland, Minnesota, Texas, Washington, and Pennsylvania.[8, 16]

Types of Traditional Female Genital Surgery

In the past, various classifications of TFGS have been used. It is now recommended that health care providers use the classifications of the World Health Organization (WHO) to provide more consistency in communication and research. Classification should be made only after careful examination. It is unlikely that women will know the classification or the extent of the alteration unless they have been examined previously and the classification communicated clearly to them.[3, 8, 9, 15, 17, 18, 19, 20]

- **Type I** (clitoridectomy): Involves excision of the prepuce, with or without excision of a portion or the entire clitoris.
- **Type II** (excision): Involves excision of the clitoris, as well as partial or total excision of the labia minora without stitching.
- **Type III** (infibulation): Sometimes called pharaonic circumcision, involves excision of a portion or all of the external genitalia and stitching/narrowing of the vaginal opening. The opening that remains may be less than one centimeter in diameter. Thus, urine and menstrual blood exits the body through this opening. After marriage, the husband enlarges the opening (sometimes over weeks or months) for sexual intercourse by attempting to penetrate the tissue with his penis. Other methods to enlarge the opening include the husband's fingers, fingernails, and sometimes a razor or knife. This type accounts for approximately 15 percent of all procedures. Women who have undergone infibulations may require repeated procedures to open and close the area for childbirth and to address issues related to sexual intercourse.
- **Type IV** (unclassified): Involves all other alterations of the female genitalia to include the following:
  - Pricking, piercing, or incising of the clitoris and/or labia.
  - Stretching of the clitoris and/or labia.
  - Cauterization of the clitoris and surrounding tissue by burning.
  - Scraping of tissue surrounding the vaginal opening (angurya cuts).
  - Cutting of the vagina using posterior or backward cuts from the vagina into the perineum for the purpose of increasing the vaginal outlet for relief of obstructed labor (gishiri cuts). These procedures may result in vesicovaginal fistulae and damage to the anal sphincter.
  - Introduction of corrosive herbs and other substances into the vagina to cause bleeding or in an attempt to tighten/narrow the opening.
  - Any other procedures used to alter the female genitalia.

Reasons for TFGS

Reasons given for TFGS vary widely among groups, but generally fall into six categories:[3, 9, 10, 15, 18, 21, 22, 23, 24]

- **Tradition**
  - Rite of transition into womanhood.
  - Prerequisite for inclusion in social activities, religious activities, or marriage to a circumcised man.
  - Physical marker of marriageability.
  - Belief that tightly infibulated women provide greater sexual pleasure for husbands.
  - Social marker of superior morality.
- **Religious significance**
  - Many people believe, erroneously, that TFGS is a religious obligation.
- **Preservation of virginity until marriage**
  - Inheritance of property and political power are guaranteed by knowing the woman was a virgin until marriage and that children are true heirs.
  - Protection against rape.
- **Control of the excessive sexuality of females**
  - Family honor is maintained. The belief is that the scar tissue barrier leads to reduced sensation and, therefore, women are less likely to engage in premarital sex.
- **Promotion of fertility**
  - Belief that spermatozoa are killed by the secretions of the genitalia in females who have not undergone TFGS.
  - Belief that women who do not undergo the procedure will be sterile or unable to give birth to a son.

- Belief that the clitoris can kill a baby if it touches the baby's head during birth.
- Belief that the clitoris can sting, poison, or kill a man if it touches the man's penis.

- **Maintenance of general body health/hygiene**
  - Belief that the female genital area is ugly and contaminated.
  - Belief that the clitoris is a masculine organ and will grow in a manner similar to the growth of the penis in males. Thus, TFGS maintains femininity.

Complications of TFGS

Complications of TFGS are typically classified as immediate/short-term, late/long-term and obstetrical. Typically, health care providers in Western society encounter long-term and obstetrical complications. Women who have undergone the procedure may not associate complications with the procedure, but attribute them to other causes. Be aware that all women who have undergone the procedure do not experience sexual problems.[4, 5, 9, 10, 12, 14, 25, 26, 27, 28]

- **Immediate Complications:** (ten percent of girls and women die from immediate complications).
  - **Hemorrhage**: Most common complication, frequently related to cutting the clitoral artery.
  - Shock.
  - Death.
  - Infection/septicemia.
  - Severe pain.
  - Anemia.
  - Abscesses.

- Tetanus.
- Gangrene of the vulvar tissue.
- Fractured long bones/clavicles (as a result of restraining measures during the procedure).

- **Late/Long-Term Complications:** (25% of women die as a result of long-term and obstetrical complications). Long-term complications are more associated with Type III and IV procedures.
  - Severe dysmenorrhea.
  - Repeated episodes of vaginitis.
  - Endometriosis.
  - Rectocele.
  - Cystocele.
  - Incontinence.
  - Keloids (may be associated with all types of procedures).
  - Hematocolpos (painful retention and accumulation of blood in the vagina).
  - Hematometra (retention of blood in the uterus).
  - Adhesions.
  - Vaginal stenosis.
  - Chronic pelvic infections leading to infertility.
  - Chronic urinary tract infections, urinary calculi, painful urination.
  - Slow urine stream (may take 5–15 minutes to urinate). If catheterization is required for monitoring urinary output and the urinary meatus is not accessible because of TFGS, defibulation may be required. Obtain appropriate consents.

- Dermoid cysts, sebaceous cysts, abscesses.
- Clitoral neuroma.
- Painful intercourse.
- Chronic anxiety and depression.
- HIV infection (related to using the same surgical tools on multiple girls/women without disinfection).
- Psychological consequences.

- **Obstetrical Complications:** (TFGS doubles the risk of the mother dying during childbirth. There is a three to four times risk of death or injury to the baby.)
  - Women may be fearful of Western obstetricians and midwives who are believed to have limited or no experience in dealing with infibulated women, particularly related to defibulation for childbirth and reinfibulation after delivery. (Some husbands divorce wives who are not reinfibulated.)[29]
  - If defibulation is necessary for delivery, Toubia recommends performing it during the second trimester using local anesthesia. Determine if the mother wishes to be reinfibulated following delivery. If the woman presents in labor and is still infibulated, it is recommended that an anterior episiotomy be performed during the second stage of labor after the head crowns. An additional postero-lateral episiotomy may be needed if the skin around the vagina has lost its elasticity because of scar tissue. Multiparas may have severely scarred and deformed perineums as a result of multiple defibulations and reinfibulations. Medical providers who are not familiar with the procedures should consult with other providers who have performed the procedures, as needed.[5,9]
    - Perineal tears.
    - Delayed perineal healing because of scar tissue.
    - Prolonged second state of labor.
    - Avascular necrosis and atrophy of genital tissue.
    - Rectovaginal/vesiculovaginal fistulae.

- Postpartum hemorrhage.
- Fetal brain damage, hypoxia or fetal death related to obstructed labor.
- Unnecessary Cesarean section.

Care Considerations

- Many of the women who have undergone TFGS have arrived as refugees and may have faced atrocities, life in refugee camps, starvation, loss of family, and other psychological/physical traumas. Refer to support services as appropriate.
- Health care providers should take steps to learn about TFGS and to become comfortable with their own feelings, emotions, and opinions prior to interacting with or caring for women who have undergone the procedure.[23]
- Health care providers should dialogue with interpreters prior to interacting with the client. Discuss how sensitive issues will be conveyed. Request that the interpreter discuss potentially offensive questions with the health care provider before interpreting them to the patient. If possible, use interpreters who are familiar with TFGS and its cultural meanings.[25]
- It is preferable that the term *female genital mutilation* not be used because most of the women will not feel that they have been "mutilated." They may also be unaware that the practice is not common worldwide and experience shame and profound embarrassment once they find that their genital area is different from other females. Health care providers will need to use a compassionate and non-judgmental approach.[7,30]
- Provide female caregivers, including physicians, if possible. The husband and male guardian may be opposed to examinations of the woman by male health care providers or demand to be present during the exam. It can be expected that the male will be heavily involved in decision-making.
- Women may not seek prenatal care and preventive gynecological services because of fear of reactions to TFGS by health care providers, breaches of confidentiality, and the desire of health care providers to "show the infibulated area to other health care providers" as a means of teaching. **Maintain absolute privacy.**[31]

- Horowitz and Jackson suggest the following questions for gaining information from women who have undergone TFGS.[9,25]
  - "Many women from your country have been circumcised or 'closed' as children. If you do not mind telling me, were you circumcised or closed?" "What is the operation called in your country?" (Document the term used in the patient's record for future reference.)
  - "Do you have any problems passing your urine?" "Does your menstrual blood get stuck?"
  - "Do you have itching or burning or discharge from your pelvic area?"
  - (If sexually active) "Do you have any pain or difficulty when having relations?"
- Women who have undergone TFGS may not perceive the appearance of the genital area as 'abnormal' but as having a more pleasing appearance than normal female anatomy. The appearance is "normal" for the women, and they may have no memory of the procedure or of non-circumcised female anatomy.[25,32] The women may have difficulty answering medical questions if unfamiliar with non-circumcised anatomy. Assess the patient's knowledge of genital anatomy and use models/pictures, when necessary, to enhance teaching methods.
- Utilize a warmed, pediatric speculum for vaginal exams. Be aware that the woman may have never undergone pelvic exams. The uterus and ovaries may be palpated by performing a bimanual exam using a single finger and rectal examination.[9]
- Parents may be unaware that TFGS is illegal in the United States and some other countries and request the procedure for their daughters in the interest of promoting cultural integration of the child, assuring virginity and marriageability of the child to men of their cultural group.
- Women will sometimes present requesting defibulation for various reasons. Extensive patient consultation and discussion to explore educational needs, psychosexual issues, etc. prior to performing the procedure. Some physicians may not want to reinfibulate women after birth. Women should be encouraged to discuss and resolve this issue with their physicians prior to labor and delivery. Prior to attempting defibulation or reinfibulation,

the medical provider who is not knowledgeable of performing the procedures should seek consultation from providers who are familiar with performing the procedures.[5,33,34]

- Treatment for vaginal yeast infections may require oral instead of vaginal medication in women who are infibulated. Vaginal suppositories and vaginal cream applicators may not fit into the opening that is left after infibulation.[25]

- Urine specimens may show the presence of bacteria in the absence of infection because of mixing of urine and vaginal secretions.[25]

- Women may be very stoic during painful procedures or during childbirth since many are taught that expressing pain brings shame and dishonor to the family.[15]

- May be reluctant to drink adequate amounts of fluid because of painful urination.[17]

- Support groups may be appropriate for those women who do not choose to have their daughters undergo TFGS.[29]

Political/Legal/Educational Issues

- Although there are major efforts to abolish the practice of traditional female genital surgery worldwide, the practice persists. Interestingly, females in countries where the procedure is practiced, often oppose abolishment of the procedure either because it is against tradition or because it decreases their opportunity to be married and have more economic security.[35]

- In 1997, WHO, the United Nations Children's Fund, and the United Nations Population Fund produced a joint plan to reduce TFGS over the next ten years and to completely eliminate it within three generations. The United Nations formally gave support of the initiative in 2008 and expanded the goal to include wider efforts to bring about abandonment of the practice. In 2010, WHO expanded its efforts to eliminate the practice through publishing strategies aimed at discouraging the performance of the procedure by health care providers. International efforts continue to support advocacy to eliminate the practice, research, and education.[8]

- Worldwide, TFGS is illegal in an increasing number of countries, including some where the procedure is widely practiced such as in African countries. The level of enforcement of laws and punishments vary widely. Examples of countries where the practice is illegal are Sweden, New Zealand, Australia, Norway, Holland, Egypt, Belgium, Canada, France, Italy, the United Kingdom, and the United States.[3, 5, 36]

- Federal laws in the United States are focused on the person performing the procedure and child protection. The law makes the practice a crime if it is performed on a female younger than eighteen years of age. Federal law also mandates that the Department of Immigration/ Naturalization and the State Department provide information to persons entering the United States about TFGS and to instruct immigrants about the penalties of the law.[14] The law prohibits exemptions based on personal conviction such as religious belief.[37] Some states have also passed legislation to punish parents or guardians who "allow" the procedures since parents may send their girls abroad to have the procedure done if they can afford it.[38]

- Twenty states in the United States have criminalized TFGS and have provisions similar to or more severe than those of federal laws.[6, 39, 40] **Health care providers should consult legal resources in their state related to TFGS and reporting laws.**

- It is imperative that curricula for health care providers include information concerning TFGS, its management, ethical, and counseling issues.[29]

---

1 Lane, S. & Rubinstein, R. (1996). Judging the other: Responding to traditional female genital surgeries. *Hastings Center Report, 26*(3), 31-40.

2 Gruenbaum, E. (2001). *The female circumcision controversy: An anthropological perspective.* Philadelphia, PA: University of Pennsylvania Press.

3 Elchalal, U., Ben-Ami, B., Gillis, R. & Brzenzinski, A. (1997). Ritualistic female genital mutilation: Current status and future outlook. *Obstetrics and Gynecology Surv., 52*(10), 643-51

4 McConville, B. (1998). A bloody tradition. *Nursing Times, 94*(3), 34-36.

5 Abdulcadir, J., Margairaz, C., Boulvain, M. & Irion, O. (2011). Care of women with female genital mutilation/cutting. *Swiss Medical Weekly, 140*(w.13137). doi:10.4414/smw.2011.13137

6 Rahman, A. & Toubia, N. (2000). *Female genital mutilation: A guide to laws and policies worldwide.* New York, NY: Zed Books.

7 Barber, G. (2010). Female genital mutilation: A review. *Practice Nursing, 21*(2), 62-69.

8 The World Health Organization. (2012). *Female genital mutilation.* Retrieved from http://www.who.int/mediacentre/factsheets/fs241/en/

9 Toubia, N. (1999). *Caring for women with circumcision: A technical manual for health care providers.* New York, NY: RAINBO.

[10] Toubia, N. (1994). Female circumcision as a public health issue. *The New England Journal of Medicine, 33*(11), 712-716.
[11] Winkel, E. (1995). A Muslim perspective on female circumcision. *Women and Health, 23*(1), 1-7.
[12] Anuforo, P., Oyedele, L. & Pacquiao, D. (2004). Comparative study of meanings, beliefs, and practices of female circumcision among three Nigerian tribes in the United States and Nigeria. *Journal of Transcultural Nursing, 15*(2), 103-113.
[13] Wright, J. (1996). Female genital mutilation: An overview. *Journal of Advanced Nursing, 24*(2), 251-257.
[14] Gibeau, A. (1998). Female genital mutilation: When a cultural practice generates clinical and ethical dilemmas. *JOGNN, 27*(1), 85-91.
[15] Reichert, G. (1998). Female circumcision: What you need to know about genital mutilation. *AWHONN Lifelines, 2*(3), 29-34.
[16] Brigham and Women's Hospital: African Women's Health Center. (2012). Female genital cutting risk in America. Retrieved from http://www.brighamandwomens.org/Departments_and_Services/obgyn/services/africanwomenscenter/FGCbystate.aspx
[17] Brady, M. (1998). Female genital mutilation. *Nursing 98, 28*(9), 50-51.
[18] Stewart, R. (1997). Female circumcision: Implication for North American Nurses. *Journal of Psychosocial Nursing and Mental Health Services, 35*(4), 35-38.
[19] Sundby, J. (1996). Genital mutilation of women–is it a concern for Gynecologists? *ACTA Obstetricia et Gynecologica Scandinavica, 75*(6), 513-515.
[20] Perez, G.M. & Namulondo, H. (2011). Elongation of labia minora in Uganda: Including Baganda men in a risk reduction education programme. *Culture, Health, & Sexuality, 13*(1), 45-57.
[21] Hicks, E. (1996). *Infibulation: Female mutilation in Islamic Northeastern Africa.* New Brunswick, NJ: Transaction Publishers.
[22] Gruenbaum, E. (1996). The cultural debate over female circumcision: The Sudanese are arguing this one out for themselves. *Medical Anthropology Quarterly, 10*(4), 455-475.
[23] Caldwell, J., Orubuloye, I. & Caldwell, P. (1997). Male and female circumcision in Africa from a regional to a specific Nigerian examination. *Social Science and Medicine, 44*(8), 1181-1193.
[24] Kallon, I. & Dundes, L. (2010). The cultural context of the Sierra Leonean Mende woman as patient. *Journal of Transcultural Nursing, 21*(3), 228-236.
[25] Horowitz, C. & Jancson, J. (1997). Female circumcision: African women confront American medicine. *Journal of General Internal Medicine, 12*(8), 491-499.
[26] Odol, A., Brody, S., & Elkins, T. (1997). Female genital mutilation in rural Ghana, West Africa. *International Journal of Gynaecology and Obstetrics, 56*(2), 179-180.
[27] Little, C. (2003). Female genital circumcision: Medical and cultural considerations. *Journal of Cultural Diversity, 19*(1), 30-34.
[28] Fernandez-Aguilar, S. & Noel, J. (2003). Neuroma of the clitoris after female genital cutting. *Obstetrics and Gynecology, 101*(5), 1053-1054.
[29] Morris, R. (1996). The culture of female circumcision. *Advanced Nursing Science, 19*(2), 43-53.
[30] Berggren, V., Bergström, S., & Edbert, A.K. (2006). Being different and vulnerable: Experiences of immigrant African women who have been circumcised and sought maternity care in Sweden. *Journal of Transcultural Nursing, 17*(1), 50-57.
[31] Forjuoh, S. & Swi, A. (1998). Violence against children and adolescents: International perspectives. *Pediatric Clinics of North America, 45*(2), 415-426.

[32] Blanton, K. (2011). Female genital cutting and the health care provider's dilemma: A case study. *Clinical Scholars Review, 4*(2), 119-124.
[33] Lightfoot-Klein, H. & Shaw, E. (1991). Special needs for ritually circumcised women patients. *JOGGN, 20*(2), 102-107.
[34] Ibe, C. & Johnson-Agbakwu, C. (2011). Female genital cutting: Addressing the issues of culture and ethics. *The Female Patient, 36*, 28-31.
[35] Islam, M. & Uddin, M. (2001). Female circumcision in Sudan: Future prospects and strategies for eradication. *International Family Planning Perspectives, 27*(2), 71-76.
[36] Abd El Hadi, A. (1997). A step forward for opponents of female genital mutilation in Egypt. *Lancet, 349*(9045), 129-130.
[37] Key, F. (1997). Female circumcision/female genital mutilation in the United States: Legislation and its implications for health providers. *Journal of the American Medical Women's Association, 52*(4), 179-180.
[38] Eyega, Z. & Conneely, E. (1997). Facts and fiction regarding female circumcision/female genital mutilation: A pilot study in New York City. *Journal of the American Medical Women's Association, 52*(4), 174-178.
[39] Morgan, M. (1997). Female genital mutilation: An issue on the doorstep of the American medical community. *The Journal of Legal Medicine, 18*(1), 93-115.
[40] AHA Foundation. (2012). *Female genital mutilation.* Retrieved from http://theahafoundation.org/issues/female-genital-mutilation/

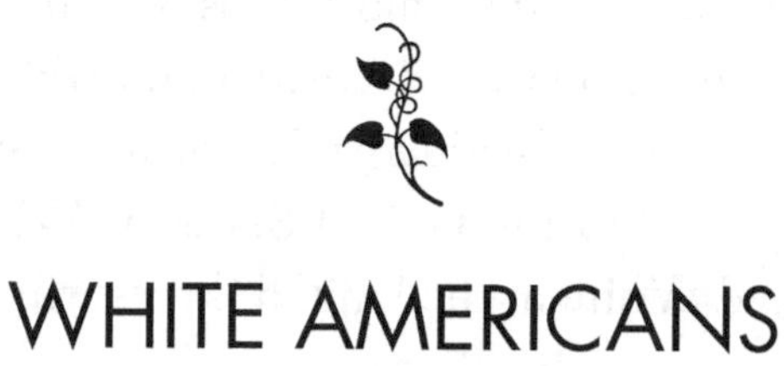

WHITE AMERICANS

Background

The early migration of English colonists and other Europeans to North America strongly influenced many of the beliefs and practices that are common today in the United States. Some of the strongest influences include language, religion, the legal system, politics, and other cornerstones of American mainstream society. Not to be forgotten are the cultural contributions of Native Americans and many other cultural groups to the development of culture in the United States. While European ancestors possessed some common physical traits, the use of the term *White* in reference to a group of people, did not emerge in American society until the late 1600s. The ancestry of Whites in the United States today includes, but is not limited to, English, German, Scottish, French, and Dutch.[3,4,5,4]

Almost 197 million people in the United States identify themselves as White. The term *non-Hispanic* is frequently added for statistical purposes to distinguish the group from light-skinned Hispanics. According to the United States Census Bureau, a White person is "an individual having origins in any of the original peoples of Europe, the Middle East, or North Africa." Historically, names such as Caucasians, Anglos, and Euro-Americans are used to broadly reference persons who identify as White in the United States. Population growth among Whites over the past decade has slowed. The majority of population growth in the United States during this timeframe is attributed to growth among other racial and ethnic groups. Whites are projected to become the minority in terms of population between 2040 and 2050.[2,5,6]

The term 'White' is commonly used in the United States in reference to ***race***. However, the use of the term "race" to define Whiteness in the United States is a topic of increasing debate. *Whiteness* in the United States has been equally used as a social construct since the term emerged in American society. Persons categorized as White have changed throughout the years. For instance, in years past, groups such as the Irish and Italians were referenced as *races*. Today, they are considered ethnic groups within the larger White population. Likewise, the long-standing "one-drop rule" deemed an individual with **any** known African ancestry *Black*. Nevertheless, many individuals of African ancestry who possessed White physical features successfully lived in the United States as White. It is predicted that the expansion of who is considered White in the United States will continue to evolve in future years.[7,8,9,10,11,12,13,14,15]

White Americans often do not think of themselves collectively as an ethnic or cultural group. Granted, as with most ethnic and cultural groups, there is a wide range of diversity among White Americans. However, middle and upper class White Americans form the dominant culture in the United States, in terms of traditionally holding the power that drives the core values and practices of mainstream society. More specifically, White men comprise approximately 38 percent of the United States population, but dominate positions of influence. Consider the following:[2,5,6,7,16,17,18,19]

- All Presidents and Vice-Presidents of the United States have been White men until President Barack Obama's election and re-election in 2008 and 2012, respectively.
- Approximately 78 percent of the seats in the United States Senate and the House of Representatives are held by White males.
- White men hold over 90 percent of senior management positions.
- Health care executive positions are dominated by White males.
- Approximately 80 percent of public school superintendents are White males.
- The majority of United States college/university presidents are White and male.
- Women earn approximately three-quarters of every dollar earned by males.

These and other powerful influences shape critical areas of United States daily life such as education, politics, economics, legalities, and of course, health care.

White Americans are found throughout the United States. According to the 2010 United States Census Bureau results, 36 percent of Whites reside in the South, 24 percent in the Midwest, 21 percent in the West, and 18 percent in the Northeast. Whites represent 90 percent or more of the population in the following states: Idaho, Iowa, Kentucky, Maine, Montana, New Hampshire, North Dakota, West Virginia, and Wyoming.[5]

White Americans have the second-highest median household incomes in the United States. Approximately 31 percent of Whites less than twenty-five years of age hold a bachelor's degree or higher. They tend to spend more than average on medical services and health care expenses. The five leading causes of death among this group are heart disease, cancer, chronic lower respiratory disease, stroke, and unintentional injuries. According to the latest CDC statistics, among new cases of HIV infections, Whites comprise approximately 16 percent. Among men who have sex with men, Whites account for the highest number of new HIV infections. Obesity is a widespread health issue in the United States. Among Whites greater than twenty years of age, approximately 72 percent of men and 59 percent of women are overweight/obese. Among children ages two to nineteen, approximately 29 percent are overweight/obese. Mortality and morbidity rates overall among Whites, tend to be lower than most other ethnic groups.[20, 21, 22, 23, 24, 25]

Language/Communication

- English is the primary language. Regional variations are common.
- Eye contact during conversations is tied to trustworthiness and attentiveness.
- A comfortable distance for conversation is approximately one arm's length unless the individual has indicated that a closer distance is needed or desired.[18, 26]
- Handshakes, regardless of gender, are acceptable. Casual touching from unfamiliar people is generally acceptable.[27]
- Communication is more verbal than non-verbal. Generally, individuals are expected to verbally communicate needs, expectations, and feelings.[18]

- Often, there are few reservations about sharing personal information.[27] Expressing feelings, talking about personal issues/problems may be seen as therapeutic.

Worldview/Religious Beliefs

- Humans are capable of exerting control over their physical, social, and natural environments.[18, 28]

- Whites are often future-oriented, believing that individuals are very capable of influencing their future and social status. Goals can be set and systematically achieved through hard work and aggressiveness toward the individual's goals.

- Success is often defined in terms of materialism and wealth. Competition and assertiveness in everyday life is seen as important to success.[1]

- There is a knowable and, usually, a measurable cause and effect for most events. These causes and effects can be discovered through the use of scientific methods and other formal means. Scientific facts, statistics, measurable outcomes, etc. add credibility to information. Ambiguity and lack of concrete answers may be difficult to accept. Health care providers may be asked to give information such as the 'odds' of recovery, etc. Second medical opinions may be sought.[5, 16, 23]

- The majority of Whites in the United States identify as Christians, with the larger number being Protestants. Sunday is recognized as the Sabbath by most. Clergy often visit church members while hospitalized or shut-in. Provide privacy during visits.

- Holidays, religious and special celebrations are primarily based on the Christian calendar. This is often reflected in health care facilities' policies and procedures.

- Time is a valuable resource and should not be "wasted." Efficiency, organization, punctuality, and 'doing' are important in daily activities. Prompt attention to requests and needs will be expected and connected to the perception of good care. Waiting past the time for scheduled appointments and clinical tests will be negatively viewed. Although productivity outcomes are important in health care businesses, patients will expect a non-rushed, but organized demeanor.[6, 18, 27]

Health Beliefs/Practices

- Mind, body, and spirit can be treated separately.
- Herbal preparations, dietary supplements, and alternative medical interventions may be used to promote health and well-being. Patient histories should include related questions to determine possible interactions with prescribed treatment regimens.
- Protection of privacy is expected. Health care facilities have a number of requirements in place to protect the privacy of individuals. Health care providers should be thoroughly familiar with the necessary documentation tools, policies, and procedures that support patient privacy and confidentiality. Private rooms are ideal.
- Individuals should be told the truth about personal health status, even if the truth is painful.[28]
- Self-care, self-reliance, self-determination, and independence are valued.[2,6] Involve family to the extent that the patient allows. Be aware that, because of the strong value of independence, individuals may not readily accept that there is a need for assistance from family or friends.
- Generally familiar with electronics and technology. Electronic and technological devices are common in the home. Often, resources such as the Internet are used to gain knowledge of diseases, treatments, etc. However, health care providers should not assume that individuals will be knowledgeable about technology found in health care facilities. Provide thorough explanations or, if the individual states that he or she has knowledge of the technology/treatment, ask him or her to share their understanding of the same.
- Skin color varies from very fair to what is often described as 'olive.' A 'healthy' appearance is often associated with tanning. Share appropriate information about precautionary measures related to sunbathing and tanning.
- Daily showers and hair shampoos are generally the norm.
- The quest for youth and beauty is a strong value. Overall, aging is less valued than among many other cultural groups. Great efforts, including cosmetic surgeries, are sometimes taken to mask signs of aging.[26]

Expression of Pain

- Generally, the individual will verbalize the need for pain relief.

Male-Female/Kinship/Social Relationships

- Informality when addressing individuals is common. Initial introductions often involve the use of first names versus more formal introductions and interactions valued among many other cultural groups.[16] In spite of this common informality, health care providers should opt for use of Mr., Mrs., etc. until given permission to address the individual by first name. Males and females are treated with equal respect during interactions.

- Handshakes are appropriate for males and females.

- *Family* often refers to nuclear family versus the inclusion of extended family. More often, other than parents and children, multiple generations do not live in the same household. Blended families are not uncommon in which the spouses/partners and children of previous marriages/relationships live in the same home as a family.[16] In recent years, same-gender households with children have become more common and accepted.[26, 27]

- Adults may plan ahead to move into assisted living facilities or nursing homes when no longer able to live independently vs. moving in with adult children to be cared for during the remainder of their lives.

- Family roles may not be as strictly defined as in some other ethnic groups since gender equality is generally supported. Spouses frequently share equally in household activities, childcare, and decision-making. Women strongly influence family health care decision-making.[18]

- Emotional control and the ability to continue regular functions under pressure or duress are often seen as an indication of strength.[2, 17]

Birth/Children

- Generally, prenatal care (including childbirth classes) is valued.
- Breastfeeding is acceptable. There are few restrictions for new mothers, and many return to daily activities very quickly following birth.
- Babies and children most often do not sleep with parents, and frequently not in the same room. A nursery is often prepared for newborns; children often have separate rooms.
- Independence is taught at an early age. Milestones toward independence such as self-feeding, brushing one's teeth, etc. are celebrated.[6] It is important for health care providers to gain information about the child's milestones that have been achieved and to explain to parents that children often regress from achieved milestones during illness.
- Children are allowed to be involved in decision-making to the extent of their development and to express their opinions. This may involve decision-making regarding choice of foods, choice of clothes, etc.[6,18] Continue these practices to the extent possible during hospitalization or treatments. However, do not offer choices that cannot be honored. For instance, the health care provider might ask the child's preference for a treat following a required treatment versus asking whether the child would like to have the treatment or not.
- Familiarity with electronic devices begins at an early age. Computer games, video games, etc. may be helpful as diversional/recreational activities, if hospitalized.
- School-age children may be home-schooled.[29]
- Behavioral changes are expected and tolerated during the teen years. These include moodiness, varying degrees of rebelliousness.[18]
- Corporal punishment is generally not supported. Non-physical methods of discipline may be employed such as "time out."

- Generally, children eighteen years of age and older are expected to continue growth in independence by being in college, working to contribute to the household, or living independently. In recent years, more young adults are returning home related to financial difficulties.

Death

- See specific religion, if individual or family identifies with a specific religious group. For those individuals not formally connected to a religious group, offer facility clergy and/or provide support from health care providers, as needed.
- Generally, all final preparation of the body is completed by the funeral home.
- **Organ Donation**: Generally, individual choice.
- **Blood Transfusions**: Generally, individual choice.

Patient Teaching/Dietary Considerations

- Usual dietary practices vary based on factors such as socioeconomic level, location of residence (rural vs. urban), accessibility to food sources such as fresh markets, etc. Fast foods and pre-packaged foods may be a major part of diet. Meals may be skipped in an effort to meet deadlines associated with work and full family schedules.
- Generally, standard patient/family teaching methods are acceptable, including group discussion. It is helpful to determine the patient/family's preferred method of learning. Assure patient/family understanding of educational material.
- Patient teaching goals can be successfully tied to the individual's future health and well-being.
- Arrange appropriate referrals for older individuals living alone and without family support.

1 Spindler, G. & Spindler, L. (1990). *The American cultural dialogue and its transmission.* New York: The Falmer Press.

2 Hitchcock, J. (2002). *Lifting the White veil: An exploration of White American culture in a multiracial context.* Roselle, NJ: Crandall, Dostie & Douglass Books, Inc.

3 Kincheloe, J. (1999). The struggle to define and reinvent Whiteness: A pedagogical analysis. *College Literature, 26*(3), 162-195.

4 Painter, N. I. (2010). *The history of white people.* New York, NY: W.W. Norton & Company.

5 United States Census Bureau. (2012). *Population estimates and projections.* Retrieved from http://www.census.gov

6 Halley, J., Eshleman, A., & Vijaya, R. M. (2011). *Seeing White: An introduction to White privilege and race.* New York, NJ: Rowman & Littlefield Publishers, Inc.

7 *American Anthropological Association.* Response to OMB directive 15. Retrieved from http://www.aaanet.org/gvt/ombsumm.htm

8 Thernstrom, S. (2000). One drop—Still. *National Review, 52*(7), 35-38.

9 Schaefer, R. (2004). *Racial and ethnic groups* (13th ed.). Upper Saddle River, NJ: Pearson Prentice Hall.

10 Davis, F. (1991). *Who is Black? One nation's definition.* University Park, PA: The Pennsylvania State University Press.

11 Will, G. (2002). Dropping the "one drop" rule. *Newsweek (Atlantic Edition), 139*(13), 13.

12 Wolfe, P. (October 2004). Race and citizenship. *OAH Magazine of History*, 66-71.

13 Cole, Y. (2005). Who is African American? *Diversity, Inc. 4*(1), 54-60.

14 Denevi, E. (2000). Whiteness. *Independent School, 6*(1). 100-109.

15 Tatum, T. (1997). *Why are all the Black kids sitting together in the cafeteria? And other conversations about race.* New York: Basic Books.

16 Diller, J. (2004). *Cultural diversity: A primer for the human services* (2nd ed.). Belmont, CA: Brooks/Cole–Thomson Learning.

17 Althen, G. (1988). *American Ways.* Yarmouth, ME: Intercultural Press, Inc.

18 Malone, R. (2001). Principal mentoring. *ERIC Digest*, July 2001.

19 Centers for Disease Control. (2012, October 26). *National vital statistics reports, 6*(11), 1-95. Retrieved from http://www.cdc.gov/nchs/data/nvsr/nvsr61/nvsr61_07.pdf

20 Centers for Disease Control. (2012). *HIV/AIDS statistics and surveillance.* Retrieved from http://www.cdc.gov/hiv/topics/surveillance/index.htm

21 Pew Research Center. (2012, June 19). *The rise of Asian Americans.* Retrieved from http://www.pewsocialtrends.org/2012/06/19/the-rise-of-asian-americans/

22 Institute of Medicine (2003). *Unequal treatment.* Washington, DC: The National Academies Press.

23 Hall, E. (1966). *The hidden dimension.* New York, NJ: Anchor Books.

24 Purnell, L.D. (2012). *Transcultural health care: A culturally competent approach* (4th ed.). Philadelphia, PA: F. A. Davis.

25 American Heart Association & American Stroke Association. (2012). *Statistical fact sheet 2012 update: Overweight & obesity.* Retrieved from http://www.heart.org/idc/groups/heart-public/@wcm/@sop/@smd/documents/downloadable/ucm_319588.pdf

[26] American Heart Association & American Stroke Association. (2011). *2011 Statistical sourcebook: Understanding childhood obesity*. Retrieved from http://www.heart.org/idc/groups/heart-public/@wcm/@fc/documents/downloadable/ucm_428180.pdf

[27] Myser, C. (2003). Differences from somewhere: The normativity of Whiteness in bioethics in the United States. *American Journal of Bioethics, 3*(2), 1-11.

[28] Bauman, J. (2001). Home schooling in the United States: Trends and characteristics. *Working Paper Series, No. 53*. United States Census Bureau.

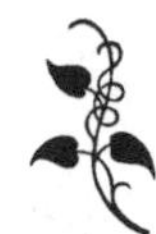

SAMPLE CULTURAL ASSESSMENT QUESTIONS

In addition to biophysical assessment, the following questions may be useful in eliciting information related to culture, but not necessarily in this order or at the same time. These and similar questions can be easily incorporated into patient assessment tools. A level of trust may need to be established with the patient/family before there is a willingness to share certain information. **Language services should be accessed to assist in conveying questions, medical information, and gaining accurate information.**

Language and Ethnohistory

- What is your country of origin?
- What ethnic/cultural group do you identify with?
- How long have you lived in this country? What led to you coming here?
- Sometimes when people are trying to leave their country, they encounter some unpleasant experiences. Is there any experience that we should know about that would be important to your care while here?

- What language is spoken in your home?
- Do you speak, read, and/or understand English or another language?
- Are there resources/equipment that you normally use to assist you with communicating?
- Tell me about any positive or negative experiences with how people communicate with you that we need to know about to better care for you.

Kinship and Social Factors

- How would you prefer to be addressed while here?
- Do you have other family members who live close to you? Do any of them live in the home with you? How would you like for them to be involved in your care?
- Are there others that you would like to be involved in your care? Who are these persons? How would you like for them to be involved?
- Will anyone other than yourself be participating in decisions affecting your care (child's care)?
- Are there any barriers related to your family getting to the hospital to visit you?
- Tell me what good care means to you. In what way would you like for nurses and other health care providers to care for you while you are ill? What can we do while you are here that will lead you to feel that you are receiving good care?
- Do you feel safe in your home? What will help you to feel safe while you are here?

Worldview

- When looking at yourself, what does the word 'healthy' mean to you?
- Share with me what you believe caused your illness.

- Why do you think that your illness started when it did?
- Since you have had this illness, do you feel any different during any particular part of the day or night or on different days of the week?
- What do you call the illness that you are here for? Have you had this illness before? When did it start? How has it made you feel?
- How will this illness/hospitalization affect your life and the life of your family?
- What made you come to the hospital (or other health care facility) now?
- It can be frightening to be in a hospital. How are you feeling about having to be in the hospital? What fears do you have about your illness?
- What disturbs you most about being here?
- Tell me about your feelings about this illness/surgery and how it might affect you as a person.

Environmental Factors

- Are you exposed to anything in the air, water that you drink, etc. where you live or work that you believe may be harmful to you and your family?
- Are you allergic to anything in the environment that you are aware of (e.g., chemicals, mold, etc.)?
- It is possible that you will need equipment of some type when you go home. Do you have the following in your home: electricity, running water/well water, indoor plumbing, stairs, etc.?
- Do you have any special item at home that would be comforting to have with you in the hospital? If so, what meaning does it have to you? If you are unable to speak for yourself, who would you like to entrust with the item?

Cultural Values, Belief, and Lifeways

- We are interested in honoring your values and beliefs. Are there any that you would like for us to know about to help you regain/maintain your health?
- How many meals per day do you normally eat? At what times?
- Tell me about the foods that you normally eat at mealtime.
- Are there foods that you do not eat ever or don't eat at certain times? Why?
- With whom do you usually eat your meals?
- What is your usual bedtime? Is there anything that helps you to sleep better or causes you to sleep worse?
- Many people have a 'routine' at home. Is there any part of your routine that you would like to keep the same, if possible, while you are here such as the time you take your shower/bath, etc.?

Religious, Philosophical, Spiritual Factors

- Both males and females work in this and other departments in the hospital, who are normally involved in caring for patients or who may be entering your room. Are there any special considerations that we should know about related to persons of the opposite gender being involved in your care?
- Tell me about any considerations that we should know about related to your religious beliefs/practices such as diet, prayer/meditation times, etc.
- Do you have any restrictions related to receiving blood/blood products?
- Is there anyone that we can call for you now to offer you spiritual/religious support?
- How can we best support you spiritually while you are here?

- Valuables (if unfamiliar items are worn such as crosses, cloth bracelets/strings, charms, medicine bag, etc.)
  - What meaning does _______ have for you? Do you feel that your well-being will be affected if _______ is removed? How?
- What normally helps you to feel better if you are feeling down/stressed?

Political and Legal Factors

- Do you have legal documents/information (Power of attorney, etc.) that we should be aware of?

Economic Factors

- How do you normally get medications that you need?
- Do you receive financial assistance/support services for any of your daily needs?

Technology Factors

- Do you use any equipment/technology at home to help you maintain your health?
- How will you get to your appointments after discharge?

Educational Factors

- How do you believe that you learn best?
- Are you able to read and write? In what language?

Generic Folk/Care Practices

- Do you seek help from anyone other than a licensed medical provider that helps you to stay well or helps you when you are not feeling well?
- What helps you to stay well?
- Tell me about things you do to help yourself feel better when you are feeling ill.
- Tell me about any herbal or vitamin supplements that you are taking. Dosage, frequency, and for what reason? How do you get the supplements? Tell me about any activities that you are involved in for your health and well-being.
- Have you taken or done anything before coming to the hospital to treat your present illness? Did it make you feel better, worse, or was there no change in how you felt?

Professional Care/Cure Practices

- Where do you most often receive care when you are feeling ill or for regular checkups?
- Tell me about any prescription drugs that you are taking. Dosage, frequency, and for what reason?
- Have you encountered any positive or negative experiences while receiving professional care that we need to know about to better care for you?

INDEX

CPSIA information can be obtained
at www.ICGtesting.com
Printed in the USA
LVHW102144110620
657890LV00008B/644